Infection Preventionist's Guide to Long-Term Care

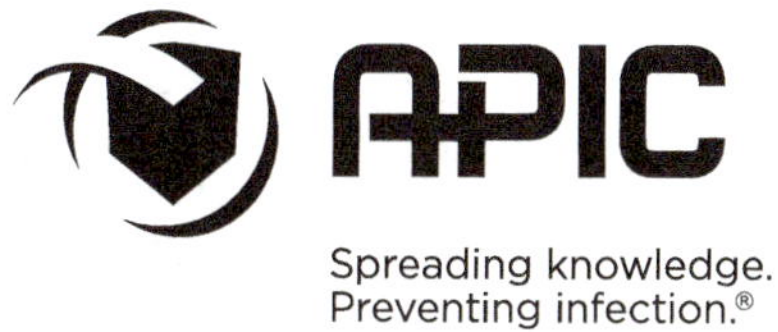

Printed in the United States of America
First edition, November 2013
ISBN: 1-933013-59-1

All inquiries about this book or other APIC products and services may be directed to:

APIC
1400 Crystal Drive, Suite 900
Arlington, VA 22202

Phone: 202-789-1890
Fax: 202-789-1899
Email: info@apic.org
Web: www.apic.org

Table of Contents

Acknowledgements

The Association for Professionals in Infection Control and Epidemiology acknowledges the valuable contributions from each of the following individuals:

Authors

Lead Author:

Steven J. Schweon, RN, MPH, MSN, CIC, HEM
Infection Prevention Consultant
Saylorsburg, PA

Contributing Authors:

Deborah Patterson Burdsall, MSN, RN-BC, CIC
Infection Preventionist
Lutheran Home/Lutheran Life Communities
Arlington Heights, IL

Dolly Greene, RN, CIC
Director of Clinical Services and Education
Diagnostic Laboratories & Radiology/ Mobilex USA
Burbank, CA

Marilyn Hanchett, RN, MA, CPHQ, CIC
Sr. Director, Professional Practice
Association for Professionals in Infection Control and Epidemiology
Washington, DC

Steven W. Hilley, RN
Infection Prevention Coordinator
Yampa Valley Medical Center
Steamboat Springs, CO

Irena Kenneley, PhD, APRN-BC, CIC
Assistant Professor/Faculty Development Officer
Case Western Reserve University
Cleveland, OH

James F. Marx, PhD, RN, CIC
Infection Preventionist Consultant
Broad Street Solutions
San Diego, CA

Patricia Rosenbaum, RN, CIC
Infection Prevention Consultant
PAR Consulting, LLC
Silver Spring, MD

Reviewers

Amy Cotton, MSN, GNP, FNP, FNGNA, FAAN
Past President, The National Gerontological Nursing Association
Eastern Maine Healthcare Systems
Brewer, ME

Sherrie Dornberger, RN, GDCN, CDP, CDONA, FACDONA
Executive Director
National Association Directors of Nursing Administration in Long Term Care
Mullica Hill, NJ

Paul Drinka, MD, AGSF, FSHEA*
Clinical Professor of Internal Medicine/ Geriatrics
University of Wisconsin and Medical College of Wisconsin
Madison, WI

Darlene Fawcett, RN**
Infection Control Practitioner
Ontario Shores Centre for Mental Health Sciences
Whitby, ON, Canada

Jill E. Holdsworth, MS, CIC, EMT-B
Infection Control Practitioner
Inova Mount Vernon Hospital
Alexandria, VA

Kathy Horn, RN, CIC
Consultant in Infection Prevention
Upper Black Eddy, PA

Jolynn Zeller, RN, BSN, CIC
Coordinator, Infection Prevention
Avera St. Luke's
Aberdeen, SD

Production Team

Executive Editor:

Marilyn Hanchett, RN, MA, CPHQ, CIC
Sr. Director, Professional Practice
Association for Professionals in Infection Control and Epidemiology
Washington, DC

Managing Editor:

Anna Conger
Sr. Manager, Practice Resources
Association for Professionals in Infection Control and Epidemiology
Washington, DC

Copyeditors:

Jim Angelo
Director, Practice Resources
Association for Professionals in Infection Control and Epidemiology
Washington, DC

Thomas Weaver, DMD
Director, Professional Practice
Association for Professionals in Infection Control and Epidemiology
Washington, DC

Cover Design:

Sarah Vickers
Art Director
Association for Professionals in Infection Control and Epidemiology
Washington, DC

Book Design and Layout:

Project Design Company
Washington, DC

Printing:

Linemark
Upper Marlboro, MD

* Paul Drinka, MD, AGSF, FSHEA reviewed on behalf of AMDA - Dedicated to Long Term Care Medicine.
** Darlene Fawcett, RN reviewed on behalf of Infection Prevention and Control Canada.

Declaration of Conflicts of Interest

Deborah Patterson Burdsall, MSN, RN-BC, CIC has nothing to declare.

Amy Cotton, MSN, GNP, FNP, FNGNA, FAAN is President and Board of Directors Chair for National Gerontological Nursing Association (volunteer).

Sherrie Dornberger, RN, GDCN, CDP, CDONA, FACDONA serves on the South Jersey Red Cross Board of Directors (volunteer).

Paul Drinka, MD, AGSF, FSHEA has nothing to declare.

Darlene Fawçett, RN has nothing to declare.

Dolly Greene, RN, CIC has nothing to declare.

Marilyn Hanchett, RN, MA, CPHQ, CIC has nothing to declare.

Steven W. Hilley, RN is a member of the State Emergency Medical and Trauma Services Advisory Council, Statewide Trauma System Committee, and Hospital Preparedness Advisory Group and is Vice Chair of the Routt County Emergency Response Coalition and Northwest Colorado Hospital Emergency Coordination System.

Jill E. Holdsworth, MS, CIC, EMT-B has nothing to declare.

Kathy Horn, RN, CIC has nothing to declare.

Irena Kenneley, PhD, APRN-BC, CIC has nothing to declare.

James F. Marx, PhD, RN, CIC is a member of the GOJO Industries consortium and speaker's bureau.

Patricia Rosenbaum, RN, CIC has nothing to declare.

Steven J. Schweon, RN, MPH, MSN, CIC, HEM has done consulting work for GOJO Industries and Crothall Healthcare and is a member of the Society for Healthcare Epidemiology of America Education Committee.

Jolynn Zeller, RN, BSN, CIC has nothing to declare.

Foreword

On behalf of APIC, I am delighted to introduce to you the *Infection Preventionist's Guide to Long-term Care*. This is the most comprehensive book that APIC has published on infection prevention and control in this unique practice setting.

With more than 15,000 long-term care facilities (LTCF) in the United States and a national priority to prevent healthcare-associated infections (HAIs), APIC has leveraged member expertise and experience specific to infection prevention and control in long-term care to produce this book.

APIC is committed to increasing its educational resources for long-term care to advance knowledge and competencies of healthcare personnel working in this setting and for the benefit of the residents under their care.

This book presents the historical context and background on LTCF as an emerging national priority for preventing HAIs. In addition, it provides detailed explanations of the requirements and the challenges in this practice setting along with recommended actions, procedures, and checklists that can be implemented to improve infection prevention programs.

When it comes to the "how-to-implement" infection prevention and control strategies and practices in this country, APIC is unparalleled. APIC is committed to patient and resident safety across the healthcare continuum. To support this commitment, APIC continues to bring forward practice resources and professional development for those working in long-term care settings.

Together, we can improve quality and prevent infections.

Katrina Crist, MBA
Chief Executive Officer
Association for Professionals in Infection Control and Epidemiology

CHAPTER 1

Understanding Infection Prevention in Long-Term Care

Deborah Patterson Burdsall, MSN, RN-BC, CIC

KEY CONCEPTS

- Infection preventionists in long-term care face unique challenges due to the nature of the care setting and its resident population.
- The aging resident population of long-term care facilities is at greater risk of infection because of deterioration of immune response.
- When developing an infection prevention and control program, the infection preventionist must understand and take into consideration the characteristics of healthcare personnel, resident populations, and work environment.

Residents and healthcare personnel (HCP) in long-term care facilities (LTCFs) have increased risk of infection for residents and direct HCP, and LTCF residents and HCP should be evaluated together when investigating the transmission of disease-causing organisms. Residents and HCP share the same environment—they breathe the same air, touch the same surfaces and objects, and often eat food from a common kitchen.

It has been estimated that 1.5 million infections occur annually in LTCFs; however, this number is likely much higher.[1,2] It is difficult to estimate the burden of infection because surveillance definitions, methods, and intensity vary widely in LTCFs. Residents in LTCFs, especially residents with dementia, are at risk for infection because of behaviors that increase the probability of contracting an infection, as well as intrinsic factors relating to aging. Contact with a resident's body and with objects in the environment by both HCP and the LTCF resident are a part of direct caregiving. This contact is a primary risk factor for both acquiring and transmitting pathogens. Secondary risk factors relate to specific population and cohort characteristics (Figure 1.1).

LONG-TERM CARE FACILITY CHARACTERISTICS

Sixty percent of LTCFs are for-profit. A profit-driven structure can produce high-resident/HCP ratios and supply restrictions as a strategy to produce profit and reduce costs. Both high-resident/HCP ratios and supply restrictions result in less time for care, a decreased ability to keep the environment clean, and encourage cutting corners when performing infection prevention activities.[3] Lapses in infection prevention activities not only increase the risk of intrafacility transmission, but also are often correlated with citations by the Centers for Medicare & Medicaid Services (CMS) Survey and Certification.[4] If nursing assistants, nursing departments, and infection prevention and control programs are not supported, and if there are insufficient supplies, outbreaks of infectious diseases can be well established before nurses or primary care providers are aware they exist.

OLDER ADULT AND RESIDENT POPULATION CHARACTERISTICS IN LTCFs

Between 1.5 and 1.7 million older adults live in LTCFs annually. With an average age of 80 years, older adult residents generally live in LTCFs because of a self-care deficit or a medical condition that requires constant and consistent support.[1,2] Residents require assistance ranging from cues and reminders to total dependence and are more likely than those who are living independently to have conditions such as:

- Increased frailty
- Dementia
- Decreased immune function
- Decreased skin integrity and wounds
- Problems with nutrition, chewing, and swallowing
- Issues with incontinence
- Decreased bowel and bladder function
- Decreased mobility[2]

These conditions create a greater likelihood of residents being partially or totally dependent on nursing assistants for activities of daily living (ADLs).[1] This support can include various levels of assistance for dressing; bathing; grooming; eating; and ambulating or assistance with wheelchairs, walkers, and canes, all of which involve close physical contact between the HCP and the resident.

The normal aging process increases vulnerability to infection because of a multitude of biopsychosocial changes. Healthcare providers, including infection preventionists, must provide a person-centered approach to maintain health and avoid preventable infection.[2,5,6] It is estimated that there are between 1.6 and 3.8 million infections annually in elderly residents of LTCFs. The population of individuals over age 85 is expected to grow to 7.3 million by 2020, and a focus on preventable infection is critical since the personal and economic expense of infection is high.[2] For instance, the attributed

FIGURE 1.1: INFECTION RISK FACTORS IN LONG-TERM CARE

OLDER ADULTS IN LTC

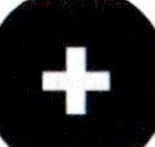

DIRECT CAREGIVERS IN LTC

- 1.5–1.7 million residents in more than 15,000 long-term care facilities (LTCFs)
- 90 percent over 65 years of age
- Mean age 80+ years
- Increased dependence on healthcare personnel (HCP) for activities of daily living (ADLs), mainly nursing assistants
- Decreased immune function "changes are of limited clinical significance in healthy elderly"[2]
- Decreased skin integrity
- Decreased swallowing/chewing ability
- Dementia/depression/apathy
- Wandering and dependence increase opportunities for transmission of pathogens
- Incontinence and decreased bladder and bowel tone
- Decreased mobility/Immobility
- Multiple medications/polypharmacy
- Increased acuity and frailty

- 1.85 million employees in facility-based and home care settings of long-term care
- Primarily paraprofessionals (nurse's aides, home health aides, attendants, orderlies, contract caregivers by families)
- Nursing assistants' (paraprofessional) certification approximately 6-8 weeks; uncertified aide training less or on the job. Foreign-born more likely to have college degree (14.6 percent) than native-born (6.0 percent)
- Nurses, primarily LPN/LVNs and associate degree RNs
- 20 percent foreign born (2005)
- 90 percent women
- Labor shortage in LTCFs provide job opportunities for immigrants: ESL, multiple cultural issues
- Turnover, multiple jobs/multiple policies/ procedures interfere with integrating into institutional culture/training
- Multiple staff from different cultures either reinforces or challenges prior beliefs, cultural taboos, teachings, and behaviors.
- Inadequate staffing levels for assistance or for proper supervision

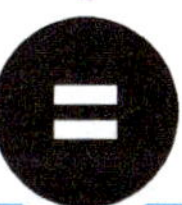

INFECTIONS IN LTCF

- **Incidence and prevalence of LTCF infections:** Literature skewed by outbreak investigations conducted by public health or investigations external to the LTCF infection prevention program. Also, lack of established surveillance systems in LTCFs which cannot distinguish between new incidence and point or period prevalence.[2]
- **Incidence:** Reported between 1.8 and 13.5 infections per 1,000 resident days.[19] Between 3 and 15 percent of 1.43 million residents acquire infections in LTCF annually.[1]
- Prevalence can include colonization as well as infection. Dutch researchers conducted an annual one-day prevalence study from 2007 to 2009 that demonstrated infection rates of 5.4 to 13.2 percent in 17 nursing homes.[18]
- Between 350,000 and 400,000 deaths from infections in LTC. Cost is between $673 million to $2 billion.
- Ranges are large primarily because surveillance and reporting are not standardized in LTCFs.
- LTCF outbreaks are 15 percent of all reported outbreaks and 19 percent of all outbreak reported deaths, and affect both residents and direct caregivers, especially respiratory and gastroenteritis outbreaks.
- **Respiratory infections:** Leading cause of resident death, and second most common LTCF infection: Incidence between 0.3 and 2.5 episodes/1,000 resident days.[2]
- **Gastroenteritis:** LTCF gastroenteritis outbreaks largest number reported to CDC. Residents four times more likely to die than community dwelling elders: Incidence between 0.004 and 1.9/1,000 bed days.[50]

median dollar cost of a methicillin-resistant *Staphylococcus aureus* (MRSA) bloodstream infection has been reported to be as high as $51,492 with an associated mortality rate more than 20 percent.[7]

Immune Response in Long-term Care Populations

The immune system is dynamic and protective and provides defense against infection. It can be divided into three areas:

(1) the physical and primary chemical and secretory barriers to infection,

(2) the innate immune system, and

(3) the adaptive immune system.[8]

Protection from infection comes from a hierarchy of defenses. The first of these are the physical barriers, such as the skin and mucous membranes. The intact skin and mucous membranes act as a physical barrier that shields inner structures from the majority of potential infectious agents. Glands in the skin secrete lactic acid, oils, and fatty acids, which acidify the skin and create a bacteriostatic environment. The enzyme lysozyme secreted in tears, saliva, and other body fluids acts against bacterial membranes, while immunoglobulin A (IgA), contained in mucosal secretions, protects the mucous membranes.[9] The human body can also rid itself of invaders, expelling them through the processes of urination, defecation, vomiting, diarrhea, coughing, and skin sloughing.[10] These macro-level mechanisms play a very important role in the primary immune system.

The *innate immune response* is the primary spontaneous and reactive portion of the immune system. It is present at birth and does not adapt through encounters with potentially destructive organisms and substances called antigens. Antigens are broadly defined as any substance identified by the human immune system as "other" or "foreign."[10] Introduction of microorganisms through a break in the mucous membranes causes the body to respond with inflammation, an increase in localized white blood cells (WBCs), and other complex automatic systems responses. Myeloid WBC leukocytes are released from the bone marrow and are responsible for initial phagocytosis. Basophilic cells and mast cells release histamine and promote an immediate inflammatory response. This response is also seen with percutaneous exposure to objects contaminated with microorganisms or other antigens. As individuals age, there is a decrease in the number and the ability of certain types of white blood cells. With the reduction in the number of white blood cells, the individual's ability to fight infections decreases.

The *adaptive immune response* comes from the part of the immune system that recognizes and reacts to antigens. When an antigen enters the body, the adaptive immune system learns to recognize the antigen as foreign and creates a defense against it. When the antigen enters the body a second time, the adaptive immune system recognizes and reacts more quickly and strongly than before. T-cells and B-cells are the WBCs that have the capability to learn from a first encounter with an antigen and then remember the antigen during subsequent encounters. A wide variety of organisms can cause an immune reaction, including organic and inorganic substances such as mold; fungus; bacteria; parasites; venom from insects, arachnids, and reptiles; and others.[10]

Changes occur in aging that affect immunity, and these changes can be thought of as a generalized blunting of the immune response and have been referred to as immunosenescence.[5,11] Changes in immune function are not the only reason for increased infection risk in the elderly.[2,12,13] The possibility of increased infection in the elderly may be due to conditions such as increased incontinence, poor hygiene, and behaviors related to dementia. Breaks in the skin, wounds, dependence upon others for hygiene, use of catheters, and decreased nutrient and fluid intake increase the chance for antigens to enter the body.[2,12,13] Once this happens, a blunted elder immune response can increase susceptibility to infection.

The age-associated changes that relate to risk of infection involve every part of a person's life. As individuals age, there are changes within all systems and all organs of the body. The ability to maintain mobility, nutritional and hydration status, cleanliness, and safety may be affected by the many changes in their lives. Comorbidities such as diabetes; congestive heart failure with dependent edema; decreased eyesight, hearing, and sense of smell; decreased thirst and hunger mechanism; pain upon movement from undertreated chronic issues such as osteoarthritis, depression, lack of sleep, and fear of falls; neuropathy; polypharmacy; and loss of transportation and financial difficulty increase the risk for infection from a practical standpoint.[2,13-16] The physical systems with the highest risk for developing infection include the urinary tract, the skin and soft tissue, the respiratory system, and the gastrointestinal system.

The elderly have significant issues with persistent colonization of multidrug-resistant organisms (MDROs). In studies of MRSA colonization, elderly individuals in long-term care were found to have colonization rates of between 5 and 60 percent.[17]

The most common types of infections in LTCF residents are:

- Urinary tract infections with asymptomatic bacteriuria
- Respiratory infections
- Skin and soft tissue infections and infestations
- Gastrointestinal infections
- Bacteremia infections and bloodborne viral illness
- Other infections such as conjunctivitis[2]

Outbreaks of highly transmissible agents such as influenza and norovirus pose a special risk in dementia care units, where persons with dementia may not be able to verbalize how they feel. They may become increasingly agitated and disoriented if they are coughing; have difficulty breathing; and have a fever, feel nauseated, or have diarrhea or vomiting. Persons with dementia may also need increased hygiene support, and the environment will need to be cleaned more frequently, which further increases the contact between resident, HCP, and infectious agent. Although outbreaks on dementia units may be more difficult to control, prevalence of infections in dementia units has been found to be lower (6.3 percent, range 5.4 to 7.2 percent) than infection prevalence in LTCF rehabilitation units (12.1 percent, range 10.8 to 13.3 percent).[18] This statistic is not surprising, considering that the population in rehabilitation units consists primarily of older adults recovering from an acute illness or procedure. Most residents in dementia units have cognitive deficits, but as long as they are provided appropriate support, they are generally in stable health.

INFECTIONS IN LTCFS AS THEY RELATE TO HCP AND RESIDENT POPULATIONS

Infectious organisms can be difficult to control when introduced into the LTCF population. This introduction may be via a resident admission, a visitor, or HCP. Transfer between different levels of community and healthcare treatment facilities increases exposure to foreign microorganisms, and increase the risk of infection with MDROs. When a vulnerable older population comes into close contact with an often under staffed, partially trained, and/or marginally supervised nursing assistant population, it may be difficult to prevent the spread of infectious agents or to control outbreaks with LTCF resources alone (Figure 1.2). Contaminated HCP hands, gloves, and equipment can spread pathogens between the resident, the environment, and the HCP. Residents with dementia can spread pathogens through contaminated hands, clothing, equipment, uncontained drainage, or uncovered wounds.

Outbreaks can be caused by breaks in technique and may have an impact on the HCP health and their ability to work, especially if the HCP acquires the illness. Outbreaks affect organizational economic well-being, regulatory status, and reputation by increasing the need for supplies and reducing admissions, which also increases the possibilities of citations and lawsuits and media exposure.

Reported prevalence of infections in LTCF literature ranges from 1.6 to 32 percent. Incidence rates have been reported ranging from 1.8 to 13.5 infections per 1,000 resident days.[19] The wide range of both prevalence percentages and incidence rates can be attributed to the lack of standardized infection definitions, surveillance, reporting, as well as the general lack of comprehensive infection prevention and control programs.[2] Infections in LTCFs are associated with HCP training and motivation, staffing patterns, HCP wellness, availability of necessary

FIGURE 1.2: HEALTHCARE PERSONNEL AND RESIDENT INTERACTION RELATED TO INFECTION

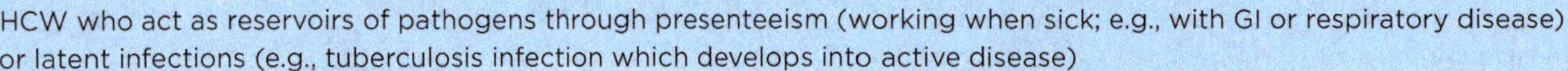

OLDER ADULT INFECTION RELATED TO CHARACTERISTICS OF RESIDENT/NURSE AIDE INFECTIONS

HCW who act as reservoirs of pathogens through presenteeism (working when sick; e.g., with GI or respiratory disease) or latent infections (e.g., tuberculosis infection which develops into active disease)

Incomplete and infrequent hygiene and perineal care from poor training/technique, cultural taboos, or language barriers that can include no hygiene, no gloves, or contaminated gloves which leads to exposure to pathogens and increased incontinence, skin breakdown/infection, and UTI	Inadequate assistance with eating related to lack of time or training or language barriers that increase risk for aspiration pneumonia and dehydration/malnutrition	Rushed or unnecessary assistance related to lack of time/training or language barriers that foster resident dependence which increases risk for infection
Inadequate staffing or cultural/gender issues about asking for help with transfers and care requiring two people Inadequate supervision/guidance of HCP includes aides and nurses Leads to "get it done and I don't care how" attitudes	Improper use of equipment (lifts, wheelchairs, restraints, glucose testing) related to lack of training/time, wrong equipment, or broken/missing equipment, or language barriers which can lead to injuries including skin tears pressure areas and BBP exposure, increasing the risk of infection	Resident immobility related to lack of time/training, language barriers on the part of HCP, leading to decreased ambulation, increased risk of pressure areas, pneumonia, incontinence

medical supplies, and environmental condition and suitability. They are also affected by the HCP and the organizational views regarding the importance of infection prevention and control. Infections may also be associated with resident level of ADL dependence, dementia, as well as increased contact with peers, HCP, and the environment. Skin condition, invasive devices, dehydration, malnutrition, chronic illness, and immobility affect the rate and susceptibility to infection.[2] For additional information, see Chapter 6 on nursing care.

Infectious disease outbreaks disturb residents, the staff's well-being, routine ADLs, resident mobility, staffing levels, visits from residents' families and significant others, and volunteer activities. Infectious disease outbreaks may be caused by transmission between HCP and residents, but a clear temporal relationship needs to be shown between the HCP illness and the resident illness. Assistance from the public health department may be requested in the case of a complaint, a spike in hospitalizations, or the realization that an infectious disease outbreak is beyond the abilities of the LTCF staff to control.

The two most common types of outbreaks in LTCFs are respiratory infections, which generally are spread by contact or by droplets (or in the case of tuberculosis, via the airborne route), and gastrointestinal outbreaks, which are spread by contaminated surfaces, food, vomit, feces, or aerosolized droplets.[2] If a nursing assistant or a resident is ill or incubating an illness such as influenza or norovirus, the close proximity of caregiving makes transmission of pathogens possible by contact (direct contact), droplet (within 3 to 6 feet if the sick person coughs or sneezes), or airborne routes if personal protective equipment is not worn. Nursing units in LTCFs may need to be closed during outbreaks, and procedures may need to be changed, causing general disruption of normal routines. These changes may have a personal impact on the residents when volunteers cannot visit and family visits are limited or when family members or HCP become ill.

Outbreaks can affect residents' well-being by restricting resident movement and participation in activities or therapy. HCP who become sick will cause extra work for healthy HCP. In addition to norovirus and influenza, outbreaks of respiratory syncytial virus (RSV), group A streptococcal disease (GAS), pertussis, and tuberculosis have been reported, involving both residents and HCP. These can result in significant morbidity for both HCP and residents, as well as mortality for residents.[20-23] Outbreaks of Hepatitis B and C, which can be caused by misuse of glucose testing supplies or inappropriate HCP technique, have also been described.[24-30]

Influenza

Respiratory infections are the leading cause of LTCF residents' death with an incidence of between 0.3 and 2.5 infections/1,000 resident days and an estimated 0.16 to 2.57 million cases annually.[31] Individuals with influenza are infectious from the day before symptoms appear to five days after symptoms occur.[32] Transmission of influenza from direct caregivers to LTCF residents is a possible cause of influenza outbreaks. Vaccinating LTCF employees for influenza reduces hospitalizations and deaths in older adult residents. Studies have shown a measurable benefit from employee influenza vaccination programs in LTCFs.[33,34] Staff may not consider influenza vaccination an infection prevention strategy, and there may be cultural resistance to vaccination.[35,36] The LTCF leadership should reinforce the importance of vaccination as a strategy for protecting both employees and residents. Vaccinations should be promoted as an employee benefit using appropriate education and understanding of cultural issues. Voluntary influenza employee vaccination rates in healthcare range from 8 to 65 percent, whereas facilities with formal employee vaccination programs and mandatory declinations have higher employee participation rates.[37]

Norovirus

Centers for Disease Control and Prevention (CDC) data from health departments of 24 states collected between October/December 2005 and 2006 reported 1,316 outbreaks of gastroenteritis. Approximately half of these occurred in LTCFs, and 26 percent were laboratory-confirmed norovirus. Published rates are between 0.1 and 2.5 per 1,000 resident days with an estimated 0.05 to 1.37 million cases annually.[31] Norovirus is considered to be the most common cause of acute gastroenteritis in LTCFs and affect both HCP and residents. Symptoms are acute onset nausea, vomiting, and diarrhea. Individuals with norovirus are infectious prior to symptoms and up to 10 days after symptoms resolve.[38] Two cases of norovirus qualify as an outbreak in a LTCF because the virus travels rapidly through both HCP and resident populations.

Bloodborne Pathogen Transmission to Dependent Diabetic Residents through HCP Actions

Transmission of Hepatitis B and Hepatitis C to dependent diabetic residents and to HCP may occur through the improper use and re-use of contaminated blood glucose testing equipment through the use of blood glucose testing equipment without gloves or unsafe injection practices. Nursing assistants may be asked to assist with blood glucose monitoring, either as an official part of their job or to assist a resident who is attempting self-monitoring of blood glucose (SMBG). Assisted monitoring of blood glucose (AMBG) requires specific facility policies and procedures and special, dedicated equipment that complies with the Occupational Safety and Health Administration (OSHA) Needlestick Safety

Act of 2004. The Act requires barrier precautions, hand hygiene, and gloves in a manner consistent with the bloodborne pathogen OSHA regulation. The nursing assistant is required to undergo specific training and retraining, and the nursing assistant must be offered Hepatitis B vaccine. Common use equipment must be appropriately cleaned and disinfected, usually with a bleach/detergent solution, before it is reused on another individual. The improper use of AMBG has been attributed to a significant number of nursing assistant and resident exposures and active cases of Hepatitis B disease and deaths. However, the numbers are believed to be vastly underreported. Lack of education and training, the rush to complete a task due to multiple tasks and inadequate staff, the practice of sharing equipment among residents, and the lack of needed supplies all contribute to increased transmission of this type of infection.[25-27]

NURSING ASSISTANT POPULATION CHARACTERISTICS IN LTCFS

There are more than 15,000 LTCFs in the United States with almost 600,000 nursing assistants who provide physical and psychosocial support to more than 1.5 million residents and patients.[2] This heterogeneous group provides the majority of hands-on care in licensed LTCFs. According to recent studies for this group:

- 92 percent of nursing assistants were female[39]
- Almost 60 percent were over 35 years of age[39]
- More than 50 percent were white[39]
- Almost 40 percent were black[39]
- 7.9 percent were of other self-described races[39]
- High physical demands/high injury rates[40]
- High job turnover can affect quality of care[41]
- More than 60 percent of nursing assistants were in lower socioeconomic categories[39]
- The typical nursing assistant has a household income of less than $30,000 at a time when the national poverty level for a family of five was $22,610, and for a family of eight was $32,390[39,42]
- More than 50 percent of nursing assistants have 6 or more years of experience[39]
- 97 percent described a primary reason for working in nursing homes as they "like helping other people"[39]
- In 28 states, nursing assistants can take additional training to pass routine oral medications, which increases nursing assistant contact with residents[43]

Nursing assistants must perform their assigned duties reliably and consistently to prevent infections and must also report changes in resident condition. The challenges that nursing assistants face in preforming their job includes language barriers, cognitive barriers, staffing levels (specifically lack of staff and lack of supervision), lack of training, a practice of floating staff from unit to unit, and facility culture. The speed required to complete all tasks in a specified period of time during a shift may decrease opportunities for reporting resident condition change and may force the nursing assistant to take shortcuts. Cultural issues or training in a different country may affect care delivery. A call for worldwide consensus and sustainable strategies for delivering quality nursing home care has been made by The International Association of Gerontology and Geriatrics, the World Health Organization, and the Society Française de Gerontologie et de Geriatrie Task Force.[44] To understand an individual nursing assistant, it is imperative to carefully consider the cultural sensibilities and prior training that each individual has had and to use that knowledge to frame the tasks and skills of each nursing assistant.

Almost 75 percent of all nursing assistants have a high school diploma or less education. Foreign-born nursing assistants have more than twice the number of college degrees (14.6 percent) as native-born nursing assistants (6 percent).[45] This leads to an interesting dichotomy. Foreign-born nursing assistants may actually have more education and may speak and understand more languages than the licensed practical nurses or associate degree nurses who supervise them. Comprehension may vary widely, as some foreign-born individuals understand far more English than they speak and have a better understanding of Latin-based words and medical terminology than they do of simple idioms and expressions. Conflict between HCP and between HCP and residents may exist if the intelligence or competency of the assistant is judged solely on the fluency of their spoken English.

With 60 percent of nursing assistants in lower socioeconomic categories, paid sick time is a luxury. Economic realities can lead to the phenomenon of presenteeism, or working while ill.[46] Nursing assistants may feel pressured to come to work when sick, either because they have no sick leave or because they believe that calling in sick will leave the unit short-staffed or with temporary help who do not know how to care for the residents. HCP may also feel pressured to work when they are sick by supervisors and coworkers. Working while sick with infectious disease may actually increase the workload when coworkers and residents fall ill, and there are fewer healthy HCP to help with the increased workload of increased resident illness.

LTCF CHALLENGES: TAKING A DEEPER DIVE

This chapter describes the broad, overarching infection prevention challenges facing LTCFs: increasingly elderly, at risk resident populations, and the need for educated and appropriately supervised HCP. Reinforcing the importance of appropriate resident assessment and care planning, appropriate training, current policies and procedures, active vaccination programs, strong supervision, clear expectations, and communication sensitive to cultural expectations and language/cognitive barriers all help reduce the spread of infectious disease.

In the following chapters, IPs knowledgeable in LTCF prevention programs can take a deeper dive into the specific content areas that support the broad challenges just presented. These chapters are ordered so that the IP can build consecutively on the information to not only design an effective infection prevention plan and program, but also to target those areas within the facility that often present special issues or potential threats to resident and HCP safety. This content will also provide a concrete context for implementing the measures outlined in the HHS National Action Plan (see a summary of this plan on page 10). For this reason, reviewing the content in the general order presented offers the greatest value to the novice user. However, this approach is not required, and individuals proficient in LTCF prevention programs may prefer to develop a personalized approach.

The authors intend this book to accomplish the following objectives:

(1) protect the resident from the most common, preventable infections;

(2) comply with guidance from the CDC and other authoritative sources; and

(3) maximize regulatory and accrediting compliance and survey outcomes for the facility.

LONG-TERM CARE: AN EMERGING NATIONAL PREVENTION PRIORITY

In 2009 the U.S. Department of Health and Human Services (HHS) introduced the *National Action Plan to Prevent Healthcare Associated Infections: Roadmap to Elimination.* Since its original focus on acute care, the National Action Plan has expanded to include additional settings, most recently a portion of long-term care providers. The eventual goal is to develop a comprehensive federal healthcare-associated infection (HAI) prevention schema that is applicable across the various types of LTCFs. Because of the heterogeneity of both facilities and their resident populations, the long-term care component is currently based on the Medicare definition that identifies four general categories of post-acute providers: long-term care hospitals, inpatient rehabilitation facilities, nursing homes/skilled nursing facilities (NH/SNF), and home health agencies. The National Action Plan currently focuses on facility-based long-term care as delivered by NH/SNFs.[47]

Not only is there a wide range of often overlapping providers, but the underlying needs and risk factors of an aging population are equally diverse. LTCF residents have limited physiologic reserve, high rates of multimorbid conditions, inconsistent use of immunizations, and exposure to multidrug-resistant pathogens. Expected symptoms of infection may be absent or present in atypical ways when compared to younger groups of individuals.[47] These and other complex risk factors, described in this book, reflect the importance and growing urgency of preventing infections in this vulnerable group. The goal of improved infection prevention is challenged by the lack of facility infrastructure. One study reported that the number of infection preventionists (IPs) in nursing homes is four times less than the number in acute care facilities or similar.[48] Those IPs in long-term care have minimal training for their roles; another study revealed that less than 10 percent of IPs in NH/SNFs had received specialized training and/or achieved infection prevention certification compared to more than 95 percent of IPs in acute care.[49]

Because the constraints are formidable, the National Action Plan's measures and metrics for long-term care have been developed to create a basis for sustainable, meaningful, and manageable change. This change process begins with a goal of enrolling 5 percent of certified nursing homes into the National Healthcare Safety Network long-term care component over the 5 years following its launch. After that, the plan proposes measures targeting (1) *Clostridium difficile* infections, (2) influenza and pneumococcal vaccinations for residents, (3) influenza vaccination for HCP, and (4) catheter-associated urinary tract infections and catheter care processes.[47]

Much work remains ahead. The burden of collecting, analyzing, validating, and reporting infection data is a major obstacle to future success. Little is known about the best methods of risk adjustment of HAI rates across long-term care settings. The use of electronic surveillance system is minimal and the reliability of the measures they report is often unclear. Because IPs in LTCFs often have multiple roles and must juggle competing operational priorities in settings under resourced for optimum prevention practice, this book seeks to offer solutions and thereby be another cornerstone in the HHS ongoing efforts to advance the National Plan and promote a higher level of health safety among LTCF residents.

REFERENCES

1. Mody L. Infection control issues in older adults. *Clin Geriatr Med* 2007; 23(3): 499-514.
2. Smith PW, Bennett G, Bradley S, Drinka P, Lautenbach E, Marx J, et al. SHEA/APIC Guideline: infection prevention and control in the long-term care facility. *Infect Control Hosp Epidemiol* 2008; 29(9): 785-814.
3. Harrington C, Olney B, Carrillo H, Kang T. Nurse staffing and deficiencies in the largest for-profit nursing home chains and chains owned by private equity companies. *Health Serv Res* 2012; 47(1pt1): 106-128.
4. Castle NG, Wagner LM, Ferguson-Rome JC, Men A, Handler SM. Nursing home deficiency citations for infection control. *Am J Infect Control* 2011; 39(4): 263-269.
5. Htwe TH, Mushtaq A, Robinson SB, Rusher RB, Khardori N. Infection in the elderly. *Infect Dis Clin North Am* 2007 Sep; 21(3): 711-743, ix.
6. Hunt KJ, Walsh BM, Voegeli D, Roberts HC. Inflammation in aging part 2: Implications for the health of older people and recommendations for nursing practice. *Biol Res Nurs* 2010; 11(3): 253-260.
7. Peterson LR. *Detection, Education, Research and Decolonization Without Isolation in Long-term Care to Control (DERAIL) MRSA.* Clinical Trials.gov website. 2009. Available at: http://clinicaltrials.gov/ct2/show/NCT01302210.
8. Kaiser G. *Innate immune response.* Doc Kaiser's Microbiology Home Page. 2009. Available at: http://student.ccbcmd.edu/courses/bio141/lecguide/unit4/innate/inflammation.html.
9. *Selective IgA deficiency.* Immune Disease website. 2010. Available at: http://www.immunedisease.com/patients-and-families/about-pi/types-of-pi/selective-iga-deficiency.html.
10. Huether SE, McCance KL, Barnette P. *Understanding pathophysiology.* St. Louis: Mosby, 2000.
11. Pittet D, Allegranzi B, Boyce J. The World Health Organization guidelines on hand hygiene in health care and their consensus recommendations. *Infect Control Hosp Epidemiol* 2009; 30(7): 611-622.
12. Nicolle LE. Infection control in long-term care facilities. *Clin Infect Dis* 2000; 31(3): 752-756.
13. Nicolle LE. Preventing infections in non-hospital settings: long-term care. *Emerg Infect Dis* 2001; 7(2): 205-207.
14. Kagan LJ, Aiello AE, Larson E. The role of the home environment in the transmission of infectious diseases. *J Community Health* 2002; 27(4): 247-267.
15. Hunt KJ, Walsh BM, Voegeli D, Roberts HC. Inflammation in aging part 1: physiology and immunological mechanisms. *Biol Res Nurs* 2010; 11(3): 245-252.
16. Hunt KJ, Walsh BM, Voegeli D, Roberts HC. Inflammation in aging part 2: Implications for the health of older people and recommendations for nursing practice. *Biol Res Nurs* 2010; 11(3): 253-260.
17. Peterson LR, Hacek DM, Robicsek A. 5 Million Lives Campaign. Case study: an MRSA intervention at Evanston Northwestern Healthcare. *Jt Comm J Qual Patient Saf* 2007; 33(12): 732-738.
18. Eikelenboom-Boskamp A, Cox-Claessens J, Boom-Poels P, Drabbe M, Koopmans R, Voss A. Three-year prevalence of healthcare-associated infections in Dutch nursing homes. *J Hosp Infect* 2011; 78(1): 59-62.
19. Fulop T, Pawelec G, Castle S, Loeb M. Immunosenescence and vaccination in nursing home residents. *Clin Infect Dis* 2009 Feb 15; 48(4): 443-448.
20. Arnold K, Schweitzer J, Wallace B, Salter M, Neeman R, Hlady W, et al. Tightly clustered outbreak of group A streptococcal disease at a long term care facility. *Infect Control Hosp Epidemiol* 2006; 27(12): 1377-1384.
21. Centers for Disease Control and Prevention (CDC). *Tuberculosis (TB).* CDC website. 2010. Available at: http://www.cdc.gov/tb/.
22. Ferson MJ, Morgan K, Robertson PW, Hampson AW, Carter I, Rawlinson WD. Concurrent summer influenza and pertussis outbreaks in a nursing home in Sydney, Australia. *Infect Control Hosp Epidemiol* 2004; 25(11): 962-966.
23. Rajagopalan S, Yoshikawa TT. Tuberculosis in long-term-care facilities. *Infect Control Hosp Epidemiol* 2000; 21(9): 611-615.
24. Centers for Disease Control and Prevention (CDC). *National Healthcare Safety Network (NHSN): Tracking infections in long-term care facilities.* CDC website. Available at: http://www.cdc.gov/nhsn/LTC/.
25. Forero S, Alvarez JE, Doyle T. *Hepatitis B outbreak associated with home health care in South Florida.* Centers for Disease Control and Prevention website. 2010. Available at: http://www.cdc.gov/hepatitis/statistics/2009surveillance/Commentary.htm.
26. Klonoff DC, Perz JF. Assisted monitoring of blood glucose: special safety needs for a new paradigm in testing glucose. *J Diabetes Sci Tech* 2010; 4(5): 1027-1031.
27. Patel AS, White-Comstock MB, Woolard CD, Perz JF. Infection control practices in assisted living facilities: a response to hepatitis B virus infection outbreaks. *Infection* 2009; 30(3): 209-214.
28. Perz JF, Fiore AE. Hepatitis B virus infection risks among diabetic patients residing in long-term care facilities. *Clin Infect Dis* 2005; 41(5): 760-761.
29. Thompson ND, Barry V, Aleli K, Cui D, Perz JF. Evaluation of the potential for bloodborne pathogen transmission associated with diabetes care practices in nursing homes and assisted living facilities, Pinellas County. *J Am Geriatr Soc* 2010; 58(5): 914-918.
30. Thompson ND, Perz JF, Moorman AC, Holmberg SD. Nonhospital health care-associated hepatitis B and C virus transmission: United States, 1998-2008. *Ann Intern Med* 2009; 150(1): 33-39.
31. Strausbaugh LJ, Sukumar SR, Joseph CL, High KP. Infectious disease outbreaks in nursing homes: an unappreciated hazard for frail elderly persons. *Clin Infect Dis* 2003; 36(7): 870-876.

REFERENCES

32. Centers for Disease Control and Prevention (CDC). *Seasonal influenza.* CDC website. Available at: http://www.cdc.gov/flu/.

33. Carman WF, Elder AG, Wallace LA, McAulay K, Walke, A, Murray GD, et al. Effects of influenza vaccination of health-care workers on mortality of elderly people in long-term care: a randomised controlled trial. *Lancet* 2000; 355(9198): 93-97.

34. Dolan GP, Harris RC, Clarkson M, Sokal R, Morgan G, Mukaigawara M, et al. Vaccination of health care workers to protect patients at increased risk for acute respiratory disease. *Emerg Infect Dis* 2012; 18(8): 1225-1234.

35. Kata A. A postmodern Pandora's box: anti-vaccination misinformation on the Internet. *Vaccine* 2010 Feb 17; 28(7): 1709-1716.

36. Stanton BF. Assessment of relevant cultural considerations is essential for the success of a vaccine. *J Health Popul Nutr* 2004 Sep; 22(3): 286-292.

37. Centers for Disease Control and Prevention (CDC). *Influenza vaccination information for health care workers.* CDC website. Available at: http://www.cdc.gov/flu/healthcareworkers.htm.

38. Centers for Disease Control and Prevention (CDC). *Novovirus.* CDC website. Available at: http://www.cdc.gov/norovirus/.

39. Centers for Disease Control and Prevention (CDC). *Table 1. Number and percent distribution of all nursing home certified nursing assistants and those currently working in nursing homes, by selected nursing assistant characteristics: United States, 2004-2005.* CDC website. Available at: http://www.cdc.gov/nchs/data/nnhsd/Estimates/nnas/Estimates_DemoCareer_Tables.pdf#01.

40. Bureau of Labor Statistics (BLS), U.S. Department of Labor. *Occupational Outlook Handbook,* 2012-13 edition. BLS website. 2013. Available at: http://www.bls.gov/ooh/healthcare/nursing-assistants.htm.

41. Castle NG, Engberg J. Staff turnover and quality of care in nursing homes. *Med Care* 2005; 43(6): 616-626.

42. U.S. Department of Health and Human Services (HHS). *2005 HHS Poverty Guidelines.* HHS website. Available at: http://aspe.hhs.gov/poverty/05poverty.shtml.

43. Medication Aides Illinois. *Life Services Network.* Med Aides Illinois website. 2008. Available at: http://www.medaidesillinois.org/index.htm.

44. Tolson D, Morley JE, Rolland Y, Vellas B. Improving nursing home practice: an international concern. *Nurs Older People* 2011; 23(9): 20-21.

45. Clearfield D, Batalova J. *Foreign-born health-care workers in the United States.* Migration Policy Institute website. 2007. Available at: http://www.migrationinformation.org/usfocus/display.cfm?ID=583#10.

46. Widera E, Chang A, Chen HL. Presenteeism: A public health hazard. *J Gen Intern Med* 2010; 25(11): 1244-1247.

47. U.S. Department of Health and Human Services (HHS). *Chapter 8: Long-Term Care Facilities.* HHS website. 2013. Available at: http://www.hhs.gov/ash/initiatives/hai/actionplan/hai-action-plan-ltcf.pdf.

48. Roup BJ, Roch JC, Pass M. Infection control program disparities between acute and long term care facilities in Maryland. *Am J Infect Control* 2006; 34(3): 122-127.

49. Roup BJ, Scaletta JM. How Maryland increased infection prevention and control activity in long term care facilities, 2003-2008. *Am J Infect Control* 2011; 39: 292-295.

50. Kirk MD, Veitch MG, Hall GV. Gastroenteritis and food-borne disease in elderly people living in long-term care. *Clin Infect Dis.* 2010 Feb 1; 50(3): 397-404.

CHAPTER 2

Regulatory Surveys and CMS F tag 441 Compliance

Deborah Patterson Burdsall, MSN, RN-BC, CIC

KEY CONCEPTS

- Long-term care regulations have evolved over the last several decades in an effort to dramatically improve the quality of care and quality of life for residents. Regulations and standards of practice have shifted from basic facility oversight to emphasize resident-centered care.
- It is important for the infection preventionists to understand the differences between regulations and guidelines and how they should be incorporated into the infection prevention program and resident care.
- The long-term care-based infection preventionist should focus on survey preparation within the framework and intent of F441: "The facility must establish and maintain an infection control program designed to provide a safe and comfortable environment and to help prevent the development and transmission of disease and infection."[1]

LONG-TERM CARE REGULATORY BACKGROUND

There was a time in United States history when nursing homes and skilled nursing facilities were not regulated. The nursing home industry developed through the 1950s and 1960s as federal, state, and local governments established assistance funding for "medically needy" older adults in need of financial and physical support. During this period, state regulation and oversight were minimal, and as early as 1956, the federal Commission on Chronic Illness expressed concerns about the quality of care being provided in nursing homes. The chronic disease program of the Public Health Service began studying state licensure programs in 1957 and worked with the states and industry to publish *Nursing Home Standards Guide* in 1963. In addition, the Senate Special Committee on Aging (Moss Committee) began holding hearings from 1963 to 1965 to investigate problems within nursing homes. In 1965, Medicare and Medicaid funding, which provides health coverage or nursing home coverage to certain categories of low-income people, was established.[2-4] With this funding, the Centers for Medicare & Medicaid Services (CMS) began to monitor the state-run programs and establish requirements for quality and eligibility standards.

In 1974, the Moss Committee published a report detailing shortcomings of the state oversight programs, including shortage of facilities, inability of state enforcers to make meaningful change to nursing home care, and shortcomings within the structure of the survey process, which emphasized building structure as opposed to staffing and resident care issues. The report identified poor care in nursing homes, including resident deaths as a result of fires and food poisoning, resident isolation, excessive and improper use of restraints, infection, and malnutrition. As a result, the Department of Health, Education, and Welfare (HEW) established offices of long-term care standards enforcement in 1974. However, the initial surveys were focused on the facility environment and processes rather than on individual, person-centered, biopsychosocial needs.[5,6] In response to increased scrutiny and an increasing number of reports of nursing home abuse and neglect, Congress passed the Nursing Home Reform Act as part of the Omnibus Reconciliation Act (OBRA) of 1987, establishing new and improved standards of practice in skilled nursing facilities (SNFs) and intermediate care facilities (ICFs). The act mandated that CMS—previously called the Health Care Financing Administration—create a survey and certification process to ensure consistent implementation of OBRA regulations and standards of care at the facility level (Figure 2.1).

The mission of CMS is "to promote quality care for beneficiaries" and improve safety and quality of care based on the objectives of the CMS Three-Part Aim[7]:

1. Improving the individual experience of care
2. Improving the health of populations
3. Reducing the per capita cost of care for populations

CMS outlined their strategy for achieving these aims in the 2012 Nursing Home Action Plan.[7] The plan is a five-part, coordinated strategy that involves engaging consumers through the use of public websites such as www.Medicare.gov, which contains information about the survey results, rating systems, and other CMS initiatives. The information comes from a variety of sources including the minimum data set (MDS) resident assessment instrument and the survey and certification process. The goal is the enhancement of resident-centered care and an enhancement of the overall individual experience of care.[2,7]

GUIDELINES VERSUS REGULATIONS

It is important that long-term care infection preventionists (IPs) understand the difference between a guideline and a regulation. Regulations must be followed by law, but guidelines are framed as recommendations. Many times guidelines, such as those created by the Centers for Disease Control and Prevention's (CDC) Healthcare Infection Control Practices Advisory Committee (HICPAC), are written to provide practice guidance. HICPAC guidelines, such as *Guideline for Hand Hygiene in Healthcare Settings, 2002; Guideline for Isolation Precautions, 2007; Management of Multidrug-Resistant Organisms in Healthcare Settings, 2006;* and *Guidelines for preventing the transmission of*

FIGURE 2.1: INFLUENCES ON LONG-TERM CARE PRACTICE

Guidelines and regulations

Calls to address biopsychosocial needs of older adult residents

LONG-TERM CARE PRACTICE

Need for consistent and improved quality of care

Long-term care research/ expert consensus

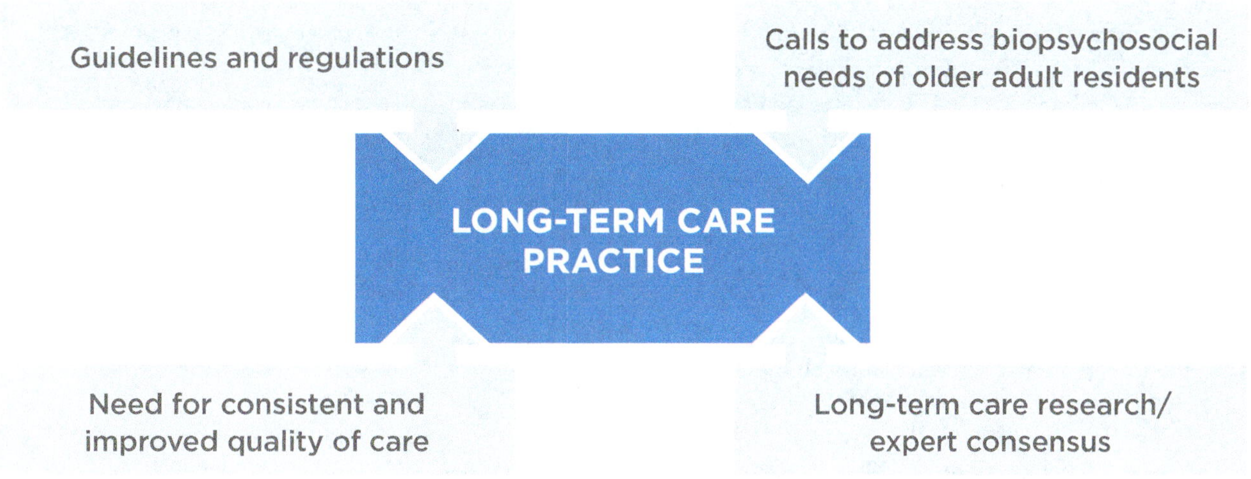

Mycobacterium tuberculosis in health-care settings, 2005, are generally formed by expert consensus using the best scientific evidence.[8-11]

The strength of the recommendations within the guidelines is based on the quality of the evidence that support the practice. Recommendations are categorized as follows:

- **Category IA:** Strongly recommended for implementation and strongly supported by well-designed experimental, clinical, or epidemiologic studies.
- **Category IB:** Strongly recommended for implementation and supported by some experimental, clinical, or epidemiologic studies and a strong theoretical rationale.
- **Category IC:** Required for implementation as mandated by federal and/or state regulation or standard.
- **Category II:** Suggested for implementation and supported by suggestive clinical or epidemiologic studies or a theoretical rationale.
- **No recommendation:** Unresolved issue. Practices for which insufficient evidence or no consensus regarding efficacy exists.[8]

Federal or state regulations can be written to include compliance with guidelines. However, there are areas of long-term care practice that have not been validated by sufficient numbers of well-designed studies. More research in long-term care infection prevention practices is needed.

REGULATIONS FOR LONG-TERM CARE INFECTION PREVENTION AND CONTROL

Long-term care facility (LTCF) regulations are published in the *Code of Federal Regulations* (CFR) Title 42 Section 483.65, and are incorporated into F tag 441, "Interpretive Guidelines for Long-Term Care Facilities." F tag 441 applies to skilled and intermediate care facilities. States may add additional regulations that require a higher standard of care to the federal requirements. State survey teams monitor compliance with both the federal and state regulations. These teams complete annual certification standard surveys and complaint surveys for both the states and for CMS. There are also federal or contracted survey teams that provide federal comparative validation surveys or "look behind" oversight for the state survey teams.[6,7]

The CMS *State Operations Manual* (SOM) and Interpretive Guidelines direct the survey process. The Interpretive Guidelines are developed through an interactive process with expert panels, stakeholder meetings, and comment periods. Interpretive Guidelines explain the intent of the regulations, define the terms utilized, and provide instruction to the surveyors as they determine compliance with regulations.[6,7,12,13]

A 2011 survey of LTCFs found that 15 percent had citations for F441.[12] To maintain compliance with (F441) 42 CFR 483.65, the LTCF's infection prevention and control program must meet the following criteria:

- The infection prevention and control program demonstrates ongoing surveillance, recognition, investigation, and control of infections to prevent the onset and the spread of infection to the extent possible.
- The facility demonstrates practices to reduce the spread of infection and control outbreaks through Transmission-based Precautions (e.g., isolation precautions).
- The facility demonstrates practices and processes (e.g., intravenous catheter care, hand hygiene) consistent with infection prevention and prevention of cross contamination.
- The facility demonstrates that it uses records of incidents to improve its infection control processes and outcomes by taking corrective action.
- The facility has processes and procedures to identify and prohibit employees with a communicable disease or infected skin lesions from direct contact with residents or their food, if direct contact will transmit the disease.
- The facility consistently demonstrates appropriate hand hygiene (e.g., hand washing) practices after each direct resident contact as indicated by professional practice.
- The facility demonstrates handling, storage, processing, and transporting of linens so as to prevent the spread of infection.[13]

The expectations are that:

- Infection prevention and control systems are put in place that promote the health of individuals within the LTCF, and maintain and sustain a healthful and clean comfortable LTCF environment. Ideal systems are economical and fit within a biopsychosocial culture change model and healthcare personnel (HCP) work flow.
- Infection prevention and control issues are correctly identified through careful surveillance, investigation, and awareness of the reality of the day-to-day situation in the LTCF.
- Quality improvement processes are utilized to correct identified infection prevention and control issues through the use of records of infection incidents to improve processes and outcomes by taking corrective actions.
- Surveillance and investigation are continuously implemented to prevent the onset and the spread of infection.
- Outbreaks are prevented and controlled and cross-contamination is avoided by using Transmission-based Precautions in addition to Standard Precautions. (See Chapter 5 for more information on Standard and Transmission-based Precautions.)
- Hand hygiene (hand washing) is consistently practiced and monitored.
- Linen is properly stored, handled, processed, and transported to minimize contamination.
- Water supply is safe.
- Surveyors are to review the following:
  - Policy and procedures manuals; however, in a change from prior regulatory guidance, "the facility's written policy alone does not confirm compliance with Federal regulatory requirements."
  - Training documents and facility systems.[13]

Although there are aspects of the entire survey process that have application in infection prevention and control, the other major F tags that relate to infection prevention and control are:

- **F272 §483.20:** Resident Assessment including Comprehensive Assessment, Care Plan, and Care Plan Revisions,
- **F315 §483.25(d):** Urinary Incontinence (and catheters),
- **F334 §483.25(n):** Influenza and pneumococcal immunizations and unnecessary drugs,
- **F371 §483.35(i):** Sanitary Conditions/Food Safety, and
- **F498 §483.75:** Proficiency of Nurses' Aides.[13]

ADDRESSING SURVEY READINESS

The survey and certification process is an important part of implementing the initiatives and regulations put forth by CMS. It allows for infection prevention and control issues to be identified and investigated any time during the course of the survey. CMS identifies the importance of updated policies and procedures to establish the expectations for infection prevention and control programs. Policies and procedures should reflect the most current applicable regulations and standards of practice. The policies of an LTCF should reflect the specific needs and characteristics of its resident population. This is important, as CMS has adopted the culture change model that encourages facilities to transform organizational values, structures, and practices from traditional instructional models to person-centered care and quality of life. The focus is on individualized plans of care instead of institutional models and set institutional policies and procedures. The facility's infection prevention and control program should include the following:

- Develop policies and procedures that reflect the most current applicable regulations and standards of practice. The policies of a specific LTCF should reflect the facility risk assessment, as well as the specific needs and characteristics of the resident/patient population.
- Ensure that direct caregivers understand the principles behind Standard Precautions and Transmission-based Precautions.
- Focus on surveillance activities that are critical to infection prevention and control.
- Process elements:
  - Hand hygiene
  - Correct glove use
  - Availability of soap, paper towels, and alcohol-based hand rub or disinfecting hand wipes
  - Availability of appropriate cleaning/disinfecting products
  - Staff trained in the proper use of cleaning/disinfecting products, including contact time requirements
  - Availability of personal protective equipment (PPE), including gloves, gowns, masks, and eye protection as a Standard Precaution
  - Staff trained in the proper and timely use of PPE
  - Medication pass monitoring
  - Treatment monitoring
  - Central line care monitoring
  - Perineal care and urinary catheter care monitoring
  - Temperature and expiration date monitoring of food and medication
  - Antimicrobial stewardship programs that reduce or prevent the unnecessary prescribing of antibiotics
- Outcome Elements
  - Infection rates
  - Antibiotic use
  - Hospital readmission rates
  - Rapid identification of condition change in residents
  - Knowledge of how to address condition change
  - Sources of surveillance data efforts including:
    a. Documentation elements
       » LTCF methods for gathering, documenting, and listing surveillance data
    b. Monitoring
       » Type and frequency of monitoring the effectiveness of infection prevention and control program
    c. Data analysis
       » How is the data analyzed and the analysis used to improve processes
    d. Communicable disease reporting
       » Identify what diseases should be reported at the state and local level
    e. Antibiotic review
       » Prescribing authority and pharmacist in combination with the IP and the interdisciplinary team (IDT)

QUALITY ASSURANCE AND PERFORMANCE IMPROVEMENT

The focus of the continual reforms has been to improve the quality of care for older adults in long-term care so that there is a consistent standard for a high level of care in all United States facilities.[6] Implementation of the Quality Indicator Survey (QIS), as well as the Quality Assurance and Performance Improvement (QAPI) process, are systems developed by CMS to continue the movement toward a person-centered model of long-term care.

The Affordable Care Act of 2010 requires that skilled and intermediate nursing facilities develop a QAPI plan. In the same way that infection prevention and control surveillance is a data and analysis based system, QAPI also relies on systematically collected data and a comprehensive system of analysis to improve quality of care. Once a well-developed QAPI plan is implemented, it should provide the structure for a competency-based, continuous quality and performance improvement system that should meet three important goals:

- Improve care for individuals
- Improve the health of populations
- Reduce per capita cost in the healthcare system[14,15]

For examples of QAPI projects for LTC, see Chapter 3.

QUALITY INDICATOR SURVEY

The survey and certification process can be one of the most challenging times for LTCFs. The goal of the CMS survey and certification process is to ensure that residents and patients of long-term care are provided a level of care that meets their biological, psychological, and social needs within a safe, sanitary, and comfortable environment. The goal of the CMS QIS is to ensure a more consistent and resident-centered survey process that is less reliant on surveyor preference and more reliant on a structured, methodical survey process (Figures 2.2 and 2.3).[14,15]

The survey team will observe infection prevention and control practices throughout the entire survey process. A member of the survey team will be assigned the overall responsibility for the completion of this task, and they will use details of F441 (Infection Control) to review the facility infection prevention and control program. Each team member will initiate the infection control observation if they were not assigned the overall responsibility. See Figure 2.4 for an excerpt from a CMS surveyor tool. Note: All surveyors must initiate this task to document concerns throughout the survey.[15]

FUTURE TRENDS

The CMS Division of Nursing Homes (DNH) is currently working with strategic partners to develop strategies to reduce preventable healthcare-associated infections. This means that the focus on infection prevention and control will increase. It is critical to have a systematic, evidence-based approach to preventing infections within long-term care.

CONCLUSION

The survey process can be one of the most stressful times of the year for long-term care staff. To successfully complete the survey process, it is important to keep in mind the reasons for infection prevention and control programs: to provide a safe and comfortable environment that reduces the risk of infection and colonization within a biopsychosocial, person-centered framework. The infection preventionist can prepare for the survey process by keeping in mind the following:

- Read the guidelines and regulations.
- Know what regulations apply to infection prevention and control and how to use the interpretive guidelines to maximize compliance.
- Evaluate the infection prevention plan to identify strengths and opportunities for improvement.
- Build a person-centered model of care to comply with the federal and state regulations in which the care community is based. For example, all healthcare settings with more than six employees need to follow the regulations from the Occupational Safety and Health Administration (OSHA). This includes offering Hepatitis B vaccine to all at-risk employees, utilizing Standard Precautions, and complying with the Needlestick Safety and Prevention Act, tuberculosis control guidelines, and vaccination requirements. See Chapter 9 for more information on OSHA bloodborne pathogens and other regulated programs.
- There will be changes. Develop the infection prevention program so that changes are easily incorporated.

FIGURE 2.2: QIS SURVEY GOAL TO BALANCE QUALITY OF LIFE WITH QUALITY OF CARE

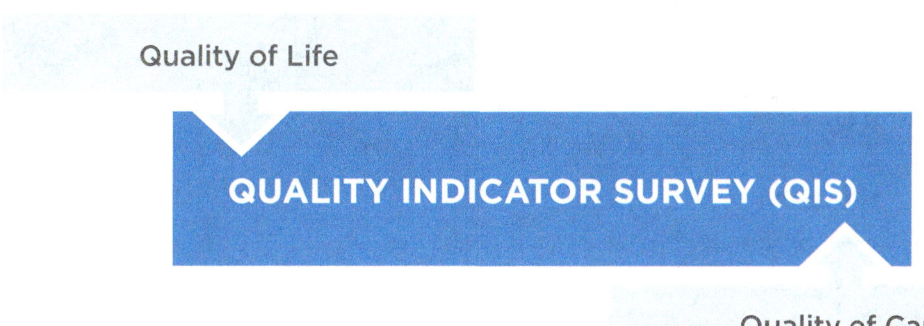

FIGURE 2.3: QIS PROCESS (ADAPTED FROM CMS QUALITY INDICATOR SURVEY)

STAGE I

Two random samples of residents/patients from MDS data

1. Select 40 residents/patients (or all in facility for facilities with less than 40) on the first day of survey
2. Select up to 30 residents/patients admitted or re-admitted within the past year (chart review)

Calculation of Quality Metrics

- Census
- Admission sample
- Quality-of-care indicators
- Quality-of-life indicators (QCLIs)
- Thresholds results calculated

Mandatory tasks: Include F441 infection prevention and control and immunizations

STAGE II

From QCLIs that exceed assigned thresholds

- Survey results
- Scope and severity of citations (F-tags)

Results of mandatory tasks: Include F441 infection prevention and control and immunizations

FIGURE 2.4: CMS SURVEYOR OBSERVATION TOOL: INFECTION PREVENTION AND IMMUNIZATIONS

Observations	Yes	No F441	Notes
1. Are proper hand washing techniques followed by the staff?	☐	☐	
2. Are gloves worn if there is contact with blood, specimens, tissue, body fluids, or excretions?	☐	☐	
3. Are gloves changed between resident contacts?	☐	☐	
4. Are staff who are providing direct care free from communicable diseases or infected skin lesions?	☐	☐	
5. Are precautions observed for the disposal of soiled linens, dressings, disposable equipment (sharps, etc.), and for the cleaning of contaminated reusable equipment?	☐	☐	
6. Are linens and laundry handled or transported in a manner to prevent the spread of infection?	☐	☐	
7. Are Isolation Precautions implemented when it is determined that a resident needs isolation?	☐	☐	

Also available on the CD-ROM.

REFERENCES

1. Centers for Medicare & Medicaid Services (CMS). *CMS Manual System Pub. 100-07 State Operations Provider Certification.* CMS website. 2009. Available at: http://www.cms.gov/Regulations-and-Guidance/Guidance/Transmittals/downloads/r55soma.pdf.

2. Committee on Nursing Home Regulation. Appendix A: History of federal nursing home regulation. In: *Improving the Quality of Care in Nursing Homes.* Washington, DC: The National Academies Press, 1986: 238-253.

3. Singh DA. *Effective management of long term care facilities.* Burlington, MA: Jones & Bartlett, 2010: 33-34.

4. ESTATE OF SMITH v. HECKLER. *747 F.2d 583 (1984)* Nos. 83-1442, 83-1466. United States Court of Appeals, Tenth Circuit. Leagle.com website. 1984. Available at: http://www.leagle.com/decision/19841330747F2d583_11232.

5. National Research Council. *Improving the Quality of Care in Nursing Homes.* Washington, DC: The National Academies Press, 1986.

6. Lin MK, Kramer KM. The Quality Indicator Survey: background, implementation, and widespread change. *J Aging Soc Policy* 2013; 25(1): 10-29.

7. Centers for Medicare & Medicaid Services (CMS). *CMS 2012 Nursing Home Action Plan Action Plan.* CMS website. 2012. Available at: http://www.cms.gov/Medicare/Provider-Enrollment-and-Certification/CertificationandComplianc/Downloads/2012-Nursing-Home-Action-Plan.pdf.

8. Centers for Disease Control and Prevention (CDC). Guideline for hand hygiene in health-care settings: recommendations of the Healthcare Infection Control Practices Advisory Committee and the HICPAC/SHEA/APIC/IDSA Hand Hygiene Task Force. *MMWR Recomm Rep* 2002; 51(RR-16): 1-45.

9. Siegel JD, Rhinehart E, Jackson M, Chiarello L, and the Healthcare Infection Control Practices Advisory Committee. *2007 Guideline for Isolation Precautions: Preventing transmission of infectious agents in healthcare settings.* Centers for Disease Control and Prevention website. 2007. Available at: http://www.cdc.gov/ncidod/dhqp/pdf/isolation2007.pdf.

10. Siegel JD, Rhinehart E, Jackson M, Chiarello L. *Management of multidrug-resistant organisms in healthcare settings, 2006.* Centers for Disease Control and Prevention website. 2006. Available at: http://www.cdc.gov/ncidod/dhqp/pdf/ar/mdroGuideline2006.pdf.

11. Jensen PA, Lambert LA, Iademarco MF, Ridzon R. Guidelines for preventing the transmission of Mycobacterium tuberculosis in health-care settings, 2005. *MMRW Recomm Rep* 2005; 54(RR-17): 1-141.

12. Castle NG, Wagner LM, Ferguson-Rome JC, Men A, Handler SM. Nursing home deficiency citations for infection control. *Am J Infect Control* 2011; 39(4): 263-269.

13. Centers for Medicare & Medicaid Services (CMS). *CMS Manual System Pub. 100-07 State Operations Manual Provider Certification. Revisions to Appendix PP – Interpretive Guidelines for Long-Term Care Facilities, Tag F441.* CMS website. 2009. Available at: http://www.cms.gov/Regulations-and-Guidance/Guidance/Transmittals/downloads/r55soma.pdf.

14. Centers for Medicare & Medicaid Services (CMS). *Updated brochure describing the Quality Indicator Survey (QIS) memorandum.* CMS website. 2008. Available at: http://www.cms.gov/Medicare/Provider-Enrollment-and-Certification/SurveyCertificationGenInfo/downloads/SCLetter08-21.pdf.

15. Centers for Medicare & Medicaid Services (CMS). *QAPI at a glance: A step by step guide to implementing quality assurance and performance improvement (QAPI) in your nursing home.* CMS website. 2012. Available at: http://www.cms.gov/Medicare/Provider-Enrollment-and-Certification/SurveyCertificationGenInfo/Downloads/Survey-and-Cert-Letter-13-05.pdf.

ADDITIONAL REFERENCES

Smith PW, Bennett G, Bradley S, Drinka P, Lautenbach E, Marx J, et al. SHEA/APIC guideline: infection prevention and control in the long-term care facility. *Infect Control Hosp Epidemiol* 2008; 29(9): 795-814.

Infection Prevention and Control Programs

Marilyn Hanchett, RN, MA, CPHQ, CIC
Patricia A. Rosenbaum, RN, CIC

KEY CONCEPTS

- The long-term care facility is an environment that presents unique challenges for the infection prevention program, including its coordination with other programs.
- The infection prevention program is described in a written plan that is based on a thorough facility risk assessment.
- The professional role of the infection preventionist, his/her competency development, and access to essential resources are necessary for the optimum success of the program.

The definition of a long-term care facility (LTCF) according to the Centers for Disease Control and Prevention (CDC) is a nursing home and/or skilled nursing facility that provides care to those people who cannot care for themselves. The CDC also estimates that 3.2 million Americans lived in Medicare- and Medicaid-participating nursing homes and skilled nursing facilities at some point during 2008.[1] Some facts about the impact of infections on the nursing home residents are[2]:

- Infections account for approximately half of all transfers to hospitals.
- Infections cause an estimated 150,000 to 200,000 hospital admissions per year.
- The cost of the transfers is estimated to be $673 million to $2 billion annually.
- Residents that are hospitalized with infections have a rate of death that can be as much as 40 percent.
- Infections per resident are estimated to average 1.6 to 3.8 annually.[3]

In recent years there has been increasing recognition of the importance of preventing healthcare-associated infections (HAIs) in the long-term care setting prompted by increasing acuity levels of residents and the increase in multidrug-resistant organisms (MDROs).

BACKGROUND OF INFECTION PREVENTION AND CONTROL PROGRAMS

Infection prevention and control programs were instituted in hospitals throughout the United States in the 1950s and 1970s in response to the CDC and the Joint Commission on Accreditation of Healthcare Organizations (JCAHO) concerns about nosocomial infections. Standards were established, and it was declared there would be an effective infection prevention and control program within hospitals. In 1970, the CDC began the National Nosocomial Infections Surveillance Systems (NNIS) to study and monitor trends of HAIs previously labeled nosocomial infections. CDC published comparative reports periodically to use in hospital benchmarking.

In 1974, the CDC initiated another study to determine the efficacy of infection prevention and control activities in reducing HAIs. The Study on the Efficacy of Nosocomial Infection Control (SENIC Project) defined an infection surveillance and control program as containing three elements: epidemiologic surveillance for the occurrence of patient infections, policies and procedures to control infections, and trained personnel to do epidemiology and collect surveillance data.

In 1986, the Institute of Medicine completed a report entitled *Improving the Quality of Care in Nursing Homes.* As a result of this report, Congress enacted the Nursing Home Reform Act as part of the Omnibus Budget Reconciliation Act (OBRA) of 1987. This law mandated quality of care standards for LTCFs that receive Medicare and Medicaid funding. It also created a survey and enforcement system with two goals:

1. To ensure compliance with specifically designed regulations; and
2. To improve the quality of care and quality of life for residents who live in nursing homes. The Centers for Medicare & Medicaid Services (CMS) is charged with the survey process. For more information, refer to Chapter 2 on survey compliance and CMS regulations.

F tag 441 provides interpretive guidelines for implementation of infection control regulations for long-term care facilities, as listed in the U.S. Code of Federal Regulations Title 42 Section 483.65, which states:[2]

> The facility must establish and maintain an infection control program designed to provide a safe, sanitary, and comfortable environment and to help prevent the development and transmission of disease and infection.
>
> A. **Infection control program.** The facility must establish an infection control program under which it:
>
> 1. Investigates, controls, and prevents infections in the facility;
> 2. Decides what procedures, such as isolation, should be applied to an individual resident; and

3. Maintains a record of incidents and corrective actions related to infections.

B. **Preventing the spread of infection:**

1. When an infection control program determines that a resident needs isolation to prevent the spread of infection, the facility must isolate the resident;
2. The facility must prohibit employees with a communicable disease or infected skin lesion from direct contact with residents or their food if direct contact will transmit the disease; and
3. The facility must require the staff to wash their hands after each direct resident contact for which hand washing is indicated by accepted professional practice.

C. **Patient linens.** Personnel must handle, store, process, and transport linens so as to prevent the spread of infection.

Other regulations and guidelines include Occupational Safety and Health Administration's (OSHA) Respiratory Protection and Bloodborne Pathogen Standards and various infection control guidelines from the CDC. It is important for infection prevention and control practices to follow current regulations and guidelines. For a quick reference, the section "Professional Practice" on the APIC website provides numerous scientific guidelines and practice resources to support an infection prevention program.

INFECTION RISK ASSESSMENT

The cornerstone of any infection prevention program is the facility-specific risk assessment. The assessment must be conducted at least annually and reviewed whenever there are significant changes or organizational prevention challenges (e.g., outbreaks, major renovation, pandemic threat, antibiotic, and/or vaccine shortages, etc.).

Assessment of facility risk must include the following basic components:

- The healthcare needs and associated infection risks of the types of individuals who receive care at the facility, including pre-admission screening and prevention of transmission among residents when infections are identified after admission.
- Community infection risks and communicable disease rates that potentially impact the facility, its staff, and residents.
- The type and frequency of utilization of invasive devices used at the facility, the baseline infection rates associated with these devices, and efforts to reduce them.
- The scope and participation in immunization and other health-promotion activities among staff and residents.
- The scope and adherence to hand hygiene programs for staff, residents, and visitors.
- Use of isolation systems, the frequency of their use, and barriers to effective implementation.
- The implementation of an antibiotic stewardship program or other antibiotic utilization management approaches.
- Cleaning and disinfecting both hard and soft surfaces throughout the facility.
- Facility readiness to respond to urgent or emergent threats, including disease outbreaks, pandemics, interruptions in power and/or water that impact resident care, weather-related emergencies, and workplace violence.

There is no preferred method of conducting the facility risk assessment, but standard scoring tools or checklists can assist in the process (see example Risk Assessment on the CD-ROM that accompanies this book). However, the overall risk assessment cannot be limited to these tools; it must be customized to reflect the needs of the facility and address its many challenges, which vary greatly between organizations. A well-constructed facility risk assessment reflects not only facility-focused issues, but also issues that are reflective of the community and overall environment of care.

The results of the risk assessment should be communicated to facility management and shared with all relevant stakeholders within the organization. A shared awareness of actual and potential risks is a crucial step in developing an effective, goal-directed prevention program. Identified risks and correlating program goals to mitigate risk are shared with and approved by relevant stakeholders. This should be accomplished annually with the Infection Prevention and Control Committee.

INFECTION PREVENTION AND CONTROL PLAN

The infection prevention and control program is described in a written plan. The plan is developed to address the needs identified in the risk assessment process, as well as:

- Identify the authoritative and guidance documents that are used to provide evidence-based direction to the facility's program (e.g., CDC guidelines are often referenced, as well as the professional and/or practice standards of the various categories of licensed healthcare employees and/or consultants who provide services at the facility).
- Identify the goals, objectives, and related metrics that will be used to analyze the effectiveness of the infection prevention program.
- Explain how the infection prevention program will collaborate and help support the facility's safety, risk mitigation, emergency preparedness, and other systems supporting a culture of safety.
- Describe reporting systems and communication processes to ensure sharing of information within the facility's team and any committees.
- Address new and ongoing educational needs for staff, residents, and visitors.
- Prioritize prevention goals and describe any special projects anticipated in order to meet them, including a description of additional resources that may be required.
- Address surveillance activities, as well as any reporting that may be required by state, provincial, or national regulations and/or compliance with voluntary accrediting standards.
- Discuss any infection challenges related to transitions in care and how resident safety will be protected during these transitions.

Because goal statements are fairly broad, they may appear similar among facilities. Common examples of goals include:

- To prevent and control the transmission of communicable infectious disease.
- To establish interventions to prevent HAIs.
- To perform surveillance to monitor the facility for infections and implement proper interventions to prevent transmission.
- To provide infection prevention education to staff, residents, and resident families.
- To establish criteria for the isolation of residents if necessary based on the CDC *Guideline for Isolation Precautions 2007*.[4]
- To implement scientific-based practice in the prevention of transmission of infectious agents.
- To implement and maintain compliance with all state and federal regulations and standards that pertains to infection prevention and control.

The objectives developed to meet these goals, however, will be specific to the facility and take into consideration the information obtained from the risk assessment, facility resources, and any other prevention issues that are unique to that institution. If the facility is part of a healthcare system, develop and implement goals that align the needs of all system providers.

SCOPE OF THE PROGRAM

The scope of the infection prevention program describes what activities will be conducted and to what extent they will be implemented. A checklist can be a useful tool in verifying that all dimensions of the program's scope are being adequately addressed (Figure 3.1). The scope

In developing a written plan, it is important to correctly differentiate program goals and objectives.

A goal is a broad statement that describes an overall aim. Objectives, written to support attainment of the goal, are specific, measurable, and time-sensitive. For example, a LTCF wants to include a project to improve participation by its employees in the seasonal influenza immunization program:

Goal: Maximize voluntary employee participation in influenza vaccination by end of [insert year]

Objective: 90 percent of all eligible employees will receive influenza vaccination by December 31, [insert year]

will vary according to the facility's risk assessment, size, resident care special needs, community threats, as well as its available resources to implement and maintain an effective program.

The scope of the infection prevention program typically includes:

- Surveillance
- Data analysis and reporting
- Implementation of prevention and control interventions
- Education of staff, residents, and families/visitors
- Environment and equipment cleaning and disinfecting procedures
- Product evaluation
- Immunizations for staff and residents
- Policy and procedure creation and annual review
- Outbreak investigation
- Committee coordination and communications
- Consultation to all services for issues related to infection prevention as well as facility-wide projects such as emergency drills, construction and/or renovation, prevention of hospital readmission, etc.
- Antibiotic stewardship program
- Disaster preparedness

If the facility offers employee health services onsite, this program component must also be identified in the scope and described in the written plan.

PROGRAM OVERSIGHT AND MANAGEMENT

The oversight and management of the infection prevention and control program should be described in the written plan. Lines of authority may vary, but usually include the Infection Prevention and Control Committee and the infection preventionist.

The Infection Prevention and Control Committee

The Infection Prevention and Control Committee is not presently required by federal regulations; however, some states require the committee and may even identify the specific members. Be sure to check state regulations for any requirements. The frequency of meetings and how committee reports are channeled to facility leadership must also be documented, as these details will be reviewed during any routine survey.

Committee members typically include the administration; medical director; director or assistant director of nursing; directors of departments for environmental services, dietary, resident activities, and the pharmacy consultant; and safety officer. The infection preventionist (IP) may lead the committee meetings or assist senior staff in coordinating them.

This committee should be incorporated into the Quality Assurance/Performance Improvement (QAPI) Committee or the Resident Safety Committee.[2] If this is done, the infection prevention portion must be clearly described in the minutes as verification that the prevention program is being adequately addressed by the team.

An executive committee consisting of the administrator, medical director, director of nursing, and the IP may be convened routinely or in response to urgent events. It is always important to keep this leadership group informed of potential problems—particularly any that may trigger reporting to public health authorities or precipitate activation of the facility's emergency response system.

The Infection Preventionist

The IP in a LTCF may be a sole practitioner or the role may be combined with another position. However, the IP's education, prior experience, and clinical background remain at the discretion of the hiring facility. If the IP lacks formal training, obtaining relevant education will be a priority immediately following hire. The IP's qualifications should be included in the human resources file as verification of competency to oversee the program. It is also important that evidence of ongoing education is included. Qualifications and experience must support the IP's ability to manage the program, assist senior leadership in making decisions, perform surveillance and reporting functions, and meet the requirements of the program described in the program plan and outlined in its scope.

FIGURE 3.1: LONG-TERM CARE PREVENTION PROGRAM CHECKLIST

Use this checklist annually to verify that all necessary elements of the long-term care facility's (LTCF) program are in place and whenever significant changes occur that may affect the infection prevention program. Not all elements listed below may apply to all LTCFs.

	Yes, Included in Program	If No, explain how improvements will be made or if not applicable
BASELINE CONSIDERATIONS		
The program defines the IP role and responsibilities		
The program addresses accreditation requirements (as needed)		
The program is aligned with the HHS National Action Plan for Long Term Care (measures and metrics)		
The program will utilize the CDC's NHSN reporting system		
The program will utilize other LTC benchmarks (as available)		
GUIDANCE DOCUMENTS		
Guidance documents for the program have been identified		
Guidance documents are referenced in the written infection prevention plan		
Current copies of identified guidance documents are readily accessible to staff		
REGULATORY COMPLIANCE, VERIFIED FOR ALL APPLICABLE AGENCIES		
CMS		
CMS CLIA (waiver program)		
OSHA		
FDA		
EPS		
State/local regulations		
COORDINATION WITH THE HEALTH DEPARTMENT		
The program includes the list of reportable disease and the methods used to report		
The program identifies outbreak reporting and health department support for investigations		
Contact information for the state/local health department is documented		
INFECTION PREVENTION RISK ASSESSMENT (RA)		
RA is completed annually and whenever new risks/emerging threats are identified		
RA includes both facility and community/area risks		
Risks are stratified for prioritization		
Comparative data are used for risk assessment (as available)		

Figure 3.1 Continued

	Yes, Included in Program	If No, explain how improvements will be made or if not applicable
THE INFECTION PREVENTION PLAN INCLUDES		
Hand hygiene, glove use		
Isolation and PPE		
Surveillance priorities, definitions, methods, analysis, and reporting		
Tuberculosis control		
Seasonal influenza immunization program		
Pneumococcal immunization program		
Public reporting (as required)		
Laboratory utilization and reporting		
Antibiotic usage and stewardship program		
Cleaning, disinfection of the environment		
Approved facility cleaning and disinfecting products (list)		
Cleaning, disinfecting isolation rooms, and prevention of MDRO transmission		
Environmental monitoring method(s)		
Cleaning, disinfecting resident care equipment		
Storage of clean and sterile supplies		

Also available on the CD-ROM.

Describing the Infection Preventionist Professional Role

The IP role must be outlined in a job description, either as a sole practitioner or as a component of another role at the facility.[2] The job description must match the needs of the infection prevention program and support its implementation. Because programs vary between facilities, job descriptions will also differ. Some common duties and responsibilities include:

- Applies scientific principles and methods to the collection and presentation of infection prevention and control data.
- Conducts surveillance following current and approved definitions of infection and standard methodologies for case identification, data collection, and reporting (see Chapter 4 for additional surveillance information).
- Prepares reports and presentations for committees.
- Investigates outbreaks of infection and implements infection prevention interventions.
- Reports outbreaks of communicable disease to the county/state health departments as needed after consultation with administration and the medical director.
- Plans and conducts educational programs.
- Develops and reviews policies and procedures; monitors their use to support optimal staff compliance and resident safety.
- Ensures compliance with county, state, and federal standards for infection prevention.

The IP role and job description should be consistent with the APIC/CHICA Professional and Practice Standards (see Additional Resources on the CD-ROM). Standards are authoritative statements that reflect the expectation, value, and priorities of the organizations that develop them. They provide a broad context for the IP role but will not explain specific functions, task, or regular/daily duties.

Competency

The IP must demonstrate competency to perform his/her role and manage the facility's program. Competency at the novice stage is frequently the focus of many new IPs, but its ongoing development is important for professional growth. This is shown in the IP competency model developed by APIC (Figure 3.2).

> Certification represents the bridging point between novice and proficient. ***The CIC® credential is the most widely recognized certification for infection preventionists in North America.***
>
> For detailed information about the examination, fees, testing procedures, and eligibility, see the CBIC website (www.cbic.org).

Patient safety is the core of the model. The essential elements that surround it include the core competencies, as identified by the Certification Board of Infection Control and Epidemiology (CBIC) through their periodic research-based practice analysis, as well as the professional and practice standards of national organizations. Within these dimensions, the model is based in science and is designed to apply to IPs in all practice settings.

Because professional competency continues to evolve, the model includes four future-oriented domains. Each of these, although rooted in science, expands outward, indicating that these are areas for ongoing professional development and are domains in which new science is needed to better define the evolving IP role. The expanding sections of the future-oriented domains have been identified through expert consensus.[5] A complete description of the model is available in the "Competency" section of APIC's website. In addition, articles from APIC's *American Journal of Infection Control* and *Prevention Strategist* are included on the CD-ROM.

There is no expectation that the IP will be equally proficient in all areas simultaneously. For example, the IP in a LTCF may be advanced in terms of infection prevention and control competencies but may have less experience with leadership and program management. Many IPs are still pursuing core competencies in the technical domain, especially related to emerging surveillance technology and various software applications. In this regard, the model is intended to help the IP begin to map his or her career stages and better identify professional areas needing administrative support for continued growth. IPs in LTCFs can also use the competency model to analyze their job description and discuss with their supervisor the descriptions of duties and responsibilities, which may need closer alignment with the domains described in the model.

PROGRAM IMPLEMENTATION

The infection prevention and control program uses a wide variety of implementation strategies, depending on its scope and overall goals. A few of the most common implementation approaches are described here. The ability to produce documentation of implementation activities, including their results and corrective actions taken when indicated, is critically important in demonstrating during a survey that the program is both active and effective in supporting a safe resident-centered care environment. Figure 3.3 is an example of a tool that was developed by the Pennsylvania Patient Safety Authority to monitor and assess a facility's implementation infection prevention best practices. The complete tool is available on the CD-ROM included with this book.

Documentation

Infection prevention reports should be reviewed per LTCF schedule or at least quarterly if infection prevention is integrated into other oversight committee meetings such as Quality or Safety. In addition to ongoing reports about surveillance results, outbreaks, investigations, and

FIGURE 3.2: APIC COMPETENCY MODEL[5]

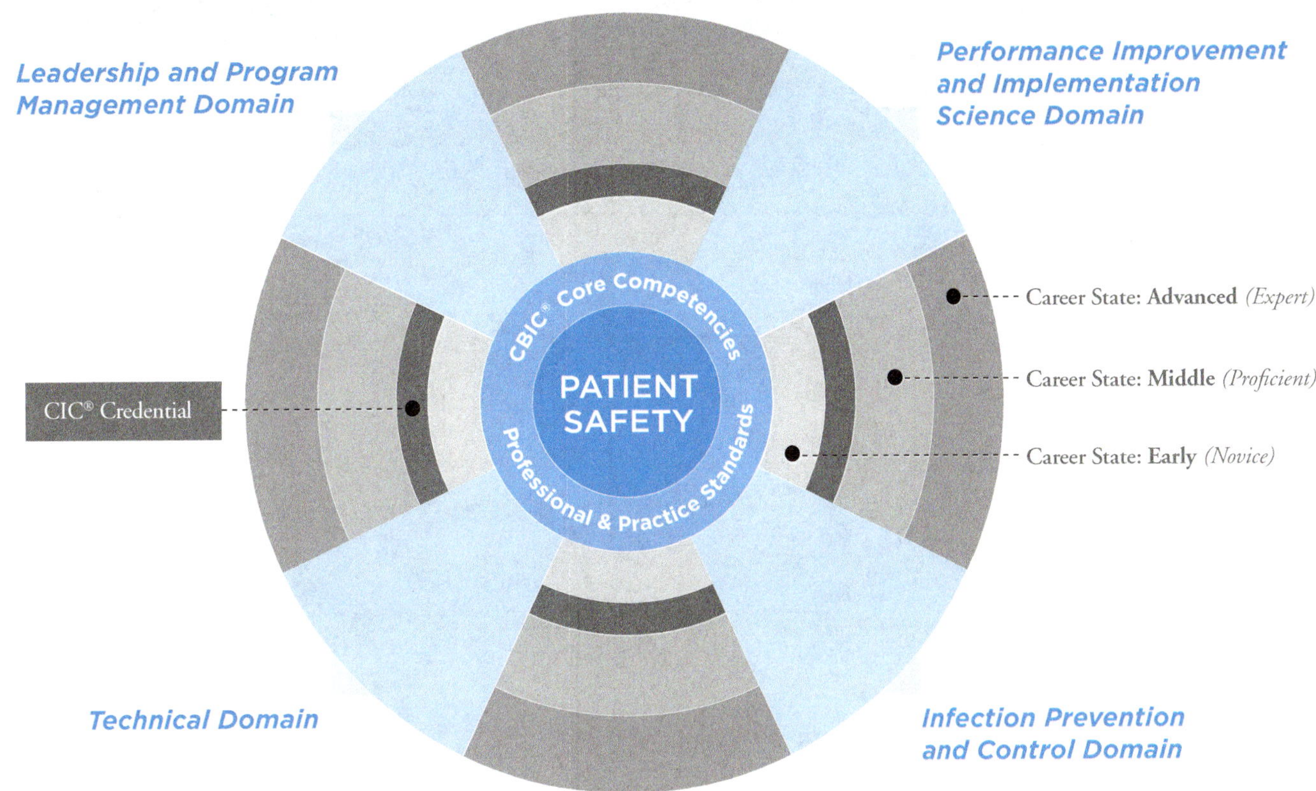

See the Quick Reference Guide on the CD-ROM for more information.

Blue areas indicate critical competencies required for the expanding IP role.
* The CIC® Credential is available from CBIC® The Certification Board of Infection Control and Epidemiology, Inc.

employee health/sharps injury issues, communications should include information about construction/renovation projects, new products or equipment, environmental issues, and emerging threats. IP documentation should include conclusions and actions taken in response to identified issues and the results of these actions. The IP should work with the pharmacy consultant and have the pharmacy provide information about antibiotic use and any updates to the antibiotic stewardship program.

Documentation should also include monthly microbiology reports of laboratory results, antibiograms, and alerts regarding epidemiologically important organisms. If a laboratory representative cannot participate in committee meetings in person or via phone, the IP may be required to summarize and submit this documentation to the committee.

Surveillance and Reporting

Surveillance systems and public reporting requirements are changing within the long-term care community. The types of surveillance conducted, reporting formats used, and electronic submission to the CDC NHSN database currently vary widely across the United States. Increased focus by regulators and payers in long-term care are expected to intensify the momentum for more standardized surveillance measures and metrics. As these

FIGURE 3.3: EXAMPLE OF AN INFECTION PREVENTION BEST PRACTICE ASSESSMENT TOOL

LONG-TERM CARE BEST-PRACTICE ASSESSMENT TOOL

4 = 100% implemented 3 = partially implemented 2 = implementation considered 1 = unknown
0 = not implemented n/a = not applicable ☐ = indicates items that can be evaluated by clinical observation

	Hand Hygiene	Infection Control Plan & Goals	Policies & Procedures	Education Process	Standard Documentation	Monitoring of Processes & Outcomes	Accountability Assigned
☐	1. Clinical staff demonstrate understanding of hand hygiene rationale, indications, and methods.						
☐	2. Alcohol-based handrub and gloves are available at the point of care.						
☐	3. Gloves are changed between residents and between clean and dirty activities on the same resident.						
☐	4. Handwashing with soap and water is performed when hands are visibly soiled.						
☐	5. Hand hygiene is performed before and after resident care.						
	6. The facility has an individualized program to monitor hand hygiene compliance.						
	7. Residents and families are knowledgeable about hand hygiene.						
	Category Subtotal	0	0	0	0	0	0

You may access the complete PDF on the CD-ROM.

Excerpted and used with permission from the Pennsylvania Patient Safety Authority.

metrics are defined, additional technological competency will be required of the IP to ensure that nationally reported data are accurate and reflect appropriate numerator and denominator data. Data validation in LTCFs is another area for future consideration.

The IP must keep a log for information about outbreaks, investigations, and disease reporting. Information should include dates, times, and the names of individuals with whom information is shared and/or consultation sought. Infection control regulations explain the requirements for keeping a record of events and corrective actions.[2]

Surveillance logs may be electronic or manual and provide the cumulative data from which reports, trend analysis, and other informational tools are developed. Resident privacy must be protected when aggregating and reporting infection information.

POLICIES AND PROCEDURE REVIEW

Policies and procedures represent the structural tools that help promote correct and consistent use of infection prevention practices. They must be developed from the most current scientific evidence or when such evidence is lacking from best practice guidelines and expert consensus documents. Policies and procedures are reviewed annually and revised when needed. Documentation must reflect an ongoing review process by the facility. Documentation of the review process is routinely inspected during a facility survey.

Infection prevention policies and procedures may be configured in a variety of ways. They may exist as a separate manual, be individual documents with a department policy manual, or be integrated into the context of specific policies throughout the facility. In large-scale long-term care companies, some or all policies may be provided through the corporate office. For LTCFs that are part of a healthcare system, policies may be developed by an inter-disciplinary team for implementation within participating facilities. In small facilities, the IP may be primarily responsible for developing and updating these documents.

Although the availability of current policies is important in any survey, their correct and consistent use by staff is also required. For that reason, policies and procedures must be supported by communications to those who are responsible for their implementation. Ongoing training must be provided and monitored to ensure optimum compliance with procedures implemented.

Rounding, Individually or by Team

Unannounced, visual inspection is a long-standing technique for identifying problems before they escalate into a serious infection threat. Rounds may be conducted by a single person or done as a small team. In some facilities, the manager whose area is being observed may accompany the team during the inspection.

Rounding is most useful to detect process failures that are readily apparent. Examples include lack of hand hygiene; incorrect use of gowns, gloves, or other appropriate personal protective equipment (PPE); breaches in the handling of soiled laundry; supplies used past their expiration date; overly full trash or sharps containers; and evidence of leaking pipes or other water damage to the facility, etc. The major drawback with this technique is that it is often perceived by staff as policing rather than an informative process. When rounding, it is essential to alert staff to variations in process or practice in a helpful, coaching manner rather than criticizing or assigning blame. Including staff in the rounding process may also encourage a more positive level of engagement.

Results of rounding activities should be compiled and included with infection prevention reports. It is important to evaluate the results of rounds for any actual or emerging trends and be prepared to proactively offer suggestions for improvement. Persistent or more serious trends noted through rounding may escalate into targeted infection prevention projects or performance improvements within the facility.

Environmental Monitoring

In addition to direct observation, new technologies now offer enhanced options for monitoring the effectiveness of environmental cleaning. All of these methods have associated costs that must be considered when moving beyond basic visual inspection.

- **Cultures:** Environmental surfaces can be cultured via swab or agar slide techniques. Cultures, due to the cost and time required to obtain a result, are not recommended for routine monitoring. They may be necessary in outbreak or other special circumstances.
- **Fluorescent Marking Systems:** In this approach, surfaces, often high-touch surfaces, are marked with a fluorescent gel that becomes transparent when it dries. After cleaning, a black light is used to detect if the gel has been removed. This is a qualitative monitoring process, most useful in helping staff recognizes when cleaning has been effective. However, it does not determine the type of organism, the colony count, or amount of reduction in bacteria present.
- **ATP Bioluminescence:** After a swab has been obtained, a handheld illuminometer is used to measure residual organic debris. Because this process does not identify specific pathogens or report a colony count, it is a surrogate marker for bacterial environmental contamination. Also, reports of residual organic matter have not been shown to correspond conclusively to infection transmission risks.

Providing Education

Educational programs remain the mainstay of improving infection prevention practices. Education can be delivered in a wide variety of ways. If online education is used, the IP should verify that the content is delivered by a provider qualified to offer accurate and relevant material. The use of newsletters, journals, inservice programs, local conferences, and webinars has enhanced the ability of the facility-based IP to encourage broader participation in educational programs. Attendance at educational programs, as well as evaluations and/or post-tests, when used, should be included with program records.

Education targeting knowledge must also be balanced with skill enhancement. Some facilities may offer skills workshops or invite specific vendors to provide demonstrations and practice sessions onsite. The availability of simulation-based training remains rare in LTCFs but is increasing in popularity in academic medical centers. One-on-one coaching or mentoring is more common in LTCFs but lacks the consistency and reliability of more formal methods. Whenever procedures are changed or new products/equipment are introduced, all staff using them must receive adequate instruction and that training must be documented. Failure to ensure that staff correctly performs resident care procedures has led to serious infections in LTCFs, especially in the misuse of lancets and injection supplies.[6] See Chapter 13 for more information on education and training.

INFECTION PREVENTION AND OTHER FACILITY PROGRAMS

Infection prevention impacts all aspects of resident care and is also essential to many aspects of employee well-being, workplace wellness, and visitor safety. LTCFs work to coordinate their infection prevention programs using simple, pragmatic approaches that align well with their operational and administrative systems and goals. But no matter what level of coordination is achieved, there are two programs for which coordination is essential.

Safety and Emergency Preparedness Program

Infection risks must be identified and addressed as part of both routine safety measures and emergency response. Although these factors will vary among facilities, common issues typically include:

- Mitigation of infectious risks from airborne contaminants
- Maintenance of perishable food and safe drinking water if utilities are disrupted
- Evacuation of residents and staff, including means of transport and assigned places of relocation
- Availability of PPE during emergency situations
- Immunization programs for staff and residents
- Restriction/redirection of facility access in response to disease outbreaks, pandemics, or other circumstances where transmission is possible

For detailed information on emergency preparedness programs for LTCFs, see Chapter 15.

Quality or Performance Improvement Program

Because issues identified through the facility risk assessment and ongoing surveillance activities must be addressed, the Quality Assessment/Performance Improvement Program (QAPI) provides an effective framework for developing, implementing, and evaluating the organization's response to actual and potential infection related threats. Infection prevention data can be extremely useful in these types of QAPI projects. Examples are shown in Figure 3.4.

CMS requires QAPI programs, but the LTCFs choose the types of improvement projects to implement. Project reports or other documentation must be maintained and include measures that quantify improvement outcomes. Graphs and other data display techniques are helpful in converting data into useful information. Facilities often post the results of their QAPI initiatives in staff areas to maximize employee awareness and, when possible, celebrate success when objectives are reached or exceeded.

PROGRAM RESOURCES

Infection prevention programs must have the resources necessary to address facility risks, contribute meaningfully to a culture of safety, and meet the goals and objectives identified in the infection prevention plan.

Although data are limited, most IPs in LTCFs are registered nurses whose duties include infection prevention. They are not considered sole practitioners.[7] There is no nationally accepted model for describing IP staffing in any type of healthcare provider setting. The complexity of determining satisfactory staffing is compounded in LTCFs where professional responsibilities so often overlap and/or may be shared. The combination of multiple roles, referred to as role compression, has not been widely studied in long-term care. In situations where role compression escalates, the time available to focus on prevention rather than response to infection risks often decreases while the difficulty in achieving desired program outcomes increases.[8]

The lack of information technology resources has also been recognized as a barrier to infection prevention programs. The availability of computers, software applications, and access to the Internet vary widely. In facilities where computers are used, the systems may be outdated.[7] The current movement toward public reporting of infections and other events in LTCFs is expected to help improve IT infrastructure in the near future.

Another evolving resource for LTC exists within state and local health departments. Public health agencies, as well as state Quality Improvement Organizations (QIOs), are increasingly directing more focus and resources to prevention activities in LTCFs. The synergies achieved by the inclusion of public health expertise and state/regional collaborative, as well as increasing resources provided by professional associations such as APIC, offer expanding options for both engagement by and assistance for the IP in LTC.

FIGURE 3.4: EXAMPLES OF QAPI PROJECTS

Example	QAPI Required Elements	Infection Prevention Program Examples
Design and Scope	A written plan addresses all services offered with emphasis on clinical care, quality of life, and resident choice. Goals are defined and measurable.	The facility's surveillance plan identifies a need to address the use of indwelling urinary catheters and (1) reduce the incidence of CAUTI* and (2) increase the prompt removal of catheters among residents who have them in place at the time of admission.
Governance and Leadership	Both the governing body and facility leadership establish the QAPI program, its goals, and priorities. They are responsible for balancing a culture of organizational safety with a culture of resident-centered rights and choice. Goals are based on the annual risk assessment.	Facility leadership prioritizes participation by all in the annual seasonal influenza vaccination program, actively participates and promotes it, recognizes facility success, and showcases facility efforts as demonstration of its commitment to wellness, health promotion, and safety.
Feedback, Data Systems, and Monitoring	Data is taken from multiple sources to determine and monitor performance indicators. Performance is measured against benchmarks and targets. Adverse events are tracked and analyzed to prevent reoccurrences.	The facility monitors hand hygiene compliances with both soap and water and alcohol-based hand rubs. Compliance rates are compared to national averages, results are tracked, and trends analyzed. Suggestions for improvement and positive behavioral change are collected and implemented in an ongoing basis. Individuals are recognized for excellent performance.
Performance Improvement Projects	A focused effort to address a problem or need within one area or through the facility. Projects are meaningful to the services and needs of the facility.	A project targets improved cleaning and disinfection of bedside commodes and wheelchairs. Products are reviewed, cleaning and disinfecting procedures clarified, and roles and responsibilities are agreed upon and shared. Additional training is provided. Staff participates in monitoring improvements and continues to offer ways to maximize the cleanliness of equipment. Results are communicated to all stakeholders regularly.
Systematic Analysis and Systemic Action	The facility applies a thorough process for improvement, including the use of root cause analysis (RCA). Failure events are analyzed in order to promote sustainable improvements throughout the facility.	A stroke patient with impaired mobility developed a sacral pressure ulcer that has become infected, requiring readmission to the acute care hospital. The team conducts a root cause analysis to identify system failures, implement corrective actions, and prevent similar occurrences. Revision of some policies and procedures are done following the RCA and education is given to all direct care staff. Pressure ulcer vigilance is increased throughout the facility.

*CAUTI: catheter-associated urinary tract infection

REFERENCES

1. Centers for Disease Control and Prevention (CDC). *Long-term care settings*. CDC website. 2010. Available at: http://www.cdc.gov/HAI/settings/ltc_settings.html.

2. Department of Health and Human Services (DHHS), Centers for Medicare & Medicaid Services (CMS). *CMS Manual System Pub. 100-07 State Operations Provider Certification, Transmittal 55. 2009.* CMS website. 2009. Available at: http://www.cms.gov/Regulations-and-Guidance/Guidance/Transmittals/downloads/r55soma.pdf.

3. Strausbaugh LJ, Joseph CL. The burden of infection in long-term care. *Infect Control Hosp Epidemiol* 2000;21:674-679.

4. Siegel JD, Rhinehart E, Jackson M, et al. Healthcare Infection Control Practices Advisory Committee (HICPAC). Guideline for Isolation Precautions: Preventing Transmission of Infectious Agents in Healthcare Settings, 2007. CDC website. 2007. Available at: http://www.cdc.gov/hicpac/2007IP/2007isolationPrecautions.html.

5. Murphy DM, Hanchett M, Olmsted RN, Farber MR, Lee TB, Haas JP, et al. Competency in infection prevention: a conceptual approach to guide current and future practice. *Am J Infect Control* 2012 May; 40(4): 296-303.

6. Centers for Disease Control and Prevention (CDC). Transmission of hepatitis B virus among persons undergoing blood glucose monitoring in long-term-care facilities-Mississippi, North Carolina, and Los Angeles County, California, 2003-2004. MMWR *Morb Mortal Wkly Rep* 2005; 54: 220-223.

7. Jones M, Samore MH, Carter M, Rubin MA. Long-term care facilities in Utah: a description of human and information technology resources applied to infection control practice. *Am J Infect Control* 2012 Jun; 40(5): 446-450.

8. Hanchett M. Performance improvement and implementation science: Infection prevention competencies for current and future role development. *Am J Infect Control* 2012 Jun; 40(5): 304-308.

CHAPTER 4

Surveillance, Epidemiology, and Reporting

Deborah Patterson Burdsall, MSN, RN-BC, CIC

KEY CONCEPTS

- Infection preventionists who are based in long-term care need to understand the purpose, methodologies, and definitions for surveillance.
- An effective surveillance program begins with engaging the interdisciplinary team, conducting a facility risk assessment, and setting goals to ensure that the data collected are consistent, useful, actionable, and timely.
- Surveillance strategies must be consistent and compliant with long-term care guidelines and regulations.
- Infection preventionists must know the reporting rationale, opportunities, and requirements for long-term care facilities.

SURVEILLANCE AND EPIDEMIOLOGY

Surveillance is "the ongoing, systematic collection, analysis, interpretation, and dissemination of data to identify infections and infection risks, to try to reduce morbidity and mortality, and to improve resident health status."[1] Surveillance is a necessary component of effective infection prevention and control in any healthcare setting,[2] and comprises systematic observation that healthcare personnel (HCP)—particularly infection preventionists (IPs) and epidemiologists—use to identify patterns of disease. It helps caregivers make informed decisions about treatments that are based on these patterns. By looking at individual resident information in a larger context, surveillance data enables the IP and other HCP to identify and analyze how the individual's condition affect the group. Surveillance involves far more than just collecting and listing infections and antibiotics. This information must translate into interventions in the delivery of care to the resident. It is important to use consistent surveillance processes and terms to improve daily practice.

Epidemiology is the study of patterns, causes, and effects of illness and disease in populations and is the science of public health. Epidemiology is defined by the World Health Organization (WHO) as "the study of the distribution and determinants of health-related states or events (including disease), and the application of this study to the control of diseases and other health problems."[3] Surveillance is a cornerstone of epidemiology and performing proper surveillance, along with learning to use epidemiological methods, is an important skill for IPs. The detection of transmission within the facility prompts staff to consider heightened secretion containment measures and/or other steps to eliminate transmission.

The U.S. Department of Health and Human Services (HHS) estimates that more than 70 percent of Americans aged 65 and older will require long-term care services, with 30 percent requiring a stay in a long-term care facility (LTCF).[4] As long-term care evolves, residents who live and stay in LTCFs will require increasingly diverse and complex care. Changes within the past 10 to 20 years have increased the variety of residents served. In place of lengthy hospitalizations for individuals on both Medicare and private insurance, many long-term care communities now serve frail older adults with chronic illnesses and rehabilitation patients as they recover from infections, orthopedic joint replacement, severe wounds, and other short-term illnesses. Home care, independent living, and assisted living in many states have taken the place of traditional residential care within nursing homes. Although the length of stay in acute care hospitals averaged 4.9 days in 2009, the average length of stay in long-term care is approximately 3 years.[5-7]

As recently as the late 1980s and early 1990s, it was possible to keep track of all resident infections and treatments by counting the number of infections or calculating simple percentages in the average LTCF of approximately 100 beds.[8,9] This process is known as whole house surveillance. However, in recent years, long-term care admissions and discharges have increased rapidly. (See example in Figure 4.1)

In the United States, while the percentage of older adults who live in nursing homes has decreased relative to the general population, the number of short-term admissions to long-term care increased to 3.2 million in 2005.[9] The increase in short-term admissions and transfers between facilities within the healthcare continuum, combined with the increasingly diverse care needs of the resident and patient populations, as well as the increased use of antimicrobials has made surveillance much more complex. Continuous monitoring within current long-term care facilities requires far greater sophistication and a more complete knowledge of established surveillance methods than previously required.

SURVEILLANCE AND REGULATORY REQUIREMENTS

The Centers for Medicare & Medicaid Services (CMS) requires that infection prevention and control programs prevent "the development and transmission of disease and infections including influenza and pneumococcal pneumonia."[1] Skilled and intermediate nursing facilities that participate in Medicare and Medicaid are reviewed under HHS CMS *Interpretive Guidelines for Long-Term*

FIGURE 4.1: LONG-TERM CARE ADMISSION AND DISCHARGE EXAMPLE 1983 TO 2009 483 MIDWESTERN LTCF

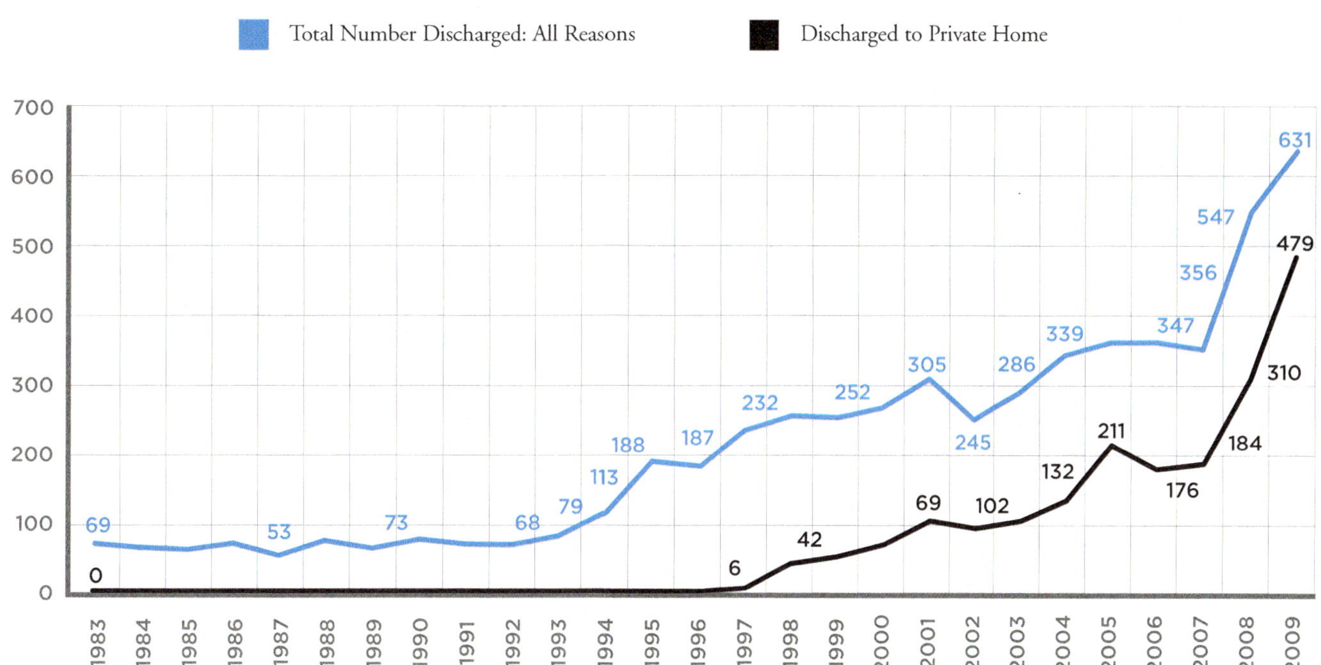

1983-1996

Discharges: All Cause
(mortality or hospital discharge)

- Average age: approx 87 years
- Average length of stay of 5 years

1997-2009

Discharges: All Cause
(to private homes, hospital discharge and mortality)

- Average age: approx 79 years
- Average length of stay:
  Long Stay: 461 days
- Average length of stay:
  Short Stay: 25 days

Mean Admissions & Discharges

- 130 admissions and discharges 1983–1993
- 465 admissions and discharges 1994–2003
- 1332 admissions and discharges 2004–2009

Care Facilities F Tag 441 (see Chapter 2 on Regulatory Surveys and CMS F Tag 441 Compliance). F Tag 441 lists the requirements for LTCFs and requires an infection prevention and control program to "perform surveillance and investigation to prevent, to the extent possible, the onset and the spread of infection."[1]

Infection prevention and control is a standards-based performance area and, in certain circumstances, The Joint Commission may have a higher standard than those reflected in other long-term care surveys. Awareness of all regulatory and guidelines is critical to comply with applicable accreditation requirements.

> Some LTCFs, ***especially beds designated as long-term care beds under a hospital license,*** may also be included in the Joint Commission Long Term Care Accreditation Program.

RISK ASSESSMENT

An effective surveillance program must collect useful, relevant, and timely information in order to identify trends and develop interventions that can help to prevent and control infections. To determine the information needed for an effective surveillance program, the IP should begin by performing a risk assessment. A complete and accurate risk assessment requires engaging the entire interdisciplinary team (IDT). This includes every department and area in the facility and must be supported by the administration. See the sample risk assessment on the CD-ROM accompanying this book.

Risk is evaluated using resident demographic data, historical infection data, known current risks, reports of infections in the community, and infection prevention and control literature. Some factors to consider when estimating the level of risk for a potential infection include:

- Historical outbreaks, and the time of year they occur—this can include facility and/or community outbreaks caused by organisms such as norovirus, *Clostridium difficile*, influenza, or West Nile virus
- Resident/patient population and any changes in their care needs, acuity, or turnover
- Vaccination rates for residents and staff
- Number of devices such as central lines, urinary catheters, ventilators
- Multidrug-resistant organisms (MDROs) that are consistently present in new admissions or colonized residents
- Historical problems or potential disruptions of supplies such as water, food, personal protective equipment, and cleaning and sanitation supplies
- Historical problems or potential disruption in medication supply, including antivirals, vaccines, or antibiotics
- Levels of hospitalization or rehospitalizations for infectious disease
- Hand hygiene and glove-use rates
- Housekeeping and laundry practices

SURVEILLANCE METHODOLOGIES: DATA COLLECTION AND INTERPRETATION

Once the risk assessment is complete, determine the surveillance methods to be employed. The methods of surveillance are used to identify conditions, practices, and processes that increase the risk of infection during the interactions between residents and HCP, families, volunteers, visitors, and the environment. The IP and IDT should consider methods that match the needs of the LTCF, the residents, and the LTCF staff and community. There are different types of surveillance activities, and each has specific benefits and challenges. Consider time and available resources when selecting the methods to be used. Collecting data without knowing what information is needed and how it may be used to improve care and prevent infection is a waste of time and effort. In addition, staff cooperation will wane if time and effort are spent collecting data that is never used. Methods chosen and data collected must fit the facility's risk assessment and goals. Infection prevention metrics should be targeted to these specific issues, and surveillance activities should be carefully selected so that the data obtained can be used to improve processes and outcomes. For example, a 65-bed LTCF in a small rural community with a population of stable residents may have an entirely different set of infection risks than a 500-bed LTCF in a suburban or urban area with a large rehabilitation population.

Table 4.1 reviews the various surveillance methodologies and the advantages and considerations for each. The use of the terminology may vary among LTCFs, and the methods described in Table 4.1 are not mutually exclusive. Surveillance methods may include simultaneously performing facility-wide (also known as house-wide), targeted, and outbreak surveillance dependent on circumstances identified at the time.

Infection surveillance information needs to be collected on a routine, systematic, and ongoing basis. It is best if surveillance is *prospective*—that is, the information is collected as it occurs—rather than trying to fit the pieces together *retrospectively*, or after the fact. Long-term care surveillance often requires the IP to collect information not only from multiple departments within the LTCF, but also from different companies and locations, as most LTCF pharmacies and laboratories are not co-located with the LTCF. Retrieving laboratory and pharmacy information from different companies held on different computers in different locations can be challenging. Having a routine delivery of the laboratory results and antimicrobial

TABLE 4.1: METHODS OF SURVEILLANCE ADVANTAGES AND DISADVANTAGES

Selected Type of Surveillance	Advantages	Disadvantages
Electronic Surveillance	• Used by most acute care hospitals with integrated electronic health records • Multiple software companies make surveillance software. Some use the CMS Quality Indicator Survey and the CMS Quality Measures • NHSN LTC component is available from CDC • Reduces the burden of paper records and storage at the facility	• Expensive • Dependent upon Minimum Data Set (MDS) or other required CMS data • Infection prevention and control surveillance requires facility, pharmacy, and lab computers to communicate together as an electronic health record
House-wide/Comprehensive Surveillance Looks at all infections, all antibiotic usage, all laboratory reports	• Can get the big picture of what is going on in a LTCF • More likely to detect infectious disease events	• Challenging in complex or large healthcare systems or LTCF • Large amount of data to collect, analyze, and interpret and disseminate • May be overwhelming • Significant resources required to implement • May be appropriate in LTCFs with stable resident populations and healthcare workers and sufficient IP staffing to collect and analyze data, and implement infection prevention interventions • May have minimal or no impact unless metrics are tied to specific areas where improvement is possible
Outbreak Surveillance • Defined in F 441 as one case of an infection that is highly communicable • Infection trends that are 10% higher than the historical rate of infection • Three or more cases of the same infection over a specific length of time on the same unit or other defined areas	• Rapid detection of an outbreak situation can prevent widespread illness and hospitalization • Requires immediate action and preestablished and well-planned interventions that can be implemented quickly • State health departments and CDC have outbreak response templates that can provide guidance • Well-presented outbreak summaries can provide public health with a clear picture of LTCF interventions.	• Requires consistent effort and accurate use of case definitions • Planning is consistent with emergency preparedness planning • Need ability to implement outbreak plans including single room isolation, close units, suspend activities, and rapidly provide prophylaxis are critical parts of an outbreak plan
Outcome Surveillance Provider rates associated with the incidence or prevalence of infections; standardized infection ratios for groups of providers	• Looks at infections which can be considered the result of the LTCF practices • When combined with process surveillance, can provide cause/effect analysis	• Can be more complex and difficult than process surveillance • Longitudinal analysis is frequently necessary
Process Surveillance Looks for adherence to steps or techniques, based on best practices, regulations, policies, and procedures	• Looks at LTCF-specific practices related to resident care • When combined with outcome surveillance, can provide cause/effect analysis	• Tendency to oversimplify the cause/effect relationship • Comparative/benchmarking data often unavailable to support conclusions • Frequently limited to before/after studies

Table 4.1 Continued

Selected Type of Surveillance	Advantages	Disadvantages
Prospective Surveillance Gathering data moving forward in real time	• Most complete access to real-time information	• Requires consistent resources for data collection
Retrospective Surveillance Gathering data by looking back at what has happened in the past	• Data collection and analysis can be done • Ready access to medical record information	• Can miss important and pertinent information • Lack of real-time information
Targeted/Priority Directed Surveillance Specific infections, procedures, or processes are selected for surveillance based upon risk assessment, quality assurance, or process improvement goals	• Based on assessment to target areas of highest infection risk	• Requires careful development and understanding of risk

prescriptions to the IP can ease the task of repeatedly requesting this information. A systematic approach can include collecting data from sources such as:

- 24-hour reports, which can contain residents on Transmission-based Precautions, new antibiotics and treatments, and acute condition changes
- Sick leave or paid time off logs
- Night supervisor reports
- Pharmacy and laboratory records (can be faxed or emailed if there is no electronic access)
- Documentation from the transferring facility
- Intake and nursing assessment data upon admission to LTCF
- Collaboration with IPs from transferring facility
- Electronic medical records (EMRs), if available

Once necessary data is collected, the information is analyzed, usually interpreted as rates, and shared with the interdisciplinary team.

> ***Confidentiality***
>
> As in all healthcare, it is critical that resident/patient/client personal and medical information is only released following applicable guidelines and regulations and on a strictly need-to-know basis, in cooperation with the resident/patient/client or their durable power of attorney for healthcare.

Tools for the collection of surveillance can range from sophisticated software programs to paper line listings. Facilities that do not have access to surveillance software programs can collect and track surveillance information in a spreadsheet that is placed on a secure LTCF shared drive, so that appropriate team members can access the information. Templates should be available to individuals who have clinical responsibilities, so that they can participate in infection prevention and data reporting. The data collection process should include multiple individuals to ensure that the absence of one individual does not interfere with the data collection. A variety of sample forms and basic software options are available on the CDC website (http://www.cdc.gov/surveillancepractice/tools.html).

USING PROCESS AND OUTCOME SURVEILLANCE

Once systems are in place to collect and analyze data, it is equally as important to have a system to monitor actual healthcare practices. This system, known as process surveillance, involves observing the individual steps of resident care and environmental interactions. Process surveillance cannot generally be based only on medical record review. To effectively implement a process surveillance program, observations need to be planned and implemented on a routine basis. Some examples may include processes listed in Table 4.2.

TABLE 4.2: PROCESS SURVEILLANCE EXAMPLES

Examples of Potential Areas for Process Surveillance	Outcomes to Avoid	Potential Infection Prevention and Control Interventions related to Process Surveillance	Monitor Results through Outcome Surveillance
How and why antibiotics are requested, ordered, and administered	• Overuse of antibiotics which increases the risk of *Clostridium difficile* and antimicrobial resistance	• Work with pharmacy, medical director, prescribers, and staff nurses • Antimicrobial stewardship program development	• Antimicrobial use
If there is evidence of employees or visitors who have been present in the care community when ill ***(presenteeism)***	• Transmission of infectious diseases outbreaks and epidemics	• Enforce regulatory and guideline-based policies and procedures relating to attendance in facility	• Infection rates • Outbreaks matching illness with high community incidence and prevalence
How and when gloves are used	• Transmission of infectious diseases outbreaks and epidemics • Use of one pair of gloves for more than one task or on more than one resident • Use of one pair of gloves moving from clean to dirty, and then back to clean	• Glove use surveillance during resident care events • Direct observation • Ensure proper supplies • Ensure competency of healthcare	• Infection rates • Colonization rates • Environmental Contamination
How and when hand hygiene is performed	• Transmission of infectious diseases outbreaks and epidemics	• Hand hygiene surveillance • Direct observation • Use of programs, sensors, and computer apps • Volume of alcohol-based hand rub used as a proxy for hand hygiene rates	• Infection rates • Colonization rates • Environmental contamination
How vascular access devices are inserted and maintained	• Sepsis • Cellulitis • Central line blood stream infections (CLABSIs)	• Ensure proper supplies • Ensure competency of nursing staff	• CLABSI rates • Intravenous site infection rates
How oral care is provided	• Oral infections • Respiratory infections	• Communication with dentist or dental technician • Scheduled dental/oral care • Ensure proper supplies • Ensure competency of nursing staff	• Oral infection rates • Respiratory infection rates
How respiratory equipment is handled	• Respiratory infections	• Ensure proper supplies • Ensure competency of nursing staff	• Respiratory infection rates • Oral infection rates
How urinary catheter care is provided	• Overuse of urinary catheters or poor care increase the risk of • Catheter-associated urinary tract infections (CAUTI)	• Ensure proper supplies, securement of device • Ensure competency of nursing staff	• CAUTI rates • Episodes of catheter obstruction or trauma
How blood glucose equipment is used and maintained	• Transmission of bloodborne pathogens (BBPs)	• Ensure proper supplies • Ensure competency of nursing staff • Avoid sharing glucometers to the extent possible	• Resident safety: no transmission of BBPs associated with blood glucose monitoring

Table 4.2 Continued

Examples of Potential Areas for Process Surveillance	Outcomes to Avoid	Potential Infection Prevention and Control Interventions related to Process Surveillance	Monitor Results through Outcome Surveillance
If single dose vials have been provided or used for multiple residents	• Transmission of bloodborne or multidrug-resistant pathogens	• Partner with pharmacy and suppliers • Enlist participation of direct care nurses	• Safe injection practices (e.g., no incorrectly used vials) • Transmission rate
If all injection supplies and equipment comply with regulations	• Use of non-safety-engineered devices increasing risk of needlestick or BBP exposure	• Partner with pharmacy and suppliers • Enlist participation of direct care nurses	• Safe injection practices (e.g., supplies and equipment complies with regulations) • Transmission rates
How the temperature is monitored for the storage of medication	• Contamination or destruction of medication through improper handling or leading to increased infection risk	• Partner with pharmacy and suppliers	• No resident complications associated with medications not maintained at correct temperature
How temperature is monitored for the storage of food items	• Contamination of food or other nutritional supplements through improper handling or leading to increased infection risk	• Partner with dining services	• No resident foodborne illness associated with dietary items not maintained at correct temperature

For example, when using process surveillance to monitor hand hygiene, observations will need to be scheduled at different times on different days to get an accurate picture of compliance. Hand hygiene surveillance is essential to all infection prevention programs, and is required to be reported in the CDC National Healthcare Safety Network (NHSN) long-term care module. There are various tools and programs that can be used for hand hygiene process surveillance, including applications for some handheld electronic devices. There are also programs available online, such as the WHO's *Clean Care is Safer Care* program. This program provides education, assessment, and surveillance tools at no cost. The program is based on the WHO's *My Five Moments for Hand Hygiene* program and now includes a long-term care module.[10,11] The WHO five moments include[12]:

1. Before touching a resident
2. Before clean/aseptic procedures
3. After body fluid exposure risk
4. After touching a resident
5. After touching resident surroundings

SURVEILLANCE DEFINITIONS

Infection surveillance definitions, also known as infection surveillance criteria, identify specific conditions that qualify as infections for the purpose of surveillance data collection, as well as calculation and reporting of infection rates. Any change in definition can affect surveillance results and make comparison of current and historical data inaccurate. Surveillance definitions are not the same as a clinical diagnosis. For example, minimum criteria for starting antibiotics may set a lower clinical threshold and be more sensitive than surveillance criteria. For this reason, it is essential to use surveillance definitions consistently and accurately.

Other important differences also exist. For example, the MDS 3.0 definitions and ICD9 or ICD10 codes for infections differ from the standard long-term care surveillance definitions.[13] In 2012, the Society for Healthcare Epidemiology of America (SHEA) and CDC released updated surveillance definitions for LTCFs (previously known as the McGeer criteria).[14] These definitions provide a reference standard for defining infections for surveillance purposes and provide the basis for any surveillance activities. See the Appendix at the end of this chapter for the full article and definitions. Figure 4.2 provides examples of decision algorithms that can assist the IP in applying the definitions to surveillance practices and processes.

CALCULATING RATES

When calculating infection rates, the denominator must accurately reflect the population being studied. For example, residents with indwelling catheters will be the population or group who are at risk for catheter-associated urinary tract infections (CAUTIs). Residents with central venous catheters will be the population or group at risk for central line-associated bloodstream infections (CLABSIs). At other times such as outbreaks of norovirus or influenza, the denominator may include all residents, staff, and visitors.

The historical incidence and prevalence rates serve as the baseline for ongoing data analysis. The rate is always for the same number of units to allow comparison between different time periods. Rates are usually expressed as rates per 1,000 units, although rates per 10,000 units or greater have also been used. The unit can be the number of days that residents were in the LTCF, and it can be used to calculate other rates such as the rate of CLABSI or CAUTI using device days. Rates are preferred to percentages as the significance of percentages can vary greatly.

Attack rates are a more specific type of incidence rate and are primarily used during outbreaks and epidemics in which a specific population is exposed to a specific infectious agent during a limited period of time.[15]

For formulas, see page 48.

STANDARDIZED INFECTION RATIO

The standardized infection ratio (SIR) is not a new measure. However, it is being increasingly used in healthcare to better measure and compare the performance of groups of similar facilities. For example, the SIR is used by the CDC when reporting healthcare-associated infection (HAI) national and/or state trends identified through NHSN.

A facility-specific SIR may be compared to a state-based SIR. In LTCFs, the SIR may be used in addition to routine surveillance measures, but does not replace the need to calculate and report standard measures such as incidence, prevalence and attack rates.

The SIR is a summary measure that describes:

$$\frac{\textit{The number of observed HAIs}}{\textit{The number of predicted HAIs}}$$

To interpret the SIR, the IP should base the analysis as follows.

- If the SIR is 1, then the number of infections reported to NHSN is the same as the number of predicted infections. For example, if the SIR for CAUTI = 1, no progress has been made in reducing CAUTIs since the baseline period.
- If the SIR is less than 1, then there were fewer infections reported than what would have been predicted given the baseline data. For example, if the CAUTI SIR = .82, it is showing improvement.
- If the SIR is greater than 1, then there were more infections reported than what was predicted given the baseline data. For example, if the CAUTI SIR = 1.15, the CAUTI rate has worsened.

General interpretive guidance is summarized in Table 4.3.

REPORTING

Once surveillance is completed, the data is collected and analyzed, and the significance is summarized. The resulting information should be shared with those who assist in prevention and control efforts. Internal reporting may include the following interdisciplinary team members:

- Resident/client/patient and their significant support systems and family members
- Nursing
- Admitting
- Therapy
- Life enrichment/activities
- Environmental services
- Maintenance
- Nutrition/dining services
- Administration
- Volunteers

FORMULAS FOR CALCULATING INCIDENCE AND PREVALENCE RATES

Formula for Calculating Incidence Rates for a Specific Population

$$\frac{\text{\# of new cases of a disease occurring during a specific period of time}}{\text{\# of people at risk for developing the disease during that period of time}} \times 1000 = \text{Incidence rate of residents}$$

Formula for Calculating Prevalence Rate for a Specific Population

$$\frac{\text{\# of cases of a disease occurring at a specific time}}{\text{\# of people at risk for developing the disease during that specific time}} \times 1000 = \text{Prevalence Rate of residents}$$

Example

Four people on a 10-resident unit develop new, symptomatic urinary tract infections during the month of March. To calculate the incidence using a percentage:

$$\frac{\text{4 new UTI cases occurring during a specific period of time}}{\text{10 people at risk for developing the disease during that period of time}} = 0.4 \times 1000 = \text{40\% of residents}$$

$$\frac{\text{4 new UTI cases occurring during a specific period of time}}{\text{10 people at risk for developing the disease March (31 days) = 310}} = \frac{4}{310} = 0.013 \times 1000 = \text{12.9 UTI per 1000 resident days}$$

Formula for Calculating Attack Rates

$$\frac{\text{The number of people at risk who develop the illness/condition}}{\text{The total number of people at risk}} \times 100 = \text{Percentage}$$

Examples

1. Respiratory outbreak with confirmed cases of influenza A that lasted 22 days. The affected unit was placed on heightened precautions, and oseltamivir was utilized according to CDC Interim Guidance for Influenza Outbreak Management in Long-Term Care Facilities. There were no hospitalizations and no related deaths.

   $$\frac{\text{33 people at risk who developed influenza}}{\text{222 total number of people at risk (includes residents, staff, and family)}} = \text{15\% Attack Rate}$$

2. Acute gastroenteritis (AGE) outbreak with confirmed norovirus that lasted 14 days. The control measures put into place were consistent with the state AGE guidelines. There were no hospitalizations and no related deaths.

   $$\frac{\text{36 people at risk who develop the influenza/condition}}{\text{158 total number of people at risk (includes residents, staff, and family)}} = \text{23\% Attack Rate}$$

FIGURE 4.2: EXAMPLE SURVEILLANCE DEFINITION ALGORITHMS

Respiratory Tract Infection (RCT) Pneumonia

At Least One Constitutional Criteria

- Fever
- Leukocytosis
- New Onset Confusion
- New Onset Functional Decline

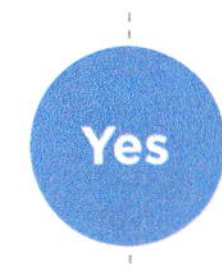

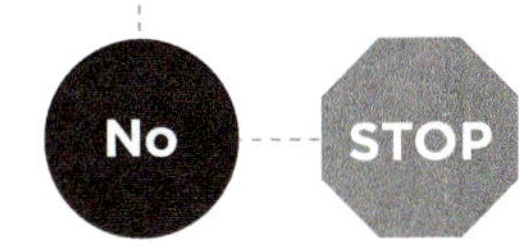

Chest X-ray new infiltrate or pneumonia?

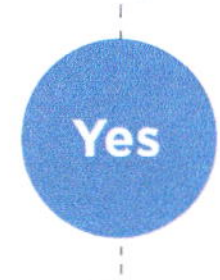

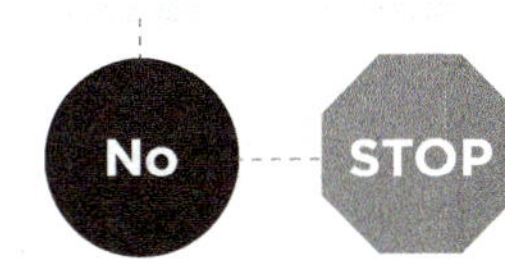

AT LEAST 1 of the following:

- New or increased cough
- New or increased sputum production
- 02 < 94% on room air OR reduction 02 of > 3% from baseline
- New or changed lung examination abnormalities
- Pleuritic Chest pain
- Respiratory rate > 25 breaths per minute

Pneumonia

Clostridium difficile infection (CDI)

Both criteria 1 and 2 must be present

1. One of the following GI subcriteria

Diarrhea: 3 or more liquid or watery stools above what is normal for the resident within a 24 hour period

Presence of toxic megacolon (abnormal dilatation of the large bowel, documented rediologically)

2. One of the following diagnostic subcriteria

A stool specimen for which *Clostridium difficile* is positively detected by PCR, or toxin test

Pseudomembranous colitis is identified during endoscopic exam or surgery, or in histopathologic exam of a biopsy specimen

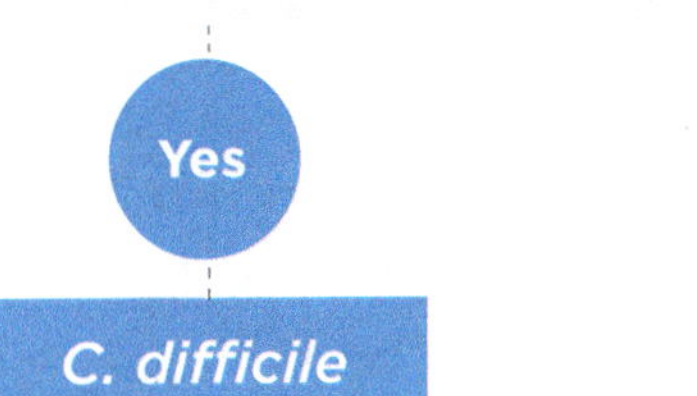

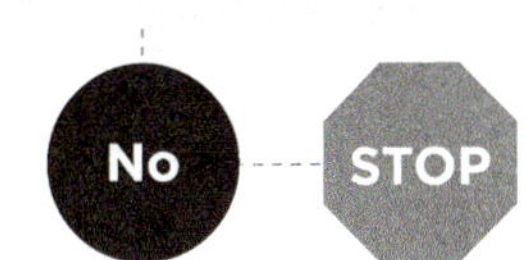

TABLE 4.3: STANDARDIZED INFECTION RATIO: INTERPRETIVE GUIDANCE

SIR LESS THAN 1	SIR GREATER THAN 1
• Fewer infections than what would have been predicted given baseline data • Infections have been prevented since the baseline period • 1 minus the SIR = percent reduction: For example, the SIR of 0.80 means that there was a 20 percent reduction from the baseline period	• More infections than what would have been predicted given baseline data • Infections have increased since the baseline period • SIR minus 1 = percent increase: For example, the SIR of 1.25 means that there was a 25 percent increase from the baseline period.

Adapted from Centers for Disease Control and Prevention. Healthcare-associated infections. CDC website. 2013. Available at: http://www.cdc.gov/HAI/surveillance/QA_stateSummary.html#a6.

Narrative summaries are important but can usually be enhanced by the use of data display techniques. These techniques include graphs, charts, and tables that can be quickly and easily created using basic software packages (see Figure 4.3). See the sample infection prevention and control report in the appendix of this chapter (a template is available on the CD-ROM included with this book).

In addition to internal reporting, IPs must know external reporting requirements and contacts including the following:

- Local/county health department
- State/provincial health department
- CDC

Reporting infectious diseases in the United States may require contacting local, state, and national public health entities, depending on the disease or the disease-causing organism. Each locality has different reporting requirements. The IP must know what to report, how to report, and who must be informed. Reporting requirements vary by state and may include reporting of healthcare-associated infections, community-associated infections, and infectious/communicable diseases. Figure 4.4 identifies states with laws requiring LTCFs to report healthcare-associated infections. As part of public reporting, it is important to make contact with public health professionals who may assist the LTCF. The surveillance program and reporting processes for the LTCF should list:

- Contact information for the local or state health department. If both exist, the process should indicate who to contact first. Communication plans should be made before there is a crisis or an outbreak.
- The specific individuals within the state or local health department who specialize in different diseases or disease categories (respiratory outbreaks, gastrointestinal outbreaks, tuberculosis, sexually transmitted diseases, immunization, etc.). Include contact information for professionals who are authorized to initiate case investigations of communicable diseases.
- State and local health departments' required forms and how they should be submitted.

State public health departments offer a broad range of services in addition to the survey process. The ten essential public health services have been identified by the Core Public Health Functions Steering Committee (see Table 4.4). The outlined duties "provide a working definition of public health and a guiding framework for the responsibilities of local public health systems."[16] When faced with an infectious disease, the state public health department can be a valuable source of information and advice.

Public health authorities are authorized to collect or receive protected health information "for the purpose of preventing or controlling disease, injury, or disability ... and the conduct of public health surveillance, public health investigations, and public health interventions."[16]

REPORTING: NATIONAL HEALTHCARE SAFETY NETWORK LONG-TERM CARE COMPONENT

The NHSN is the nation's most widely used HAI tracking system. NHSN provides facilities, states, regions, and the nation with data needed to identify problem areas, measure progress of prevention efforts, and ultimately eliminate HAIs.[17] NHSN's standard surveillance definitions allow for comparison of infection rates across time and localities. NHSN is considered the recognized gold-standard surveillance system for HAIs. NHSN recently released a LTCF component. In the same way the minimum data sheet (MDS) has been utilized to collect data, the purpose of the NHSN is to provide a secure "Internet-based surveillance system that monitors patient, resident, and healthcare personnel safety."[17]

The focus of the surveillance activities required by NHSN is to use standardized definitions and collection techniques to improve the quality and consistency of the data. There is no cost for participation. NHSN's long-term care component has been developed to include all types of LTCFs, including skilled nursing, chronic care, assisted living, and residential care facilities.

FIGURE 4.3: SAMPLE GRAPH FROM INFLUENZA AND INFLUENZA AND INFLUENZA LIKE ILLNESS OUTBREAK LOG

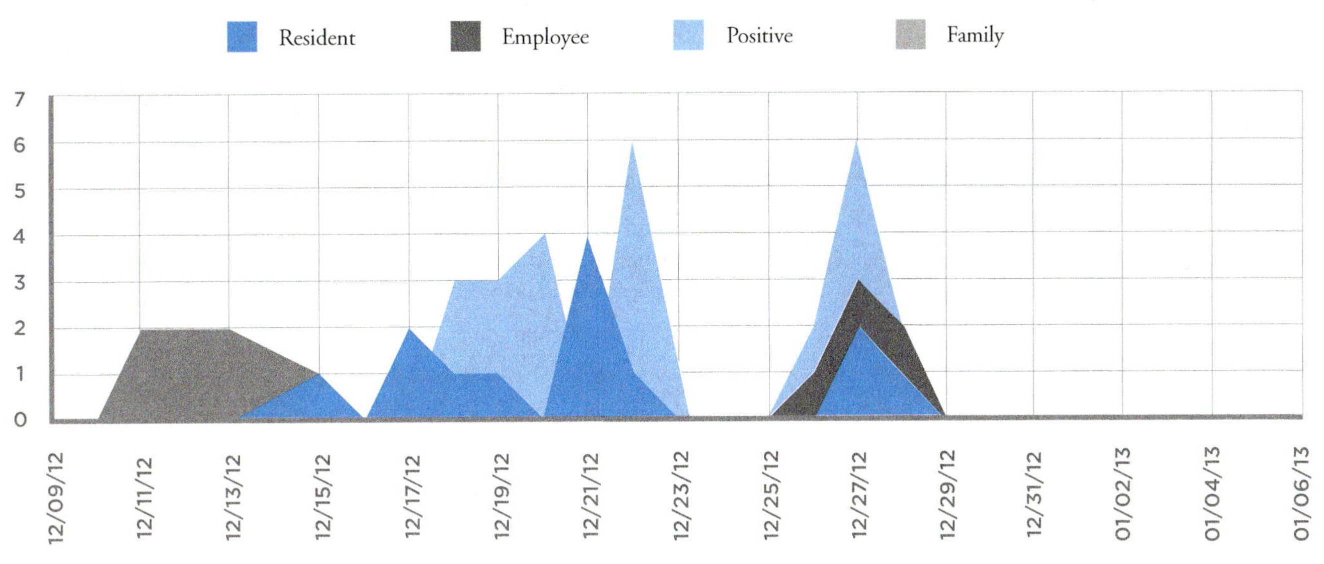

FIGURE 4.4: STATE HEALTHCARE-ASSOCIATED INFECTION LAWS THAT INCLUDE REPORTING BY LONG-TERM CARE FACILITIES

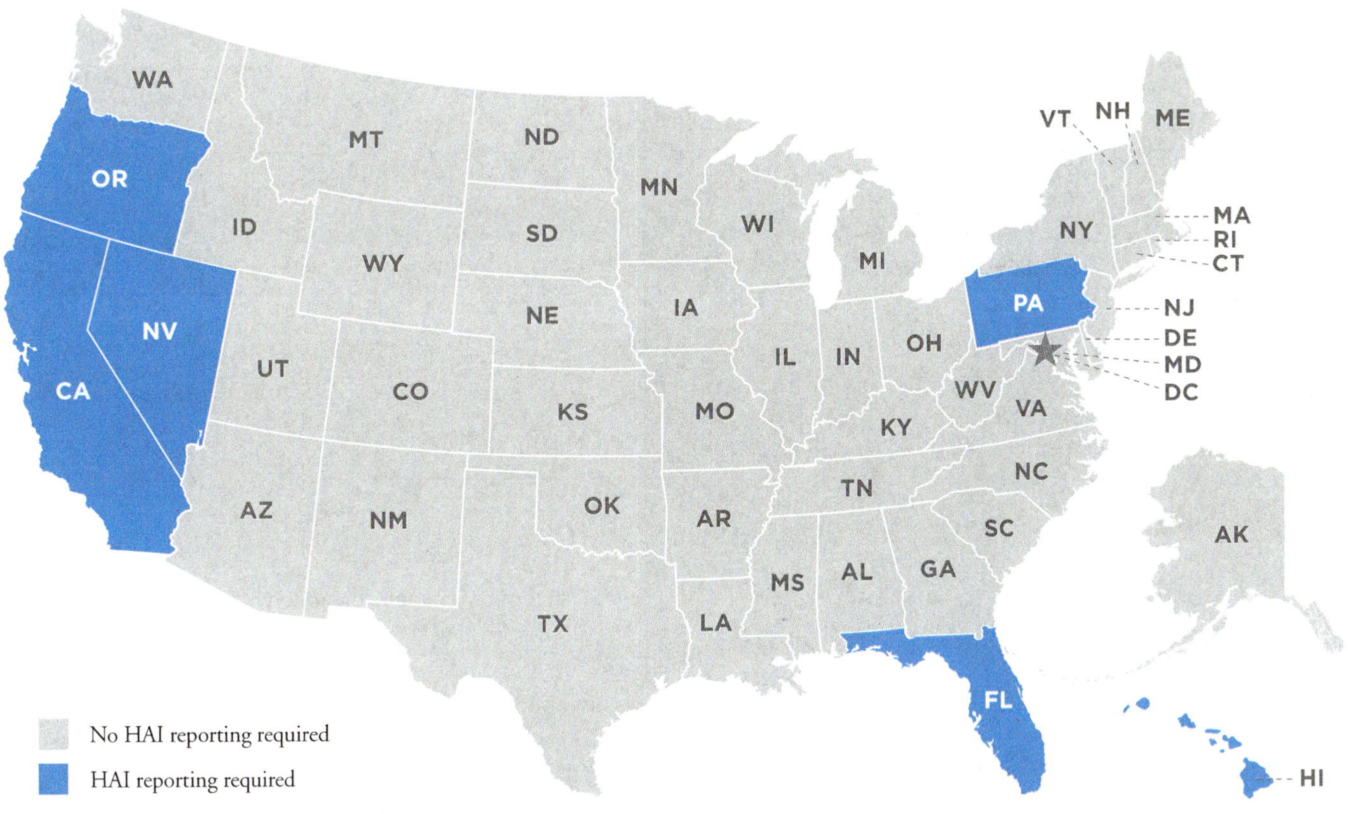

TABLE 4.4: TEN ESSENTIAL PUBLIC HEALTH SERVICES

Monitor	Health status to identify and solve community health problems
Diagnose and investigate	Health problems and health hazards in the community
Inform and educate	To empower people about health issues
Mobilize	Community partnerships and action to identify and solve health problems
Develop policies and plans	To support individual and community health efforts
Link	People to needed personal health services and ensure the provision of healthcare when otherwise unavailable
Enforce	Laws and regulations that protect health and ensure safety
Ensure	Competent public and personal healthcare workforce
Evaluate	The effectiveness, accessibility, and quality of personal and population-based health services
Research	New insights and innovative solutions to health problems

Adapted from Centers for Disease Control and Prevention. National Public Health Performance Standards Program (NPHPSP). CDC website. 2013. Available at: http://www.cdc.gov/nphpsp/essentialservices.html.

LTCFs can enroll in the *Long-term Care Facility Component* at the CDC website. The component includes the following modules:

- Healthcare-associated Infection Module
  - Catheter and non-catheter associated urinary tract infection events
- Laboratory Identified (Lab-ID) Event Module
  - *Clostridium difficile* infections (CDI)
  - MDROs
- Prevention Process Measures Module
  - Hand Hygiene
  - Gown and Glove Use

The LTCF component requires the following:

- Annual facility survey
- Monthly reporting plan for the LTCF
- Understanding of calculating the denominator for the LTCF
- Prevention process measures monthly monitoring (Process Surveillance)
- Events (e.g., UTI or Lab-ID event)

LTCFs may also enroll in the *Healthcare Personnel Safety Component* that includes the following modules:

- Healthcare Worker Exposure Module
  - Bloodborne pathogen exposure
  - Influenza exposure and antiviral use
  - Vaccination program

The goal is a uniform national infection reporting system that represents the long-term care community in both a clinically relevant and statistically significant way. In order to accomplish this, it is necessary that a large number of LTCFs submit data. However, unless required by state legislation, NHSN reporting is a voluntary process for most LTCFs. As more attention is focused on care transitions, including the threat of MDRO transmissions to and from LTCFs, the number of states requiring NHSN reporting is expected to increase. IP competency in NHSN surveillance systems will eventually become a critical skill in LTC. For more information about the risk of transmission during care transitions, see Chapter 13.

Reporting is done using standardized surveillance definitions. LTCF reporting to NHSN requires familiarity with three categories of information:

- The 2012 surveillance definitions for LTCFs published by SHEA and CDC (previously referred to as the McGeer criteria and available at the end of this chapter)
- CDC/NHSN surveillance definition of HAI and the specific modules included in the NHSN LTC component.
- Criteria for specific types of infections in the acute care setting such as for CLABSI and surgical site infections (SSIs) if these are included in the LTCF's surveillance program.[18]

NHSN Technical Requirements

A digital certificate must be obtained from NHSN in order to access the Web-based program. The LTCF information technology personnel can assist with installation. Because this is a Web-based program, it does not require specialized computer equipment or additional software. The NHSN requires an *Agreement to Participate and Consent* NHSN 308(d) document. This document requires the signature of the chief operating officer (COO), chief executive officer (CEO), or the chief financial officer (CFO) of the organization and the signature of the HCP safety primary contact person. The document notifies the LTCF that the CDC can share LTCF data with "state health departments, at their request, with access to HAI data for surveillance and prevention purposes only (*not* for regulatory purposes)."[17]

Administration and Use

A person must be designated as the NHSN facility administrator and the NHSN LTCF contact person. (Note: The person who actually enrolls the LTCF in NHSN—this is not necessarily the administrator of the LTCF). The NHSN facility administrator is responsible for the following:

- Managing NHSN users and user rights and permissions
- Adding, editing, and deleting LTCF data
- Nominating data sharing arrangements (groups)

The NHSN LTCF contact person works closely with the CDC. The facility administrator may also be the contact person. NHSN users may be given administrator roles as well. The CDC does not share the name of any individual program administrator or user.

OTHER NATIONAL MEASURES AND METRICS

In 2009 HHS published the *National Action Plan to Prevent Healthcare Associated Infections,* also known as the HHS National Action Plan. This roadmap initially targeted HAI reduction in acute care but now includes a variety of providers including long-term care.

An important component of the HHS National Action Plan is a framework to assess measures of progress toward HAI prevention. In LTCFs, these measures reflect the National Quality Strategy and HHS priorities. At this time, two HAIs that are nationally burdensome in LTC, have high prevalence and/or high cost, and are known to be preventable through implementation of evidence based practices include (1) UTIs, including CAUTI and urinary catheter care processes and (2) *C. difficile* infections. Two process measures address the need for vaccination (influenza and pneumonia) among residents and staff. The final measure seeks to increase the number of certified nursing homes enrolled in the NHSN LTC component.[19]

IPs in LTCF should be aware of national HAI initiatives and include the HHS National Action Plan measures and metrics into infection prevention surveillance programs. For more information, including the most recent results, see the *National Action Plan to Prevent Health Care-Associated Infections: Road Map to Elimination* at www.hhs.gov. Additional information on the HHS National Action Plan is also available in Chapter 1.

CONCLUSION

An infection prevention and control surveillance program for long-term care is a team effort. In planning the surveillance program, the IP should keep the following in mind:

- Develop a plan for data usage that aligns with the priorities of the LTCF's infection prevention program and identified goals.
- Collaborate with the state health department and CDC to maximize the LTCF's surveillance program effectiveness.
- Use a team approach to:
  - Assess, monitor, and reduce infection risks
  - Implement evidence-based strategies for long-term care
  - Keep track of new guidelines and regulations
  - Develop and implement an effective surveillance program
  - Share surveillance results and identify areas for improvement
  - Use comparative data, including state and national targets, as much as possible
  - Plan to enroll in NHSN, if such planning has not already started
  - Prioritize surveillance activities within the LTCF infection prevention and control plan

INFECTION CONTROL AND HOSPITAL EPIDEMIOLOGY OCTOBER 2012, VOL. 33, NO. 10

SHEA/CDC POSITION PAPER

Surveillance Definitions of Infections in Long-Term Care Facilities: Revisiting the McGeer Criteria

Nimalie D. Stone, MD;[1] Muhammad S. Ashraf, MD;[2] Jennifer Calder, PhD;[3] Christopher J. Crnich, MD;[4] Kent Crossley, MD;[5] Paul J. Drinka, MD;[6] Carolyn V. Gould, MD;[1] Manisha Juthani-Mehta, MD;[7] Ebbing Lautenbach, MD;[8] Mark Loeb, MD;[9] Taranisia MacCannell, PhD;[1] Preeti N. Malani, MD;[10,11] Lona Mody, MD;[10,11] Joseph M. Mylotte, MD;[12] Lindsay E. Nicolle, MD;[13] Mary-Claire Roghmann, MD;[14] Steven J. Schweon, MSN;[15] Andrew E. Simor, MD;[16] Philip W. Smith, MD;[17] Kurt B. Stevenson, MD;[18] Suzanne F. Bradley, MD[10,11] for the Society for Healthcare Epidemiology Long-Term Care Special Interest Group*

(See the commentary by Moro, on pages 978–980.)

Infection surveillance definitions for long-term care facilities (ie, the McGeer Criteria) have not been updated since 1991. An expert consensus panel modified these definitions on the basis of a structured review of the literature. Significant changes were made to the criteria defining urinary tract and respiratory tract infections. New definitions were added for norovirus gastroenteritis and *Clostridum difficile* infections.

Infect Control Hosp Epidemiol 2012;33(10):965-977

When McGeer and colleagues proposed the first set of infection surveillance definitions specifically for use by long-term care facilities (LTCFs), their intent was to provide standardized guidance for infection surveillance activities and research studies in nursing homes and similar institutions.[1] These definitions were adapted from existing surveillance definitions (such as those of the Centers for Disease Control and Prevention [CDC] National Nosocomial Infection Surveillance) that are used in acute care hospitals and with modifications determined by consensus discussions among infectious diseases physicians, geriatricians, and infection control nurses with experience in LTCFs,[1,2] using an unstructured review of the limited literature available at the time. These consensus definitions, also known as the McGeer Criteria, have not been validated or updated despite their ongoing use by infection prevention and control programs and in research studies of nursing homes.

The original surveillance definitions[1] were specifically developed for use in LTCFs with older adults who required (1) supervision and care for impaired cognition, (2) assistance with activities of daily living (ADLs), or (3) skilled nursing care, such as the use of indwelling devices (eg, urinary catheters or enteral feeding tubes). At the time the McGeer Criteria were developed, these facilities rarely provided intravenous therapy or had on-site laboratory or radiology services for the diagnosis of new clinical problems. Now, 20 years later, these definitions should still be applied in skilled nursing facilities and nursing homes that care for the postacute and frail elder populations, as well as in other long-term residential care environments that deliver medical and skilled nursing services if appropriate clinical and diagnostic evaluations can be provided. However, the McGeer Criteria were not designed for use in long-term acute care hospitals, acute inpatient rehabilitation facilities, or pediatric LTCFs.

In March 2009, members of the Society for Healthcare Epidemiology of America (SHEA) Long-Term Care Special Interest Group (LTCSIG) agreed that the surveillance definitions of infections in LTCFs should be updated in light of

Affiliations: 1. Centers for Disease Control and Prevention, Atlanta, Georgia; 2. East Carolina University, Greenville, North Carolina; 3. New York Medical College, Valhalla, New York; 4. University of Wisconsin and William S. Middleton VA Medical Center, Madison, Wisconsin; 5. University of Minnesota and Minneapolis VA Medical Center, Minneapolis, Minnesota; 6. Medical College of Wisconsin, Milwaukee, Wisconsin; 7. Yale University School of Medicine, New Haven, Connecticut; 8. University of Pennsylvania School of Medicine, Philadelphia, Pennsylvania; 9. McMaster University, Hamilton, Ontario, Canada; 10. University of Michigan Medical School, Ann Arbor, Michigan; 11. Geriatric Research Education and Clinical Center, VA Ann Arbor Healthcare System, Ann Arbor, Michigan; 12. University at Buffalo School of Medicine and Biomedical Sciences, Buffalo, New York; 13. University of Manitoba, Winnipeg, Manitoba, Canada; 14. University of Maryland School of Medicine and Baltimore VA Medical Center, Baltimore, Maryland; 15. Pleasant Valley Manor Nursing Home, Stroudsburg, Pennsylvania; 16. University of Toronto School of Medicine, Toronto, Ontario, Canada; 17. University of Nebraska Medical Center, Omaha, Nebraska; 18. Ohio State University Hospitals, Columbus, Ohio.

*Members of the Society for Healthcare Epidemiology Long-Term Care Special Interest Group are listed at the end of the text.

Received May 4, 2012; accepted May 7, 2012; electronically published September 6, 2012.

 0899-823X/2012/3310-0001$15.00. DOI: 10.1086/667743

(1) a substantial increase in the body of evidence-based literature about infections in the elderly in LTCF settings, (2) the availability of improved diagnostics for infection surveillance, (3) the changing populations of patients who are cared for in nonhospital settings, and (4) the updated acute care hospital surveillance definitions of the CDC's National Healthcare Safety Network (NHSN). The process of updating the McGeer Criteria included an evidence-based structured review of the literature in addition to consensus opinions from industry leaders including infectious diseases physicians and epidemiologists, infection preventionists, geriatricians, and public health officials.

METHODS

Review of Clinical Syndromes

We systematically reviewed the definitions of clinical syndromes that commonly occur in LTCF residents, including respiratory tract infections (RTIs), urinary tract infections (UTIs), skin and soft tissue infections (SSTIs), and gastrointestinal (GI) tract infections. Because of a lack of recent, relevant research pertaining to systemic infections (bloodstream infections [BSIs] and unexplained febrile episodes), revisions to the definitions in these categories were not pursued. Specific criteria for defining nasal and otic infections have been removed; categorizing these events should be based on evaluation by a clinical provider. Oropharyngeal and conjunctival infections were included with SSTIs as mucosal infections. For the infection surveillance definitions of each clinical syndrome undergoing revision, a team of SHEA LTCSIG members was assigned to review the literature and provide updated surveillance criteria. The definitions were reviewed, modified where appropriate on the basis of the review, and approved by the LTCSIG and a panel of outside reviewers selected by the SHEA Board of Directors.

Search Procedure

First we searched for relevant guidelines, using Medline, National Guideline Clearinghouse, Cochrane Health Technology Assessment, National Institutes of Health Consensus Development, and the US Preventative Services Task Force. On the basis of a review of those guidelines, each team developed a series of key questions. Examples of these key questions are "What is the utility of examination of urine for pyuria for the diagnosis of symptomatic urinary tract infection?" and "What is the diagnostic accuracy of pulse oximetry for nursing home pneumonia?" These key questions further guided the evidence review used to revise the existing surveillance criteria. Next, a search of the primary literature was performed, using Medline, CINAHL, Embase, Cochrane Systematic Reviews, and the Cochrane Controlled Clinical Trials Registry. Examples of key search terms include the following: nursing home, long-term care, aged, skilled nursing facility, older adults, elderly, fever, healthcare-associated infection, pneumonia, influenza, respiratory tract infection, functional impairment, confusion, leukocyte count, pulse oximetry, urinary tract infection, bacteriuria, urine culture, gastroenteritis, diarrhea, *Clostridium difficile*, norovirus, cellulitis, soft tissue infection, pressure ulcer, scabies. A line listing of articles that met the search criteria and were included in the final analyses is available upon request from the authors.

Evidence Review

A reference was included if it was (1) relevant to key questions; (2) a systematic review, meta-analysis, or primary research report; and (3) written in English. For each clinical syndrome, a standardized evidence table was prepared that summarized the data from each relevant article. Information on the type(s) of LTCF and the specific resident population(s) was included in the evidence tables. The strategy for review of the literature by asking key questions and summarizing the evidence was based on a standard methodology developed by the CDC's Healthcare Infection Control Practices Advisory Committee and the University of Pennsylvania Center for Evidence-Based Practice.[3] When evidence was limited or unavailable to inform changes to the definitions, expert consensus guided any modifications.

Most of the studies we evaluated were small observational or uncontrolled case series that primarily addressed questions related to the utility of signs and symptoms for the purpose of diagnosing infection in older people. The majority of these studies did not clearly address questions about the utility of 1 or more clinical findings in the context of infection detection and surveillance in LTCFs or other healthcare facilities. Because the evidence was generally indirect and judged to be of low quality, a decision was made to not grade proposed additions or changes in clinical parameters according to standardized methods that are typically applied to recommendations and guidelines.

GUIDING PRINCIPLES

The criteria that define infections for surveillance purposes were selected to increase the likelihood that the events captured by application of the definitions are true infections. Presentations of infection in older residents of LTCFs may be atypical, so failure to meet surveillance definitions may not fully exclude the presence of infection. For this reason, the surveillance definitions presented here may not be adequate for real-time case finding, diagnosis, or clinical decision making (eg, antibiotic initiation). Separate clinical guidelines address early identification of infections and appropriate initiation of antibiotic therapy in LTCF residents,[4,5] which are both important for impacting resident outcomes.

The syndromes included here represent a variety of clinically relevant infections that can occur in the LTCF population. Surveillance should be performed for infections for which there are clear strategies that can be implemented for prevention and control of transmission (Table 1). However, for completeness and consistency with the original surveil-

TABLE 1. Considerations for Inclusion of Infections in Long-Term Care Facilities (LTCFs) into Facility Infection Surveillance Programs

Points to consider	Infections	Comments
A. Infections that should be included in routine surveillance		
1. Evidence of transmissibility in a healthcare setting 2. Processes available to prevent acquisition of infection	Viral respiratory tract infections, viral gastroenteritis, and viral conjunctivitis	Associated with outbreaks among residents and healthcare personnel in LTCFs.
3. Clinically significant cause of morbidity or mortality	Pneumonia, urinary tract infection, gastrointestinal tract infections including *Clostridium difficile*, and skin and soft tissue infections	Associated with hospitalization and functional decline in LTCF residents.
4. Specific pathogens causing serious outbreaks	Any invasive group A *Streptococcus* infection, acute viral hepatitis, norovirus, scabies, influenza	A single laboratory-confirmed case should prompt further investigation.
B. Infections that could be considered in surveillance		
1. Infections with limited transmissibility in a healthcare setting 2. Infections with limited preventability	Ear and sinus infections, fungal oral and skin infections, and herpetic skin infections	Associated with underlying comorbid conditions and reactivation of endogenous infection.
C. Infections for which other accepted definitions should be applied in LTCF surveillance (may apply to only specific at-risk residents)	Surgical site infections, central-line-associated bloodstream infections, and ventilator-associated pneumonia	LTCF-specific definitions were not developed. Refer to the National Healthcare Safety Network's criteria (http://www.cdc.gov/nhsn/TOC_PSCManual.html).

lance definitions,[1] several infections that may occur because of underlying host factors rather than transmission within the facility have also been included in this document, so that both infection prevention programs and research studies have a standard set of criteria. Given the limited infection prevention and control resources that are currently available in most LTCFs, surveillance activities may need to target those infections in a facility that have the most potential for prevention. In addition, some infections are associated with a high likelihood of transmission and development of outbreaks (eg, norovirus, influenza, group A *Streptococcus*, acute viral hepatitis). For these infections, identification of even a single case in a LTCF should trigger a more intensive investigation.[6,7]

For infection surveillance purposes, infections should be attributed to a LTCF onset if (a) there is no evidence of an incubating infection at the time of admission to the facility (on the basis of clinical documentation of appropriate signs and symptoms and not solely on screening microbiologic data) and (b) onset of clinical manifestation occurs >2 calendar days after admission. Although debate exists about the use of this time frame to determine a LTCF onset for *C. difficile* infections,[8] it is consistent with acute care infection surveillance reporting and surveillance methodology, and there is currently no evidence to support changing this standard for LTCFs.

As outlined in the original McGeer Criteria, 3 important conditions should be met when applying these surveillance definitions:

1. All symptoms must be new or acutely worse. Many residents have chronic symptoms, such as cough or urinary urgency, that are not associated with infection; however, a new symptom or a change from baseline may be an indication that an infection is developing.

2. Alternative noninfectious causes of signs and symptoms (eg, dehydration, medications) should generally be considered and evaluated before an event is deemed an infection.

3. Identification of infection should not be based on a single piece of evidence but should always consider the clinical presentation and any microbiologic or radiologic information that is available. Microbiologic and radiologic findings should not be the sole criteria for defining an event as an infection. Similarly, diagnosis by a physician alone is not sufficient for a surveillance definition of infection and must be accompanied by documentation of compatible signs and symptoms.

The feasibility of implementation and the validity of these surveillance definitions would benefit from further assessment in different types of LTCFs. As with the original article by McGeer and colleagues,[1] these definitions have not been tested in advance of their publication. Data from a French study demonstrated that application of the original surveillance definitions underestimated the number of nursing home–associated infections when compared with provider diagnoses of infection.[9] This finding highlights the need for future studies to determine the sensitivity and specificity of criteria used within the surveillance definitions and to validate their application in this setting.

DEFINITIONS

Constitutional Criteria for Infection

In an effort to standardize terminology across the clinical syndromes defined in this article, we agreed on common definitions for fever, acute change in mental status, and acute functional decline (Table 2). The definition of fever was changed from a temperature of greater than 38°C (100.4°F), as in the original McGeer Criteria, to a definition consistent with the 2008 Infectious Diseases Society of America (IDSA) guideline for evaluating fever and infection in older adults residing in LTCFs: either (1) a single oral temperature greater than 37.8°C (100°F) or (2) repeated oral temperatures greater than 37.2°C (99°F) or rectal temperatures greater than 37.5°C (99.5°F) or (3) a single temperature greater than 1.1°C (2°F) over baseline from any site.[4] The rationale for this recommendation includes:

1. A desire to maintain consistency across different guidelines.
2. Recognition that although the IDSA guideline is based on data from small numbers of participants in studies performed nearly 2 decades ago, no recent evidence has provided any rationale to modify them.
3. The lower threshold will increase sensitivity for detecting infection given the greater likelihood of a lower febrile response in the elderly.[10,11]

Although both the IDSA guideline and the original McGeer Criteria note that "worsening mental or functional status" can be a nonspecific manifestation of acute infection in an elderly resident of a LTCF,[1,4] there are relatively few studies that have defined a standard assessment of mental status or functional change in the context of acute infection. Mehr et al, in their prospective study involving 36 nursing homes and 2,334 episodes of pneumonia in 1,474 residents, showed that residents with either probable or possible pneumonia were more likely to be somnolent and confused when compared with those with no pneumonia.[12] Lim and MacFarlane[13] compared 397 patients with community-acquired pneumonia (CAP) with 40 patients who had nursing home–acquired pneumonia and found that the patients with nursing home–acquired pneumonia were more likely to be confused when compared with patients who had CAP. Integrated into the recently released Minimum Data Set (MDS), version 3.0, is an assessment of delirium that is based on the confusion assessment method (CAM) criteria.[14,15] In order to standardize an assessment of acute mental status across LTCFs, the CAM criteria are adopted here for the definition of acute confusion or altered mental status (Table 3). For similar reasons, the definition of acute functional decline is also based on changes in ADLs according to the scoring system in MDS 3.0.[16]

Respiratory Tract Infections

Relative to the original surveillance definitions,[1] few changes were made to the definitions of RTIs, which include 4 subcategories: (1) common cold syndromes or pharyngitis, (2)

TABLE 2. Definitions for Constitutional Criteria in Residents of Long-Term Care Facilities (LTCFs)

A. Fever
- 1. Single oral temperature >37.8°C (>100°F)
  OR
- 2. Repeated oral temperatures >37.2°C (99°F) or rectal temperatures >37.5°C (99.5°F)
  OR
- 3. Single temperature >1.1°C (2°F) over baseline from any site (oral, tympanic, axillary)

B. Leukocytosis
- 1. Neutrophilia (>14,000 leukocytes/mm^3)
  OR
- 2. Left shift (>6% bands or ≥1,500 bands/mm^3)

C. Acute change in mental status from baseline (all criteria must be present; see Table 3)
- 1. Acute onset
- 2. Fluctuating course
- 3. Inattention
  AND
- 4. Either disorganized thinking or altered level of consciousness

D. Acute functional decline
- 1. A new 3-point increase in total activities of daily living (ADL) score (range, 0–28) from baseline, based on the following 7 ADL items, each scored from 0 (independent) to 4 (total dependence)[14]
  - a. Bed mobility
  - b. Transfer
  - c. Locomotion within LTCF
  - d. Dressing
  - e. Toilet use
  - f. Personal hygiene
  - g. Eating

influenza-like illness, (3) pneumonia, and (4) lower RTI (Table 4). No changes were made to the definitions of cold syndromes or pharyngitis.

The only change to the definition of influenza-like illness was the removal of seasonal restrictions for the identification of this infection. In the past, seasonal influenza activity in the United States typically peaked in January or February. However, on occasion, seasonal influenza activity has extended into May. In 2009, the H1N1 influenza A virus strain caused increased hospitalization, morbidity, and mortality from influenza-related illnesses during the summer months.[17] Because of increasing uncertainty surrounding the timing of the start of influenza season, the peak of influenza activity, and the length of the season, "seasonality" is no longer a criterion to define influenza-like illness.

Changes to the surveillance definitions of pneumonia and lower RTI were made to increase the specificity of the criteria. Several recent studies have used at least 1 respiratory and 1 constitutional sign or symptom, along with radiographic findings, to define pneumonia.[13] The definition of lower RTI requires the presence of 2 respiratory criteria and 1 constitutional sign or symptom without radiographic findings that is suggestive of pneumonia. The respiratory signs and symptoms are unchanged in this article from the original criteria except for the addition of oxygen saturation in the lower RTI and pneumonia definitions, because of increased access to pulse oximeters in most facilities.

Given that the initial respiratory examination of a LTCF resident who has suspected pneumonia is rarely performed by a physician, the literature was reviewed to determine the role of a physical examination by a nurse or paramedic in predicting pneumonia. Mehr et al[12] demonstrated that a nurse's assessment for the presence of crackles and the absence of wheezing was highly predictive of identifying radiographic evidence of pneumonia. Ackerman and Waldron[18] retrospectively reviewed 244 ambulance reports of breathing difficulty to determine whether paramedic physical examinations, patient history, and clinical judgment correlated with emergency room physician diagnoses. In that study, the classification of respiratory disease included aspiration, asthma, chronic obstructive pulmonary disease, dyspnea, pleurisy, pneumonia, and upper respiratory tract infection (URI). The paramedic respiratory diagnoses had a sensitivity of 71% (range, 58%–82%) and a specificity of 94% (range, 89%–96%). These 2 studies suggest that nonphysician assessments can assist with the determination of pneumonia, and therefore we retained in our definitions the criterion of abnormal findings on lung examination.

The structure of the new pneumonia and lower RTI definitions should facilitate surveillance by segregating criteria into 3 categories (radiography results, respiratory signs or symptoms, and constitutional criteria) and explicitly requiring the exclusion of alternative explanations for respiratory signs or symptoms such as congestive heart failure, atelectasis, and other noninfectious respiratory conditions.

Urinary Tract Infections

The definitions for UTI presented here differ substantially from the original surveillance definitions[1] for both (A) residents without an indwelling catheter and (B) residents with an indwelling catheter (Table 5). The revised definitions take into account the low probability of UTI in residents without indwelling catheters if localizing symptoms are not present, as well as the need for microbiologic confirmation for diagnosis.[19]

For residents without an indwelling catheter, the clinical criterion "acute dysuria" and the urinary tract subcriteria are derived from Loeb et al's[5,20] consensus criteria, which require localizing genitourinary findings and have been validated in a prospective randomized trial showing efficacy and safety. The criterion "acute pain, swelling, or tenderness of the testes, epididymis, or prostate" was added by expert consensus during the review. Fever or leukocytosis plus 1 localizing urinary tract subcriterion or the presence of 2 or more new or increased localizing urinary tract subcriteria could be used to meet the definition for symptomatic UTI. Acute change in mental status and change in the character of the urine (eg, change in color or odor) were each independently associated with bacteriuria ($\geq 10^5$ colony-forming units [cfu]/mL) plus pyuria ($\geq$10 white blood cells per high-power field) in a prospective study of LTCF residents with clinically suspected UTI;[21] however, these 2 symptoms are frequently demonstrated in the presence of asymptomatic bacteriuria[22] due to other confounding clinical

TABLE 3. Confusion Assessment Method Criteria

Acute onset	Evidence of acute change in resident's mental status from baseline
Fluctuating	Behavior fluctuating (eg, coming and going or changing in severity during the assessment)
Inattention	Resident has difficulty focusing attention (eg, unable to keep track of discussion or easily distracted)
Disorganized thinking	Resident's thinking is incoherent (eg, rambling conversation, unclear flow of ideas, unpredictable switches in subject)
Altered level of consciousness	Resident's level of consciousness is described as different from baseline (eg, hyperalert, sleepy, drowsy, difficult to arouse, nonresponsive)

NOTE. Criteria are adapted from a study by Lim and MacFarlane.[13]

TABLE 4. Surveillance Definitions for Respiratory Tract Infections (RTIs)

Criteria	Comments
A. Common cold syndrome or pharyngitis (at least 2 criteria must be present) 1. Runny nose or sneezing 2. Stuffy nose (ie, congestion) 3. Sore throat or hoarseness or difficulty in swallowing 4. Dry cough 5. Swollen or tender glands in the neck (cervical lymphadenopathy)	Fever may or may not be present. Symptoms must be new and not attributable to allergies.
B. Influenza-like illness (both criteria 1 and 2 must be present) 1. Fever 2. At least 3 of the following influenza-like illness subcriteria a. Chills b. New headache or eye pain c. Myalgias or body aches d. Malaise or loss of appetite e. Sore throat f. New or increased dry cough	If criteria for influenza-like illness and another upper or lower RTI are met at the same time, only the diagnosis of influenza-like illness should be recorded. Because of increasing uncertainty surrounding the timing of the start of influenza season, the peak of influenza activity, and the length of the season, "seasonality" is no longer a criterion to define influenza-like illness.
C. Pneumonia (all 3 criteria must be present) 1. Interpretation of a chest radiograph as demonstrating pneumonia or the presence of a new infiltrate 2. At least 1 of the following respiratory subcriteria a. New or increased cough b. New or increased sputum production c. O_2 saturation <94% on room air or a reduction in O_2 saturation of >3% from baseline d. New or changed lung examination abnormalities e. Pleuritic chest pain f. Respiratory rate of ≥25 breaths/min 3. At least 1 of the constitutional criteria (see Table 2)	For both pneumonia and lower RTI, the presence of underlying conditions that could mimic the presentation of a RTI (eg, congestive heart failure or interstitial lung diseases) should be excluded by a review of clinical records and an assessment of presenting symptoms and signs.
D. Lower respiratory tract (bronchitis or tracheobronchitis; all 3 criteria must be present) 1. Chest radiograph not performed or negative results for pneumonia or new infiltrate 2. At least 2 of the respiratory subcriteria (a–f) listed in section C above 3. At least 1 of the constitutional criteria (see Table 2)	(See comment for section C above.)

conditions, such as dehydration. Other nonspecific signs and symptoms (eg, falls) without localizing lower urinary tract findings were not associated with bacteriuria plus pyuria.

For residents with an indwelling catheter, the first clinical criterion, "fever, rigors, or new-onset hypotension with no alternate site of infection" is consistent with the criteria of Loeb et al.[5] Localizing urinary tract symptoms for residents with an indwelling catheter include "new-onset suprapubic pain," "costovertebral angle tenderness," and "purulent discharge from around the catheter." "Acute pain, swelling, or tenderness of the testes, epididymis, or prostate" is included for both catheterized and noncatheterized men as recognized complications of UTI in males, particularly when an indwelling urinary catheter is present.[23] The additional criterion "acute change in mental status or acute functional decline with no alternate diagnosis and leukocytosis" has been included. Acute mental status change and functional decline are nonspecific manifestations of many conditions including hypoxia, dehydration, and adverse effects of medication. The additional requirement of concomitant leukocytosis, a marker of a systemic inflammatory reaction, provides support that the clinical deterioration has an infectious etiology. However, symptomatic UTI in the catheterized resident should always be a diagnosis of exclusion in the absence of localizing urinary tract findings.

A positive urine culture is necessary for diagnosis of UTI[4] and is applied in the revised surveillance definitions for both subcategories (residents without and with an indwelling catheter). For individuals without an indwelling catheter, at least 10^5 cfu/mL of no more than 2 species of microorganisms is the recommended quantitative count from a voided specimen, and for a specimen collected by in-and-out catheteri-

TABLE 5. Surveillance Definitions for Urinary Tract Infections (UTIs)

Criteria	Comments
A. For residents without an indwelling catheter (both criteria 1 and 2 must be present) 1. At least 1 of the following sign or symptom subcriteria a. Acute dysuria or acute pain, swelling, or tenderness of the testes, epididymis, or prostate b. Fever or leukocytosis (see Table 2) and at least 1 of the following localizing urinary tract subcriteria i. Acute costovertebral angle pain or tenderness ii. Suprapubic pain iii. Gross hematuria iv. New or marked increase in incontinence v. New or marked increase in urgency vi. New or marked increase in frequency c. In the absence of fever or leukocytosis, then 2 or more of the following localizing urinary tract subcriteria i. Suprapubic pain ii. Gross hematuria iii. New or marked increase in incontinence iv. New or marked increase in urgency v. New or marked increase in frequency	UTI should be diagnosed when there are localizing genitourinary signs and symptoms and a positive urine culture result. A diagnosis of UTI can be made without localizing symptoms if a blood culture isolate is the same as the organism isolated from the urine and there is no alternate site of infection. In the absence of a clear alternate source of infection, fever or rigors with a positive urine culture result in the noncatheterized resident or acute confusion in the catheterized resident will often be treated as UTI. However, evidence suggests that most of these episodes are likely not due to infection of a urinary source.
2. One of the following microbiologic subcriteria a. At least 10^5 cfu/mL of no more than 2 species of microorganisms in a voided urine sample b. At least 10^2 cfu/mL of any number of organisms in a specimen collected by in-and-out catheter	Urine specimens for culture should be processed as soon as possible, preferably within 1–2 h. If urine specimens cannot be processed within 30 min of collection, they should be refrigerated. Refrigerated specimens should be cultured within 24 h.
B. For residents with an indwelling catheter (both criteria 1 and 2 must be present) 1. At least 1 of the following sign or symptom subcriteria a. Fever, rigors, or new-onset hypotension, with no alternate site of infection b. Either acute change in mental status or acute functional decline, with no alternate diagnosis and leukocytosis c. New-onset suprapubic pain or costovertebral angle pain or tenderness d. Purulent discharge from around the catheter or acute pain, swelling, or tenderness of the testes, epididymis, or prostate	Recent catheter trauma, catheter obstruction, or new-onset hematuria are useful localizing signs that are consistent with UTI but are not necessary for diagnosis.
2. Urinary catheter specimen culture with at least 10^5 cfu/mL of any organism(s)	Urinary catheter specimens for culture should be collected following replacement of the catheter (if current catheter has been in place for >14 d).

NOTE. Pyuria does not differentiate symptomatic UTI from asymptomatic bacteriuria. Absence of pyuria in diagnostic tests excludes symptomatic UTI in residents of long-term care facilities. cfu, colony-forming units.

zation it is at least 10^2 cfu/mL of any number of organisms. Although a small proportion of female residents in LTCFs who have UTI have voided specimens with quantitative counts of less than 10^5 cfu/mL, these specimens were usually evidence of contamination.[24] Before urine samples for culture are obtained from individuals with a chronic indwelling catheter (in place for more than 14 days), the original urinary catheter should be replaced and the specimen should be obtained from the new catheter.[25] Again, a small number of individuals with symptomatic UTI may have lower counts, but a value of at least 10^5 cfu/mL is recommended for increased specificity for surveillance criteria,[26] and it is also consistent with current NHSN acute care definitions for symptomatic UTI.[27] Repeat urine cultures following treatment as a "test of cure" are not recommended because of the high prevalence of asymptomatic bacteriuria in the LTCF population.

A diagnosis of UTI can be made without localizing urinary tract symptoms if a blood culture isolate is the same as the organism isolated from the urine and there is no alternate site of infection. This secondary BSI provides definitive evidence of the existence of systemic infection; in the absence of an alternate source, a UTI becomes the presumptive diagnosis.

Skin, Soft Tissue, and Mucosal Infections

Consistent with the original surveillance definitions,[1] this section includes definitions for (A) skin (cellulitis/soft tissue/wound) infections, (B) scabies, (C) fungal oral/perioral and skin infections (fungal mucocutaneous infections), (D) herpesvirus skin infections, and (E) conjunctivitis (Table 6). The review of the literature revealed that because diagnoses of infections of the skin, soft tissue, and mucous membranes are heavily dependent on clinical criteria, developing definitions with specificity is challenging. Additionally, there was no original research literature that described the validation of a surveillance definition for soft tissue infections.

The original definitions for SSTIs include clinical but not microbiological criteria, whereas the definitions used by NHSN for infection surveillance include a laboratory component.[27] At this time, there is insufficient evidence to support changing the criteria. However, for LTCF residents who have undergone recent surgical procedures, it would be appropriate to utilize the NHSN criteria for defining surgical site infections.

The review of the literature did not identify studies describing the validation of a surveillance definition for scabies. A criterion for identification of an epidemiological linkage to a known case has been added to the definition because (a) residents with scabies, particularly heavily infested residents, are highly infectious and (b) skin scraping, which remains the dominant diagnostic test, has low sensitivity.[28]

The original surveillance definitions of fungal mucocutaneous infections, including those caused by *Candida* species, require diagnosis by a physician or dentist.[1] Definitions of mucocutaneous candidiasis are based on vague clinical descriptions, and there is insufficient basis for changing the criteria; however, a description of typical lesions has been added to increase the specificity of the definition. Although fungal skin infections other than mucocutaneous candidiasis are rare, the original definition for these required both a maculopapular rash and either physician diagnosis or laboratory confirmation. The minor change in the definition substitutes "characteristic rash or lesions" for "maculopapular rash," since dermatophyte lesions may be macular.[29] No data were found to support revisions in the definitions of herpesvirus skin infections (herpes simplex and herpes zoster) or conjunctivitis.

Gastrointestinal Tract Infections

This section includes infection definitions for (A) gastroenteritis, (B) norovirus gastroenteritis, and (C) *C. difficile* infection (Table 7). The general surveillance definition for gastroenteritis was unchanged from that proposed in the original surveillance definitions.[1] Two new surveillance definitions have been added: (a) criteria for determining the presence of norovirus gastroenteritis and (b) criteria for *C. difficile* infection. These new GI infection definitions were developed because it is now recognized that norovirus is highly transmissible, causing frequent and often large outbreaks in healthcare institutions including LTCFs,[30] and *C. difficile* is the major infectious cause of healthcare-associated and antibiotic-associated diarrhea, contributing to significant morbidity and mortality among elderly institutionalized individuals.[31,32]

The gastroenteritis criteria were deemed appropriate and adequate for identifying sporadic or outbreak-associated cases of GI infection caused by common bacterial enteric pathogens. A minor change in the definition of diarrhea substitutes "liquid or watery stools" for "loose or watery stools," since the concept of liquid stools (ie, conforming to the shape of the specimen collection container) is consistent with other surveillance definitions for diarrheal illness.[27,33] Additionally, the definition of diarrhea as "3 or more stools above what is normal for a resident in a 24-hour period" was standardized across GI infections to simplify surveillance activity.

The definition for norovirus gastroenteritis requires the presence of both a compatible clinical presentation and a laboratory confirmation with detection of the infectious agent by one of several accepted laboratory methods. This definition is based on numerous descriptions of norovirus outbreaks and studies of the clinical manifestations of norovirus gastroenteritis in healthcare settings.[34] The norovirus definition can be used to identify either sporadic or outbreak-associated cases. However, sporadic cases would require laboratory confirmation, whereas outbreak cases may not if either a subset of cases involved in the outbreak have laboratory-confirmed diagnosis or the "Kaplan Criteria" are met.[35] The Kaplan Criteria, which have been useful in identifying outbreaks of acute gastroenteritis due to norovirus,[36] provide a surveillance definition to detect a presumed norovirus-like outbreak in a LTCF even in the absence of laboratory confirmation.

C. difficile has been associated with severe, life-threatening disease, especially in the elderly, and infection with this organism can be acquired or transmitted in LTCFs.[32] *C. difficile* infection may be endemic in some healthcare facilities, as well as a cause of outbreaks. Consequently, it is recommended that surveillance for *C. difficile* infection should be done in LTC settings.[31] Surveillance should include prompt clinical and appropriate laboratory evaluation of LTCF residents who have antibiotic-associated diarrhea or an acute diarrheal illness that is not otherwise explained. A surveillance definition for *C. difficile* infection is proposed that includes clinical and microbiology laboratory test criteria. Importantly, because LTCF residents may be colonized with this organism, tests for *C. difficile* or its toxins should be performed only on diarrheal (liquid) stool specimens, unless ileus is suspected. Laboratory surveillance of asymptomatically colonized residents or repeat testing for the presence of *C. difficile* toxins following treatment is not recommended.[31,32] The proposed definition includes criteria for determining whether the *C. difficile* infection is a primary episode or whether it represents

TABLE 6. Surveillance Definitions for Skin, Soft Tissue, and Mucosal Infections

Criteria	Comments
A. Cellulitis, soft tissue, or wound infection (at least 1 of the following criteria must be present) 1. Pus present at a wound, skin, or soft tissue site 2. New or increasing presence of at least 4 of the following sign or symptom subcriteria a. Heat at the affected site b. Redness at the affected site c. Swelling at the affected site d. Tenderness or pain at the affected site e. Serous drainage at the affected site f. One constitutional criterion (see Table 2)	Presence of organisms cultured from the surface (eg, superficial swab sample) of a wound is not sufficient evidence that the wound is infected. More than 1 resident with streptococcal skin infection from the same serogroup (eg, A, B, C, G) in a long-term care facility (LTCF) may indicate an outbreak.
B. Scabies (both criteria 1 and 2 must be present) 1. A maculopapular and/or itching rash 2. At least 1 of the following scabies subcriteria a. Physician diagnosis b. Laboratory confirmation (scraping or biopsy) c. Epidemiologic linkage to a case of scabies with laboratory confirmation	An epidemiologic linkage to a case can be considered if there is evidence of geographic proximity in the facility, temporal relationship to the onset of symptoms, or evidence of common source of exposure (ie, shared caregiver). Care must be taken to rule out rashes due to skin irritation, allergic reactions, eczema, and other noninfectious skin conditions
C. Fungal oral or perioral and skin infections	
1. Oral candidiasis (both criteria a and b must be present) a. Presence of raised white patches on inflamed mucosa or plaques on oral mucosa b. Diagnosis by a medical or dental provider	Mucocutaneous *Candida* infections are usually due to underlying clinical conditions such as poorly controlled diabetes or severe immunosuppression. Although they are not transmissible infections in the healthcare setting, they can be a marker for increased antibiotic exposure.
2. Fungal skin infection (both criteria a and b must be present) a. Characteristic rash or lesions b. Either a diagnosis by a medical provider or a laboratory-confirmed fungal pathogen from a scraping or a medical biopsy	Dermatophytes have been known to cause occasional infections and rare outbreaks in the LTCF setting.
D. Herpesvirus skin infections 1. Herpes simplex infection (both criteria a and b must be present) a. A vesicular rash b. Either physician diagnosis or laboratory confirmation 2. Herpes zoster infection (both criteria a and b must be present) a. A vesicular rash b. Either physician diagnosis or laboratory confirmation	Reactivation of herpes simplex ("cold sores") or herpes zoster ("shingles") is not considered a healthcare-associated infection. Primary herpesvirus skin infections are very uncommon in a LTCF except in pediatric populations, where it should be considered healthcare associated.
E. Conjunctivitis (at least 1 of the following criteria must be present) 1. Pus appearing from 1 or both eyes, present for at least 24 h 2. New or increased conjunctival erythema, with or without itching 3. New or increased conjunctival pain, present for at least 24 h	Conjunctivitis symptoms ("pink eye") should not be due to allergic reaction or trauma.

NOTE. For wound infections related to surgical procedures, LTCFs should use the Centers for Disease Control and Prevention's National Healthcare Safety Network Surgical Site Infection criteria and report these infections back to the institution where the original surgery was performed.

TABLE 7. Surveillance Definitions for Gastrointestinal (GI) Tract Infections

Criteria	Comments
A. Gastroenteritis (at least 1 of the following criteria must be present) 1. Diarrhea: 3 or more liquid or watery stools above what is normal for the resident within a 24-h period 2. Vomiting: 2 or more episodes in a 24-h period 3. Both of the following sign or symptom subcriteria a. A stool specimen testing positive for a pathogen (eg, *Salmonella*, *Shigella*, *Escherichia coli* O157 : H7, *Campylobacter* species, rotavirus) b. At least 1 of the following GI subcriteria i. Nausea ii. Vomiting iii. Abdominal pain or tenderness iv. Diarrhea	Care must be taken to exclude noninfectious causes of symptoms. For instance, new medications may cause diarrhea, nausea, or vomiting; initiation of new enteral feeding may be associated with diarrhea; and nausea or vomiting may be associated with gallbladder disease. Presence of new GI symptoms in a single resident may prompt enhanced surveillance for additional cases. In the presence of an outbreak, stool specimens should be sent to confirm the presence of norovirus or other pathogens (eg, rotavirus or *E. coli* O157 : H7).
B. Norovirus gastroenteritis (both criteria 1 and 2 must be present) 1. At least 1 of the following GI subcriteria a. Diarrhea: 3 or more liquid or watery stools above what is normal for the resident within a 24-h period b. Vomiting: 2 or more episodes of in a 24-h period 2. A stool specimen for which norovirus is positively detected by electron microscopy, enzyme immunoassay, or molecular diagnostic testing such as polymerase chain reaction (PCR)	In the absence of laboratory confirmation, an outbreak (2 or more cases occurring in a long-term care facility [LTCF]) of acute gastroenteritis due to norovirus infection may be assumed to be present if all of the following criteria are present ("Kaplan Criteria"): (a) vomiting in more than half of affected persons; (b) a mean (or median) incubation period of 24–48 h; (c) a mean (or median) duration of illness of 12–60 h; and (d) no bacterial pathogen is identified in stool culture.
C. *Clostridium difficile* infection (both criteria 1 and 2 must be present) 1. One of the following GI subcriteria a. Diarrhea: 3 or more liquid or watery stools above what is normal for the resident within a 24-h period b. Presence of toxic megacolon (abnormal dilatation of the large bowel, documented radiologically) 2. One of the following diagnostic subcriteria a. A stool sample yields a positive laboratory test result for *C. difficile* toxin A or B, or a toxin-producing *C. difficile* organism is identified from a stool sample culture or by a molecular diagnostic test such as PCR b. Pseudomembranous colitis is identified during endoscopic examination or surgery or in histopathologic examination of a biopsy specimen	A "primary episode" of *C. difficile* infection is defined as one that has occurred without any previous history of *C. difficile* infection or that has occurred >8 wk after the onset of a previous episode of *C. difficile* infection. A "recurrent episode" of *C. difficile* infection is defined as an episode of *C. difficile* infection that occurs 8 wk or sooner after the onset of a previous episode, provided that the symptoms from the earlier (previous) episode have resolved. Individuals previously infected with *C. difficile* may continue to remain colonized even after symptoms resolve. In the setting of an outbreak of GI infection, individuals could have positive test results for presence of *C. difficile* toxin because of ongoing colonization and also be coinfected with another pathogen. It is important that other surveillance criteria be used to differentiate infections in this situation.

a recurrence (relapse or reinfection). Published recommendations for surveillance for *C. difficile* infection have also attempted to determine the setting in which the infection was likely to have been acquired;[33] however, there is controversy about how to apply these attribution criteria in LTCFs.[8]

Systemic Infections

The original surveillance definitions included BSI and unexplained febrile episodes in this section.[1] However, there has been scant literature to better define approaches to the diagnosis or routine surveillance of these clinical entities in LTCFs. In 2008, the IDSA guideline did not recommend performing blood cultures as part of the evaluation for infection in "most" residents in LTCFs, but they qualified this by saying that in facilities with quick access to laboratory facilities, physicians available to respond to results, and capacity to administer parenteral antibiotics, diagnostic blood cultures would be appropriate.[4]

There have been limited studies assessing the utility and reliability of blood cultures in LTCFs. In 2005, Mylotte[37] reviewed several studies evaluating nursing home–associated BSI. Only 1 reported on the total numbers of blood cultures obtained during the study period,[38] and 1 reported the proportion of contaminated blood cultures ("false positives").[39] None of the studies in the review had data more recent than from 2000. Since the Mylotte review, a single study from Israel has reported on results from blood cultures performed on samples from a multilevel geriatric facility over a 2-year period from 2002 to 2004.[40] In this study, 252 (15.8%) of 1,588 cultures had positive results, which indicates an incidence of BSI of 0.46 per 1,000 resident-days. The study did not provide data on episodes of suspected contaminated cultures. However, in a cohort of 100 bacteremic residents, only 58% had received adequate empiric antibiotic therapy and the mortality rate was 34%, compared with 13% in nonbacteremic matched controls. The incidence of BSI and the prevalence of positive cultures were much higher in this study compared with earlier studies, suggesting that those LTCFs with the capacity to perform blood cultures and respond to results should include blood cultures in the diagnostic evaluation of infection.

Given the limited evidence addressing the effectiveness of blood cultures in LTCFs, we did not attempt to propose a revised surveillance definition for BSI. Instead, consideration should be given to an application of the NHSN criteria for central line–associated BSI in those LTCFs who care for residents with indwelling vascular catheters including peripherally inserted central catheters (PICCs) and hemodialysis catheters.[27]

CONCLUSIONS

These infection surveillance definitions for LTCFs update the consensus definitions proposed by McGeer et al, incorporating evidence published over the interim 20 years. The majority of definitions and criteria were retained with only minor revisions except for those for UTI, where the criteria were made more specific, and GI infection, where 2 new infections were added to the surveillance definitions (norovirus and *C. difficile*).

These updated definitions are intended to serve as a national standard for infection surveillance in LTCFs. Because they are implemented in this setting, feedback from providers and efforts to validate the definitions will guide subsequent modifications as appropriate.

CONTRIBUTORS

McGeer Study Steering Committee

Nimalie D. Stone and Suzanne F. Bradley (co–project leaders), Lindsay E. Nicolle, Andrew E. Simor, Philip W. Smith, Kurt B. Stevenson; *Gastrointestinal Writing Group*: Andrew E. Simor (group leader), Muhammad S. Ashraf, Carolyn V. Gould, Taranisia MacCannell, Preeti N. Malani; *Respiratory Tract Infection Writing Group*: Mark Loeb and Lona Mody (co–group leaders), Christopher Crnich, Joseph P. Mylotte, Steven J. Schweon; *Skin and Soft Tissue Writing Group*: Philip W. Smith (group leader), Jennifer Calder, Kent Crossley, Mary-Claire Roghmann; *Urinary Tract Infection Writing Group*: Lindsay E. Nicolle (group leader), Paul J. Drinka, Ebbing Lautenbach, Manisha Juthani-Mehta; *Fever and Delirium Standards Subcommittee*: Suzanne F. Bradley, Kent Crossley, Paul Drinka, Preeti Malani, Lona Mody, Lindsay Nicolle, Mary-Claire Roghmann, Nimalie D. Stone.

SHEA Long-Term Care Special Interest Group

Kurt B. Stevenson (chair; Ohio State University Hospitals, Columbus, OH), Nimalie D. Stone (vice-chair; Centers for Disease Control and Prevention, Atlanta, GA), Muhammad S. Ashraf (East Carolina University, Greenville, NC), Suzanne F. Bradley (University of Michigan Medical School and Geriatric Research Education and Clinical Center [GRECC], VA Ann Arbor Healthcare System, Ann Arbor, MI), Mike Brown (Evergreen Hospital Medical Center, Kirkland, WA), Chris Cahill (California Department of Public Health [retired], Richmond, CA), Jennifer Calder (New York Medical College, Valhalla, NY), Christopher J. Crnich (University of Wisconsin and William S. Middleton VA Medical Center, Madison, WI), Kent Crossley (University of Minnesota and Minneapolis VA Medical Center, Minneapolis, MN). Paul J. Drinka (Medical College of Wisconsin, Milwaukee, WI), Jon P. Furuno (Oregon State University, Portland, OR), Rosemary Ikram (Christchurch, New Zealand), Jennie Johnstone (McMaster University, Hamilton, ON), Manisha Juthani-Mehta (Yale University School of Medicine, New Haven, CT), Keith S. Kaye (Wayne State University School of Medicine, Detroit, MI), Ebbing Lautenbach (University of Pennsylvania School of Medicine, Philadelphia, PA), Donna R. Lewis (Atlanta Veterans Affairs Medical Center, Atlanta, GA), Mark Loeb (McMaster University, Hamilton, ON), Anurag N. Malani (St. Joseph Mercy Hospital, Ypsilanti, MI), Preeti N. Malani (University of Michigan Medical School and GRECC, VA Ann Arbor Healthcare System, Ann Arbor, MI), James Marx (University of Phoenix, San Diego, CA), Allison McGeer (University of Toronto School of Medicine, Toronto, ON), Lona Mody (University of Michigan Medical School and GRECC, VA Ann Arbor Healthcare System, Ann Arbor, MI), Joseph P. Mylotte (University at Buffalo School of Medicine and Biomedical Sciences, Buffalo, NY), Lindsay E. Nicolle (University of Manitoba, Winnipeg, MB), Joseph F. Perz (Centers for Disease Control and Prevention, Atlanta, GA), Chesley Richards (Centers for Disease Control and Prevention, Atlanta, GA), Mary-Claire Roghmann (University of Maryland School of Medicine and Baltimore VA Medical Center, Baltimore, MD), Brenda J. Roup (Maryland Department of Health and Mental Hygiene, Baltimore, MD), Steven J. Schweon (Pleasant Valley Manor Nursing Home, Stroudsburg, PA), Joseph Segal (Drake Center, Cincinnati, OH), Andrew E. Simor (University of Toronto School of Medicine, Toronto, ON), Michael R. Spence (Kalispell Regional Medical Center, Kalispell, MT), Philip W. Smith (University of Nebraska Medical Center, Omaha, NE), Lauri D. Thrupp (University of California, Irvine, CA), Kavita Trivedi (California Department of Public Health, Richmond, CA), Constanze Wendt (University of Heidelberg, Heidelberg, Germany).

ENDORSEMENTS

These definitions have been endorsed by the American Medical Directors Association, the Association of Medical Microbiology and Infectious Disease–Canada, the Association for Professionals in Infection Control and Epidemiology, the Community and Hospital Infection Control Association–Canada, and the National Association of Directors of Nursing Administration in Long Term Care.

ACKNOWLEDGMENTS

Special thanks to Malinda McCarthy and Elizabeth Bolyard from the Centers for Disease Control and Prevention for their administrative and organizational support of this writing project.

Potential conflicts of interest. All authors report no conflicts of interest relevant to this article. All authors submitted the ICMJE Form for Disclosure of Potential Conflicts of Interest, and the conflicts that the editors consider relevant to this article are disclosed here.

Address correspondence to Dr. Nimalie D. Stone, 1600 Clifton Road NE, DHQP/CDC, Mailstop A-31, Atlanta, GA 30333 (nstone@cdc.gov).

The findings and conclusions in this report are those of the authors and do not necessarily represent the official position of the Centers for Disease Control and Prevention or the Department of Veterans Affairs.

REFERENCES

1. McGeer A, Campbell B, Emori TG, et al. Definitions of infection surveillance in long-term care facilities. *Am J Infect Control* 1991; 19:1–7.
2. Peppler C, Campbell B, Prince K, Rivera A, Scully D; Cooperative Infection Control Committee. *A surveillance protocol for long term-care facilities.* Markham, Ontario, Canada: Ontario Nursing Home Association, 1988:8–14.
3. Umscheid CA, Agarwal RK, Brennan PJ; Healthcare Infection Control Practices Advisory Committee. Updating the guideline development methodology of the Healthcare Infection Control Practices Advisory Committee (HICPAC). *Am J Infect Control* 2010;38:264–273.
4. High K, Bradley SF, Gravenstein S, et al. Clinical practice guideline for the evaluation of fever and infection in older adult residents of long term care facilities. *Clin Infect Dis* 2009;48: 149–171.
5. Loeb M, Bentley DW, Bradley S, et al. Development of minimum criteria for the initiation of antibiotics in residents of long-term–care facilities: results of a consensus conference. *Infect Control Hosp Epidemiol* 2001;22:120–124.
6. Schwartz B, Ussery XT. Group A streptococcal outbreaks in nursing homes. *Infect Control Hosp Epidemiol* 1992;13:742–747.
7. Centers for Disease Control and Prevention. Transmission of hepatitis B virus among persons undergoing blood glucose monitoring in long-term-care facilities: Mississippi, North Carolina, and Los Angeles County, California, 2003–2004. *Morb Mortal Wkly Rep* 2005;54:220–223.
8. Mylotte JM. Surveillance for *Clostridium difficile*–associated diarrhea in long-term care facilities: what you get is not what you see. *Infect Control Hosp Epidemiol* 2008;29:760–763.
9. Rothan-Tondeur M, Piette F, Lejeune B, de Wazieres B, Gavazzi G. Infections in nursing homes: is it time to revise the McGeer criteria? *J Am Geriatr Soc* 2010;58:199–201.
10. Castle SC, Yeh M, Toledo S, Yoshikawa TT, Norman DC. Lowering the temperature criterion improves detection of infections in nursing home residents. *Aging Immunol Infect Dis* 1993;4: 67–76.
11. Roghmann M-C, Warner J, Mackowiak PA. The relationship between age and fever magnitude. *Am J Med Sci* 2001;322:68–70.
12. Mehr DR, Binder EF, Kruse RL, Zweig SC, Madsen RW, D'Agostino RB. Clinical findings associated with radiographic pneumonia in nursing home residents. *J Fam Pract* 2001;50: 931–937.
13. Lim WS, MacFarlane JT. A prospective comparison of nursing home acquired pneumonia with community acquired pneumonia. *Eur Respir J* 2001;18:362–368.
14. Minimum Data Set, version 3.0. Nursing Home Comprehensive (NC), version 1.00.2 10/01/2010, section C, p. 7.
15. Inouye SK, van Dyck CH, Alessi CA, Balkin S, Siegal AP, Horwitz RI. Clarifying confusion: the confusion assessment method: a new method for detection of delirium. *Ann Intern Med* 1990; 113:941–948.
16. Minimum Data Set, version 3.0. Nursing Home Comprehensive (NC), version 1.00.2 10/01/2010, Section G, p. 14.
17. The 2009 H1N1 pandemic: summary highlights, April 2009–April 2010. Centers for Disease Control and Prevention website. http://www.cdc.gov/h1n1flu/cdcresponse.htm.
18. Ackerman R, Waldron RL. Difficulty breathing: agreement of paramedic and emergency physician diagnoses. *Prehosp Emerg Care* 2006;10:77–80.
19. Orr PH, Nicolle LE, Duckworth H, et al. Febrile urinary infection in the institutionalized elderly. *Am J Med* 1996;100:71–77.
20. Loeb M, Brazil K, Lohfeld L, et al. Effect of a multifaceted intervention on number of antimicrobial prescriptions for suspected urinary tract infections in residents of nursing homes: cluster randomized controlled trial. *Br Med J* 2006;351:669–671.
21. Juthani-Mehta M, Quagliarello V, Perrelli E, Towle V, Van Ness P, Tinetti M. Clinical features to identify urinary tract infection in nursing home residents: a cohort study. *J Am Geriatr Soc* 2009;57:963–970.
22. Nicolle LE. Symptomatic urinary tract infection in nursing home residents. *J Am Geriatr Soc* 2009;57:1113–1114.
23. Weld KJ, Dmochowski RR. Effect of bladder management on urological complications in spinal cord injured patients. *J Urol* 2000;163:768–772.
24. Ouslander JG, Schapira M, Schnelle JF. Urine specimen collection from incontinent female nursing home residents. *J Am Geriatr Soc* 1995;43:2;79–81.
25. Hooton TM, Bradley SF, Cardenas DD, et al. Diagnosis, prevention, and treatment of catheter-associated urinary tract infection in adults: 2009 international clinical practice guidelines from the Infectious Diseases Society of America. *Clin Infect Dis* 2010;50:625–663.
26. Tenney JH, Warren JW. Long term catheter-associated bacteriuria: species at low concentration. *Urology* 1987;30:444–446.
27. Horan TC, Andrus M, Dudeck MA. NHSN definitions: CDC/NHSN surveillance definition of health care–associated infection and criteria for specific types of infections in the acute care setting. *Am J Infect Control* 2008;36:309–332.
28. Cahill CK, Rosenberg J, MD, Schweon SJ, Smith PW, Nicolle

LE. Scabies surveillance, prevention, and control. *Ann Long-Term Care* 2009;17:31–35.

29. Laube S. Skin infections and ageing. *Ageing Res Rev* 2004;3: 69–89.
30. Said MA, Perl TM, Sears CL. Gastrointestinal flu: norovirus in health care and long-term care facilities. *Clin Infect Dis* 2008; 47:1202–1208.
31. Simor AE, Bradley SF, Strausbaugh LJ, Crossley K, Nicolle LE; SHEA Long-Term-Care Committee. SHEA Position Paper: *Clostridium difficile* in long-term-care facilities for the elderly. *Infect Control Hosp Epidemiol* 2002;23:696–703.
32. Simor AE. Diagnosis, management, and prevention of *Clostridium difficile* infection in long-term care facilities: a review. *J Am Geriatr Soc* 2010;58:1556–1564.
33. McDonald LC, Coignard B, Dubberke E, et al. Recommendations for surveillance of *Clostridium difficile*-associated disease. *Infect Control Hosp Epidemiol* 2007;28:140–145.
34. Lopman BA, Reacher MH, Vipond IB, Sarangi J, Brown DWG. Clinical manifestations of norovirus gastroenteritis in health care settings. *Clin Infect Dis* 2004;39:318–324.
35. Kaplan JE, Gary GW, Baron RC, et al. Epidemiology of Norwalk gastroenteritis and the role of Norwalk virus in outbreaks of acute nonbacterial gastroenteritis. *Ann Intern Med* 1982;96: 756–761.
36. Turcios RM, Widdowson M-A, Sulka AC, Mead PS, Glass RI. Reevaluation of epidemiologic criteria for identifying outbreaks of acute gastroenteritis due to norovirus: United States, 1998–2000. *Clin Infect Dis* 2006;42:964–969.
37. Mylotte JM. Nursing home–acquired bloodstream infection. *Infect Control Hosp Epidemiol* 2005;26:833–837.
38. Nicolle LE, McIntyre M, Hoban D, Murray D. Bacteremia in a long term care facility. *Can J Infect Dis* 1994;5:130–132.
39. Richardson JP, Hricz L. Risk factors for the development of bacteremia in nursing home patients. *Arch Fam Med* 1995;4: 785–789.
40. Raz R, Ben-Israel Y, Gronich D, Granot E, Colodner R, Visotzky I. Usefulness of blood cultures in the management of febrile patients in long-term care facilities. *Eur J Clin Microbiol Infect Dis* 2005;24:745–748.

SAMPLE INFECTION PREVENTION AND CONTROL REPORT

Infection Type	# of New Infections	Average Census	# of Days in Reporting Period	# of Resident Days per Reporting Period	Infection Rate
Facility Associated	99	371.5	31	11,518	8.6 infections per 1,000 resident days

Infection Category (*Sort by risk, or historical frequency, or by alphabetical order*)	# of New Infections	Comments	Infection Rate per 1000 resident days		
			Current	Last Month	Prior Year*
Cellulitis, Soft Tissue, or Wound Infection	2	Dressing change technique reviewed Feb	0.15	3.0	NA*
Central Line Bloodstream Infection (CLABSI)	0	No CLABSI	0	1.9	NA*
Conjunctivitis	1	1 viral conjunctivitis	0.07	0	NA*
Fungal Infection: Oral, Perioral, or Skin	1	1 case oral thrush	0.07	1.2	NA*
Gastroenteritis	14	See acute gastroenteritis (AGE) report	1.2	0	NA*
Norovirus	8	See AGE report	0.7	0	NA*
Respiratory tract infection: common cold or pharyngitis	22	Sporadic clusters of respiratory illness on 1A, 2A, 3H/J Respiratory controls put in place	1.9	2.1	NA*
Respiratory tract infection: influenza-like illness (ILI)	23	Sporadic clusters of respiratory illness on 1A, 2A, 3H/J Respiratory controls put in place	2.0	3.1	NA*
Respiratory tract infection: pneumonia	4	1 aspiration pneumonia	0.3	1.0	NA*
Respiratory tract infection: lower respiratory tract infection	2	Sporadic clusters of respiratory illness on 1A, 2A, 3H/J Respiratory controls put in place	0.15	0	NA*
Surgical site infection	0	0	0	0	NA*
Scabies	0	0	0	0	NA*
Urinary tract infection (no urinary catheter)	17	No clusters of related organisms	1.46	1.2	NA*
Urinary tract infection (catheter-associated [CAUTI])	0	No CAUTI	0	0	NA*

Clostridium difficile (CDI) per 10,000 resident days is standard for CDI rates	# of New Infections	Comments	Infection Rate per 1000 resident days		
	3	2 associated CDI enhanced cleaning Antimicrobial	2.6	3.0	3.8

See the CD-ROM for Template.

Courtesy of Deborah P. Burdsall, MSN, RN-BC, CIC.

SAMPLE INFECTION PREVENTION AND CONTROL REPORT BY CARE UNIT

Optional Approach to Data Presentation: Consider using a unit-specific graph as a substitute for the table in this document to reduce the risk of redundant data collection.

Resident Care Area	# of New Infections	Infection Rate per 1,000 resident days	Comments
1	14	11.2	• Cluster of colds and ILI with • 2+ influenza • 6+ RSV
1H	5	3.99	• 3 colds • 2 ILI with • 1 RSV+
2	16	13.5	• 5 colds • 2 ILI with • 2 influenza+ and 3 RSV+ • 1 pneumonia • 2 lower resp tract infections • 2 UTI • 1 wound infection • 2 *C. difficile* • 1 norovirus
2E	3	8.37	• 1 pneumonia • 2 UTI separate organisms
2F	0	0	• No reportable infections
2H	2	6.9	• 2 colds
3	5	4.12	• 1 cold • 3 UTI • 1 norovirus
3H	14	11.52	• 9 gastroenteritis • 3 UTI • 2 ILI

Sample Summary

March had an overall infection rate of 8.6 infections per 1,000 resident days. This rate is a result of an increase in sporadic mixed respiratory illness caused primarily by RSV, influenza A and B and unknown etiology, and two clusters of gastroenteritis on two different units with no common staff. Only one of the cases of nausea, vomiting, or diarrhea met the definition of acute gastroenteritis per the state health department acute gastroenteritis (AGE).

An increase in the rate of wound infections was addressed by inservicing the nurses on dressing change techniques and products used for different stages and types of wounds. The wound infection rate decreased from 3.0 infections per 1,000 resident days to 0.15 infections per 1,000 resident days. Monitoring of dressing change techniques will be targeted for the next 6 months.

There were no confirmed cases of scabies or tuberculosis. There were multiple cases of upper and lower respiratory infections, caused primarily by RSV, influenza, and unknown etiology. County Department of Public Health was consulted for both the respiratory illness and gastroenteritis outbreaks.

See the CD-ROM for Template.

REFERENCES

1. Centers for Medicare & Medicaid Services (CMS). CMS Manual System Pub. 100-07 State Operations Provider Certification, Transmittal 55. December 2, 2009. Available at: http://www.cms.gov/Regulations-and Guidance/Guidance/Transmittals/downloads/R51SOMA.pdf.

2. Carrico R, ed. *APIC Text of Infection Control and Epidemiology,* 3rd ed. Washington, DC: Association for Professionals in Infection Control and Epidemiology, 2009.

3. World Health Organization (WHO). *Health Topics: Epidemiology.* WHO website. 2012. Available at: http://www.who.int/topics/epidemiology/en/.

4. Centers for Disease Control and Prevention (CDC). *Hospital Utilization (in non-Federal short-stay hospitals).* CDC website. 2013. Available at: http://www.cdc.gov/nchs/fastats/hospital.htm.

5. American Hospital Association (AHA). *Fast Facts on US Hospitals.* AHA website. 2013. Available at: http://www.aha.org/research/rc/stat-studies/fast-facts.shtml.

6. Genworth. *Financial Planning for Long-term care—statistics.* Genworth website. 2012. Available at: http://www1.genworth.com/content/lets_talk/united_states/english/planning_for_long/statistics.html.

7. Centers for Disease Control and Prevention (CDC). *National Hospital Care Survey.* CDC website. 2012. Available at: http://www.cdc.gov/nchs/nhcs.htm.

8. Moody EF. *Nursing Home Statistics (AHCA).* EF Moody website. 2012. Available at: http://www.efmoody.com/longterm/nursingstatistics.html.

9. Centers for Medicare and Medicaid Services (CMS). *Nursing Home Data Compendium.* CMS website. 2012. Available at: https://www.cms.gov/Medicare/Provider-Enrollment-and-Certification/CertificationandComplianc/downloads/nursinghomedatacompendium_508.pdf.

10. Sax H, Allegranzi B, Chra ti MN, Boyce J, Larson E, Pittet D. The world health organization hand hygiene observation method. *Am J Infect Control* 2009; 37(10): 827-834.

11. World Health Organization (WHO). *Hand Hygiene in Outpatient and Home-based Care and Long-term Care Facilities: A Guide to the Application of the WHO Multimodal Hand Hygiene Improvement Strategy and the "My Five Moments For Hand Hygiene" Approach.* WHO website. 2012. Available at: http://apps.who.int/iris/bitstream/10665/78060/1/9789241503372_eng.pdf.

12. World Health Organization (WHO). *WHO Guidelines on Hand Hygiene in Health Care.* WHO website. 2009. Available at: http://whqlibdoc.who.int/publications/2009/9789241597906_eng.pdf.

13. Centers for Medicare & Medicaid Services (CMS). *MDS 3.0 Quality Measures User's Manual* (v5.0 03-01-2012) (RTI Project Number 0211942.001.100.004). CMS website. 2012. Available at: http://www.cms.gov/Medicare/Quality-Initiatives-Patient-Assessment-Instruments/NursingHomeQualityInits/downloads/MDS30QM-Manual.pdf.

14. Stone ND, Ashraf MS, Calder J, Crnich CJ, Crossley K, Drinka PJ, et al. SHEA/CDC Position Paper: Surveillance definitions of infections in long-term care facilities: revisiting the McGeer Criteria. *Infect Control Hosp Epidemiol* 2012; 33(10): 965-977.

15. Potts A, Wilson AC. Use of statistics. In: Carrico R, ed. *APIC Text of Infection Control and Epidemiology,* 3rd ed. Washington, DC: Association for Professionals in Infection Control and Epidemiology, 2009: 5-1–5-20.

16. Centers for Disease Control and Prevention (CDC). *National Public Health Performance Standards (NPHPS).* CDC website. 2012. Available at: http://www.cdc.gov/nphpsp/essentialservices.html.

17. Centers for Disease Control and Prevention (CDC). *National Healthcare Safety Network (NHSN) Overview.* CDC website. 2013. Available at: http://www.cdc.gov/nhsn/PDFs/pscManual/1PSC_OverviewCurrent.pdf.

18. Horan TC, Andrus M, Dudeck MA. CDC/NHSN surveillance definition of health care-associated infection and criteria for specific types of infections in the acute care setting. *Am J Infect Control* 2008; 36(5): 309-332.

19. U.S. Department of Health and Human Services (HHS). *Chapter 8: Long-Term Care. In National Action Plan to Prevent Healthcare-Associated Infections: Roadmap to Elimination.* HHS website. 2013. Available at: http://www.hhs.gov/ash/initiatives/hai/actionplan/hai-action-plan-ltcf.pdf.

ADDITIONAL RESOURCES

1. Gordis L. *Epidemiology,* 3rd ed. Philadelphia: Elsevier Sanders, 2004.

2. Mody L. Infection control issues in older adults. *Clin Geriatr Med* 2007; 23(3): 499-514.

3. Smith PW, Bennett G, Bradley S, Drinka P, Lautenbach E, Marx J, et al. SHEA/APIC guideline: Infection prevention and control in the long-term care facility. *Am J Infect Control* 2008; 36(7): 504-535.

Isolation Precautions

Dolly Greene, RN, CIC

KEY CONCEPTS

- Provide a consistent approach to prevent the risk of transmission of infectious agents among residents, healthcare personnel, families and visitors, as well as from contact with the long-term care facility environment and equipment.
- Standard Precautions (once referred to as Universal Precautions and Body Substance Isolation) are based on the principle that blood and/or body fluids may contain transmissible pathogens and are therefore applicable in all resident care situations.
- Transmission-based Precautions (also known as Isolation Precautions) are used to manage specific, highly transmissible, or epidemiologically important pathogens based on the mode of transmission: contact, droplet, and airborne.

The goal of the long-term care facility (LTCF) is to provide a safe and sanitary environment for residents, visitors, and employees. Isolation systems are an integral component of the infection program in preventing interfacility transmission. These measures are outlined in the 2007 Centers for Disease Control and Prevention (CDC) *Guideline for Isolation Precautions: Preventing Transmission of Infectious Agents in Health Care Settings.*[1] Because the CDC considers LTCFs nonacute healthcare settings, resident placement into either a shared or private room should be based on individual risk assessment.[2] Restricting residents to their room when colonized or infected with certain organisms includes both advantages and disadvantages. Isolation, even for a brief period, may have unintended psychological risks such as depression, anxiety, and fear of healthcare personnel (HCP) and may pose a greater risk of adverse events.[3] Therefore, there must be a balance between the consequences of social isolation and the need to prevent the possible spread of disease within the LTCF. The assessment should also include clinical risk factors such as wounds, indwelling devices, secretion containment, the ability to follow instructions, and personal hygiene. The least restrictive approach, including the use of a private room as available, that balances these multiple priorities should be used.

A facility should implement Transmission-based Precautions (TBP) when the resident is known or suspected to be infected or colonized based on the route of transmission with an infectious agent. Transmission-based Precautions should be maintained as long as the resident has clinical signs of an infection. Once the signs and symptoms of infection have resolved, precautions may be discontinued. Maintaining Transmission-based Precautions longer than necessary may adversely affect the psychosocial well-being of the resident.[4]

Facilities should follow a three-tier system for precautions:

- Standard Precautions
- Transmission-based Precautions
- Intensified Interventions

STANDARD PRECAUTIONS [1,5,6]

Standard Precautions (SP) are based on the principle that blood, all body fluids and secretions, excretions (not including sweat), nonintact skin or lesions, and mucous membranes may contain transmissible infectious organisms. Standard Precautions should be practiced by all LTCF staff and should be used for all resident care at all times. Standard Precautions include: hand hygiene and use of gloves, gown, mask, and eye protection or face shield depending on the anticipated exposure. Standard Precautions also include safe injection practices. For additional information on safe injection practices, see Chapter 9. HCP need to determine if any, or all, of these elements of SP are needed during specific resident interactions. Table 5.1 provides a summary of components and recommendations for Standard Precautions.

TRANSMISSION-BASED PRECAUTIONS[1,5,6]

Transmission-based Precautions should be implemented for residents known or suspected to be infected or colonized with an infectious agent requiring additional control measures based on the route of transmission:

- Contact
- Droplet
- Airborne

TBP are initiated according to facility policy and procedure. Commonly, TBP are initiated by a physician, infection preventionist (IP), the director of nursing, the assistant director of nursing, or by the nursing supervisor. Staff nurses may also initiate precautions if permitted by policy or protocol. When TBP are initiated, the IP should be notified so that surveillance, monitoring, and other follow-up can begin as soon as possible. In most situations, follow-up monitoring of any resident requiring TBP is a shared responsibility between the IP and the nursing team.

Generally, TBP are discontinued only by senior clinical staff. Limiting staff that can discontinue precautions helps to ensure that TBP are terminated only when the risk of transmission is no longer a safety threat to others at the LTCF.

TABLE 5.1: RECOMMENDATIONS FOR APPLICATION OF STANDARD PRECAUTIONS FOR THE CARE OF ALL RESIDENTS IN ALL HEALTHCARE SETTINGS

Component	Recommendations
HAND HYGIENE	
Hand Hygiene	After contact with blood, body fluids, secretions, excretions, contaminated items; immediately after removing gloves; between resident contacts, before and after food preparation and service
PERSONAL PROTECTIVE EQUIPMENT (PPE)	
Gloves	For contact with blood, body fluids, secretions, excretions, and contaminated items; for touching mucous membranes and nonintact skin; for contact with intact skin when infection risks are identified
Gown	During procedures and resident care activities when HCP uniform or clothing may contact blood/body fluids, secretions, and excretions
Mask, eye protection (goggles), face shield*	During procedures and resident care activities likely to generate splashes or sprays of blood, body fluids, and secretions, such as suctioning, tracheostomy care
OTHER COMMON APPLICATIONS	
Soiled resident care equipment	Handle in a manner that prevents transfer of microorganisms; physically separate clean and soiled holding areas, wear gloves if visibly contaminated or handling equipment removed from an isolation room; perform hand hygiene
Environmental hygiene	Develop procedures for routine cleaning and disinfection of environmental surfaces, especially frequently touched surfaces and common areas of the facility; if a contractor provides this service, verify that procedures, chemicals, safety measures, and cleaning schedules are maintained
Textiles and laundry	Handle in a manner that prevents transfer of microorganisms to others and to the environment; soiled linen must be contained; store clean linen so that it does not become contaminated
Needles and other sharps	Follow the "one needle-one syringe-only one vial" rule and other safety practices outlined by the CDC; use safety engineered products; dispose of used needles and other contaminated sharps per OSHA requirements; determine need for PPE before using needles and other sharps/injection supplies
Resident resuscitation	Use mouthpiece, resuscitation bag, or other ventilation devices to prevent contact with mouth and oral secretions
Resident placement	Consider private room if resident is at increased risk of transmission, likely to contaminate the environment, unable to follow instructions, does not maintain appropriate hygiene, or at increased risk of acquiring infection
Respiratory hygiene/ cough etiquette (source containment of infectious respiratory secretions in symptomatic residents, beginning at initial point of encounter)	Instruct symptomatic persons to cover mouth/nose when sneezing/coughing; use tissues and dispose in no-touch receptacle; perform hand hygiene after contaminating hands with respiratory secretions; wear surgical mask if unable to follow basic respiratory hygiene practices; maintain spatial separation >3 feet between residents' beds if possible

* During aerosol-generating procedures on residents with suspected or proven infections transmitted by respiratory aerosols (e.g., SARS), wear a fit-tested N95 or higher respirator in addition to gloves, gown, and face/eye protection.

Adapted from Siegel JD, Rhinehart E, Jackson M, Chiarello L, and the Healthcare Infection Control Practices Advisory Committee. *Guideline for isolation precautions: Prevention of transmission of infectious agents in healthcare settings,* June 2007. CDC website. 2007. Available at: http://www.cdc.gov/hicpac/pdf/isolation/Isolation2007.pdf.

INTENSIFIED INTERVENTIONS[1,7]

Intensified Interventions (II) is the third tier suggested for implementation by the CDC under any of the following circumstances:

- When a highly transmissible pathogen is circulating in the LTCF (influenza, norovirus)
- When transmission of known pathogens has been documented within the LTCF (methicillin-resistant *Staphylococcus aureus* [MRSA], *Clostridium difficile*)
- When a pathogen with an unusual resistance pattern has been identified and confirmed by the laboratory
- When the incidence of a specific pathogen is either increasing or fails to decrease despite the implementation of and adherence to routine infection prevention and control procedures

What is Cohorting?

According to the CDC, cohorting is the ***practice of grouping residents infected or colonized with the same infectious agent together to confine their care to one area and prevent contact with susceptible individuals*** (cohorting residents). During outbreaks, HCP may be assigned to a cohort of residents to further limit opportunities for transmission (cohorting staff).

These conditions may occur during outbreaks. The following Intensified Interventions are instituted in a tiered response and as needed, based on careful evaluation of the specific situation and its associated risks:[1,6,7]

- Cohorting infected and colonized residents
- Dedicating staff to care for isolated and/or cohorted residents
- Restricting new admissions or closing affected nursing units
- Increasing environmental cleaning and disinfection procedures
- Performing active surveillance cultures

PROCEDURE FOR TRANSMISSION-BASED PRECAUTIONS

Before initiating TBP, the IP (or individual responsible for initiating isolation) should determine the category of TBP required by CDC.[1,6] Table 5.2 lists the type and duration of precautions recommended for common infections in long-term care.

Preparation and Education

The resident, family, and visitors should be advised about the reason and use of Transmission-based Precautions. The IP may need to assist in teaching and coaching the resident, family, and visitors about hand hygiene and the correct use and disposal of any required personal protective equipment (PPE). It is important to allow time for all to ask questions about TBP and to identify any concerns. The resident and family should be reassured that TBP will neither disrupt normal care routines nor decrease the frequency of contact with LTCF staff. The IP may also help reinforce these key messages and help allay any concerns related to the possible risk of social isolation during the time that TBPs are required.

Concurrently, the IP should explain and inform staff members about the need for TBP. Post appropriate isolation signage (Figures 5.1 to 5.4) outside the resident's room; provide education, as appropriate, on TBP policies and procedures; and perform periodic observations/audits to ensure accurate implementation. Reinforcing the importance of removing all PPE before exiting the resident's room is often necessary. The IP should also carefully observe glove use not only to verify that they are used correctly, but also to confirm that incorrect practices (e.g., attempting to clean gloves with an alcohol-based hand rub [ABHR] rather than removing them; wearing two pair of gloves in lieu of hand washing) are not deemed acceptable by the direct care staff. Figures 5.5 and 5.6 depict the correct procedure for donning and removing PPE and may be used for training or may be posted as visual reminders for staff. Table 5.4 is a sample audit tool that may be used when observing TBP-related practices.

TABLE 5.3: SUPPLIES FOR TRANSMISSION-BASED PRECAUTIONS

PPE SUPPLY
Provide table, cart, dispensing units, etc. for 24-hour access to a supply of PPE (e.g., masks, gowns, gloves, etc.) to maintain Transmission-based Precautions. These items must be covered and/or stored in a clean environment (covered cart, closed cabinet, over the floor hanging dispenser).
SIGNAGE
Provide signage and post outside the resident room where the sign may be easily seen. **The resident name or name of organism should NOT appear on the sign.*** (See Figures 5.1 to 5.4 for sample isolation signs.)
HAND HYGIENE AND PERSONAL CARE ITEMS
Check the resident's room for personal hygiene supplies, toiletries, alcohol-based hand rub, hand washing soap, and paper towels. Encourage the use of small dispensers and disposable containers to the extent possible.
NONCRITICAL CARE EQUIPMENT
Provide thermometer and any other noncritical care equipment, such as stethoscope, sphygmomanometer, or gait belt that will be dedicated to the resident's care. Equipment owned by facility must be thoroughly cleaned and disinfected when it is removed from the isolation room. Equipment owned by the resident (walker, wheelchair) should remain inside the room and be cleaned and disinfected per a scheduled determined by the facility and consistent with manufacturer's recommendations. Bleach solution should only be used in situations where it will not damage equipment and other noncritical surfaces.

* Signage should be in accordance with CMS F Tag 241, section 483.15(a) and adhere to facility policy.

> The use, style, type, and specific verbiage of isolation signage in the long-term care setting is a complex, evolving issue. Any isolation signage used should be in compliance with CMS F tag 241 section 483.15(a), state requirements, and specific facility policy.

Notify other departments that the resident is in Transmission-based Precautions. For example, environmental services should be notified to ensure that appropriate daily and terminal cleaning is performed. Depending on the infectious agent, changes in cleaning routine, as well as changes of types of cleaners and disinfectants, may be required. The IP should follow up with environmental services (EVS) staff to ensure their readiness to work in isolation situations, compliance with the different requirements of TBP, and disposal of cleaning products and/or supplies to reduce the risk of room-to-room transmission.

Provide supplies and equipment needed for maintaining Transmission-based Precautions (Table 5.3). Be sure to replenish PPE and hand hygiene products such as paper towels, soap, and ABHR to ensure that supplies are sufficient for all personnel. In some high demand situations, replenishing supplies may be needed more frequently than every 24 hours. Monitoring the availability and accessibility of these supplies should be included in the regular facility rounds conducted by the IP.

Initiating Transmission-based Precautions: Contact Precautions

In addition to Standard Precautions, use Contact Precautions for residents known or suspected to be infected with microorganisms that can be easily transmitted by direct or indirect contact. This includes touching environmental surfaces or handling resident care items. The use of Contact Precautions in LTCFs may differ from the criteria used in hospitals. For residents, Contact Precautions may be needed based on a clinical assessment of secretion containment or infection syndrome rather than culture results. These types of situations may include a draining wound that cannot be contained, a resident who exhibits noncompliant behaviors with stool or other body fluids, or a resident who has very poor personal hygiene.

Contact Precautions should be used when there is evidence of multidrug-resistant organisms (MDROs) or other epidemiologically significant organisms causing clinical symptoms. Because Contact Precautions pose a variety of implementation challenges, facilities should consider the clinical status of the resident as well as the prevalence or incidence of MDRO in the facility before initiating this level of isolation.[6] Organisms included in this category are, but are not limited to, MRSA; vancomycin-resistant enterococci (VRE); extended spectrum beta-lactamase (ESBL); multidrug-resistant, gram-negative bacteria (MDR-GNB); carbapenem-resistant Enterobacteriaceae (CRE); *C. difficile*; norovirus; impetigo; herpes simplex or zoster (shingles); and other conditions such as a rash of unknown origin, conjunctivitis, scabies, pediculosis, and draining wounds.[8]

Residents on Contact Precautions may be allowed to go to the dining room area or activity room if the site of the infection can be covered and secretions contained. The resident's personal hygiene and behavior should be assessed to minimize the risk of transmission to others. A resident on Contact Precautions should perform hand hygiene before leaving his or her room. If the resident should require any care after leaving his or her room, the care team should assist the individual in returning prior to providing any interventions. Staff should not perform care procedures or utilize PPE in common areas of the LTCF. The only exception to this may include emergency life support services. Residents who are symptomatic with an active respiratory infection caused by an MDRO or with active *C. difficile* infection diarrhea should not be allowed to attend group dining or activities as long as symptoms persist.

Initiating Transmission-based Precautions: Droplet Precautions

In addition to Standard Precautions, use Droplet Precautions when microorganisms are transmitted by large droplets generated by sneezing, coughing, or talking. Although potential distance of transmission is only 3 to 6 feet, it is still a significant threat. Spatial separation and drawing the privacy curtain between resident beds is especially important in multibed rooms. Diseases spread via large droplets include bacterial infections such as invasive *Haemophilus influenzae*, invasive *Neisseria meningitides*, *Mycoplasma pneumonia*, *Streptococcus* infection, and some viral infections, including adenovirus, influenza, mumps, and rubella.[1,9]

Initiating Transmission-based Precautions: Airborne Precautions

In addition to Standard Precautions, Airborne Precautions are initiated when pathogenic organisms can remain suspended in the air and be widely dispersed by air currents within a room or over a long distance. Examples of infectious diseases that require Airborne Precautions are tuberculosis, measles, varicella (chickenpox), and disseminated herpes zoster (disseminated shingles). HCP must wear an N95 respirator or powered air purifying respirator (PAPR) upon entering the room. These protective items must be approved by the National Institute for Occupational Safety and Health (NIOSH). HCP using a N95-style respirator must receive initial and annual training on its use. N95 respirators are single use devices; they should not be removed outside the resident's room and reused by the same staff member at a later time.

In addition, the N95 must be "fit tested" for each user by an individual qualified to perform this task. The Occupational Safety and Health Administration (OSHA)-accepted fit test protocols can be found at 29 CFR 1910.134 appendix A. Although there are both approved quantitative and qualitative methods for fit testing, the most commonly used method in LTCFs is qualitative and is completed according to the following general procedure:

1. The first step determines the HCP's ability to detect the test agent (e.g., saccharin, isoamyl acetate, denatonium benzoate) at a sensitivity level that corresponds to less than an acceptable fit before put on (donning) the tight-fitting face piece respirator (N95). The HCP enters an exposure chamber, has a test enclosure placed on his/her head, or is positioned somewhere in

an open test area and the test agent is generated around him/her. The HCP signals when the test agent is sensed. The fit test operator proceeds with the fit test only if the demonstrated sensitization level is low enough to ensure the test agent will be sensed at all levels representing a failure to achieve an acceptable fit. (Note: Isoamyl acetate, being an organic vapor, cannot be used as a test agent for particulate respirators.)

2. Next, the HCP follows the manufacturer's instructions to put on what initially seems to be the best fitting respirator provided by the LTCF. This is usually accomplished by visually matching the size and shape of the available respirators to the HCP's face.
3. The HCP then completes a user "seal check" to confirm that the respirator is properly positioned on the face.
4. The HCP then enters an exposure chamber and has a test enclosure placed on his/her head or is positioned somewhere in an open test area. The test agent is generated at the designated test level around the subject.
5. The fit test operator observes the HCP during exposure while directing him/her through a series of exercises. The fit test operator notes involuntary coughing (irritant smoke) during the test or asks the HCP at the end of the test if he or she smelled or tasted anything at any time during the test. From the test subject's response and the fit test operator's observations, the fit test operator determines a pass/fail judgment by which the respirator make, model, and size may be assigned to the HCP.[10]

How often must fit testing be done?

According to NIOSH, each brand, model, and size of particulate face piece (N95) respirators will fit slightly differently, the LTCF should engage in a fit test for staff every time a new model, manufacture type/brand, or size is worn. Also, if HCP weight fluctuates or facial/dental alterations occur, a fit test should be done again to ensure the respirator remains effective. Otherwise, fit testing should be completed at least annually to ensure continued adequate fit.

The Airborne Infection Isolation Room (AIIR), formerly called a negative pressure isolation room, is a single occupancy, resident care room used to isolate individuals with a suspected or confirmed airborne infectious disease. AIIRs should provide negative pressure in the room (i.e., the air should flow under the door and into the room). The door of the room should be closed at all times. An airflow rate of six air changes per hour (ACH) is required for existing buildings. For new construction or renovation, 12 ACH is required. Direct exhaust of air from the room to the outside of the building or recirculation of air through a high efficiency particulate air (HEPA) filter is required.[11] If the LTCF does not have an AIIR, arrangements should be made to transfer the resident to a facility that is equipped to provide isolation in a negative pressure room. During the transfer HCP should wear a fitted N95 mask respirator, and the resident should use a surgical mask.

POINTS TO CONSIDER FOR RESIDENTS IN ANY TYPE OF ISOLATION

Hand Hygiene

Hand hygiene is the single most important practice for preventing the transmission of potentially infectious microorganisms from one person to another. According to the CDC:[12]

- Studies have found hand hygiene reduces the incidence of healthcare-associated infections.
- Hands should be washed with soap and water before and after each resident contact and after contact with resident's belongings and environmental surfaces and patient/resident care equipment.
  - ABHRs can be used as an adjunct to hand washing at times when soap and water are not easily accessible.
  - ABHR should NOT be used when hands are visibly soiled or when preparing food.
- When caring for a resident during an outbreak of *C. difficile* infection diarrhea or norovirus diarrhea, hand washing is usually recommended over ABHR because of the theoretical advantage of rinsing the organisms off the hands. However, no increase in

C. difficile infection has been reported in the scientific literature as a result of using hand washing instead of ABHR in these cases.[13]

Equipment and Supplies

- Gather all equipment and supplies needed before entering the resident's room. Only take needed supplies into the room.
- No special precautions or equipment (e.g., disposable trays) are needed for dishes, cups, glasses, or eating utensils for a resident requiring Transmission-based Precautions.[7]
- A dedicated thermometer should be left in the room. It should be cleaned and disinfected after each use until Transmission-based Precautions are discontinued and then be discarded.

Resident Environment

- All faucets, handles, sinks, and hoppers and any other fixtures or dedicated equipment in the isolation room are considered contaminated.
- Do not shake or agitate soiled linen; instead, fold it upon itself and hold linen away from the body. Place into appropriate receptacle. Do not allow soiled linen to drop onto the floor. If soiled linen must be removed from the room for rinsing, transport these items in a plastic bag to prevent contamination of the environment.
- All PPE should be used **once** and discarded in either the trash or used linen (e.g., when cloth gowns are used) receptacle before leaving the room.
- Dispose of any soiled water or body fluids in the toilet in the room. Do not use common area restrooms or soiled utility room sinks for this purpose. Disposable supplies, such as dressings from a draining and/or infected wound, can be disposed of in regular trash. Red bagging is needed only if a dressing is saturated with fresh blood and may leak or drip onto environmental surfaces or the clinician's uniform/clothing. Otherwise, place contaminated disposable items in a trash bag and discard as the facility's procedure for routine waste removal. Refer to local and state regulations for defining and disposing of infectious waste.
- Verify that maintenance of air handling systems discharging to the outdoors from negative pressure rooms or using recirculated HEPA filtration are monitored according to facility policy and manufacturer specifications.

Additional Clinical Considerations

- Do not place residents with different types of active infections in the same room. For example, a resident with MRSA infection should not share a room with a resident being treated for VRE.
- Infected residents who have difficulty with excretion/secretion containment (*C. difficile* diarrhea, any respiratory infection, including MRSA, that triggers coughing and sneezing) should be restricted to their rooms until the acute symptoms have subsided and their infectious risk status within the LTCF is clinically improved.[1]
- It is not necessary to perform a "test for cure" or "clearance cultures" when antimicrobial treatment has been completed and the resident no longer shows signs or symptoms of infection.[14,15]
- Following resolution of active infection, the resident may remain colonized with the pathogenic organism. These residents require frequent and careful clinical monitoring, as colonization increases the risk of further active infection.[6]
- Residents infected with airborne pathogens such varicella, rubeola, or rubella should be assigned HCP who have documented immunity to these diseases or who have been immunized.
- No matter what the HCP's prior exposure has been, all staff must use respiratory protection when caring for a resident with pulmonary tuberculosis.
- Residents with disseminated herpes zoster (disseminated shingles) require Airborne Precautions. If this is not possible and/or the resident is awaiting transfer, the LTCF should implement combined Contact and Droplet Precautions as an interim safety measure.

TABLE 5.2: TYPE AND DURATION OF PRECAUTIONS RECOMMENDED FOR SELECTED INFECTIONS AND CONDITIONS

INFECTION/CONDITION	PRECAUTIONS		
	Type*	Duration†	Comments
Abscess:			
Draining, minor	C	DI	No dressing or containment of drainage; until drainage stops or can be contained by dressing
Draining, minor or limited	S		Dressing covers and contains drainage
Candidiasis, all forms including mucocutaneous	S		
Clostridium perfringens:			
Food poisoning	S		Not transmitted from person to person
Conjunctivitis:			
Acute bacterial:	S		
Chlamydia	S		
Gonococcal	S		
Acute viral (acute hemorrhagic)	C	DI	Adenovirus most common; enterovirus 70, Coxsackie virus A24) also associated with community outbreaks. Highly contagious; outbreaks in eye clinics, pediatric and neonatal settings, institutional settings reported. Eye clinics should follow Standard Precautions when handling patients with conjunctivitis. Routine use of infection control measures in the handling of instruments and equipment will prevent the occurrence of outbreaks in this and other settings.
Gastroenteritis:			
Campylobacter species	S		Use Contact Precautions for diapered or incontinent persons for the duration of illness or to control institutional outbreaks.
C. difficile	C	DI	Discontinue antibiotics if appropriate. Do not share electronic thermometers; ensure consistent environmental cleaning and disinfection. Hypochlorite solutions may be required for cleaning if transmission continues. Handwashing with soap and water preferred because of the absence of sporicidal activity of alcohol in waterless antiseptic handrubs.
E. coli:			
Enteropathogenic O157:H7 and other shiga toxin-producing Strains	S		Use Contact Precautions for diapered or incontinent persons for the duration of illness or to control institutional outbreaks.
Other species	S		Use Contact Precautions for diapered or incontinent persons for the duration of illness or to control institutional outbreaks.
Noroviruses:	S		Use Contact Precautions for diapered or incontinent persons for the duration of illness or to control institutional outbreaks. Persons who clean areas heavily contaminated with feces or vomitus may benefit from wearing masks since virus can be aerosolized from these body substances; ensure consistent environmental cleaning and disinfection with focus on restrooms even when apparently unsoiled). Hypochlorite solutions may be required when there is continued transmission. Alcohol is less active, but there is no evidence that alcohol antiseptic handrubs are not effective for hand decontamination. Cohorting of affected patients to separate airspaces and toilet facilities may help interrupt transmission during outbreaks.

Table 5.2 Continued

INFECTION/CONDITION	PRECAUTIONS		
	Type*	Duration†	Comments
Noroviruses Continued...			
Rotavirus	C	DI	Ensure consistent environmental cleaning and disinfection and frequent removal of soiled diapers. Prolonged shedding may occur in both immunocompetent and immunocompromised children and the elderly.
Salmonella species (including S. typhi)	S		Use Contact Precautions for diapered or incontinent persons for the duration of illness or to control institutional outbreaks
Shigella species (Bacillary dysentery)	S		Use Contact Precautions for diapered or incontinent persons for the duration of illness or to control institutional outbreaks
Hepatitis, viral:			
Type A:	S		Provide hepatitis A vaccine post-exposure as recommended
Diapered or incontinent patients	C		Maintain Contact Precautions in patients >14 yrs. of age for 1 week after onset of symptoms.
Type B-HBsAG positive; acute or chronic	S		See specific recommendations for care of patients in hemodialysis centers
Type C and other unspecified non-A, non-B	S		See specific recommendations for care of patients in hemodialysis centers
Herpes simplex (Herpesvirus hominis):			
Encephalitis	S		
Mucocutaneous, disseminated or primary, severe	C		
Mucocutaneous, recurrent (skin, oral, genital)	S	Until lesions dry and crusted	
Herpes zoster (varicella-zoster) (shingles):			
Disseminated disease in any patient. Localized disease in immunocompromised patient until disseminated infection ruled out.	A, C	DI	Susceptible HCP should not enter room if immune caregivers are available; no recommendation for protection of immune HCP; no recommendation for type of protection, i.e. surgical mask or respirator; for susceptible HCP.
Localized in patient with intact immune system with lesions that can be contained/covered.	S	DI	Susceptible HCP should not provide direct patient care when other immune caregivers are available.
Human immunodeficiency virus (HIV)	S		Post-exposure chemoprophylaxis for some blood exposures.
Impetigo	C	U 24 hrs	
Influenza:			
Human (seasonal influenza)	D	5 days except DI in immuno-compromised persons	Single patient room when available or cohort; avoid placement with high-risk patients; mask patient when transported out of room; chemoprophylaxis/vaccine to control/prevent outbreaks. Use gown and gloves according to Standard Precautions. Duration of precautions for immunocompromised patients cannot be defined; prolonged duration of viral shedding (i.e. for several weeks) has been observed; implications for transmission are unknown.
Avian (e.g., H5N1, H7, H9 strains)			See www.cdc.gov/flu/avian/professional/infect-control.htm for current avian influenza guidance.
Pandemic influenza (also a human influenza virus)	D	5 days from onset of symptoms	See http://www.pandemicflu.gov for current pandemic influenza guidance.

Table 5.2 Continued

INFECTION/CONDITION	PRECAUTIONS		
	Type*	Duration†	Comments
Lice:			
Head (pediculosis)	C	U 24 hrs	
Body	S		Transmitted person to person through infested clothing. Wear gown and gloves when removing clothing; bag and wash clothes according to CDC guidance above
Pubic	S		Transmitted person to person through sexual contact
Listeriosis (listeria monocytogenes)	S		Person-to-person transmission rare; cross-transmission in neonatal settings reported
Measles (rubeola)	A	4 days after onset of rash; DI in immunocompromised	Susceptible HCP should not enter room if immune care providers are available; no recommendation for face protection for immune HCP; no recommendation for type of face protection for susceptible HCP, i.e., mask or respirator. For exposed susceptibles, post-exposure vaccine within 72 hrs. or immune globulin within 6 days when available. Place exposed susceptible patients on Airborne Precautions and exclude susceptible healthcare personnel from duty from day 5 after first exposure to day 21 after last exposure, regardless of post-exposure vaccine.
Meningitis:			
Aseptic (nonbacterial or viral; also see enteroviral infections)	S		Contact for infants and young children
Bacterial, gram-negative enteric, in neonates	S		
Fungal	S		
Haemophilus influenzae, type b known or suspected	D	U 24 hrs	
Listeria monocytogenes (See Listeriosis)	S		
Neisseria meningitidis (meningococcal) known or suspected	D	U 24 hrs	See meningococcal disease below
Streptococcus pneumoniae	S		
M. tuberculosis	S		
Other diagnosed bacterial	S		
Multidrug-resistant organisms (MDROs), infection or colonization (e.g., MRSA, VRE, VISA/VRSA, ESBLs, resistant S. pneumoniae)	S/C		MDROs judged by the infection control program, based on local, state, regional, or national recommendations, to be of clinical and epidemiologic significance. Contact Precautions recommended in settings with evidence of ongoing transmission, acute care settings with increased risk for transmission or wounds that cannot be contained by dressings. See recommendations for management options in Management of Multidrug-Resistant Organisms In Healthcare Settings, 2006. Contact state health department for guidance regarding new or emerging MDRO.
Mumps (infectious parotitis)	D	U 9 days	After onset of swelling; susceptible HCP should not provide care if immune caregivers are available. *Note:* Recent assessment of outbreaks in healthy 18-24 year olds has indicated that salivary viral shedding occurred early in the course of illness and that 5 days of isolation after onset of parotitis may be appropriate in community settings; however the implications for healthcare personnel and high-risk patient populations remain to be clarified.
Pediculosis (lice)	C	U 24 hrs after treatment	

Table 5.2 Continued

INFECTION/CONDITION	PRECAUTIONS		
	Type*	Duration†	Comments
Pertussis (whooping cough)	D	U 5 days	Single patient room preferred. Cohorting an option. Post-exposure chemoprophylaxis for household contacts and HCP with prolonged exposure to respiratory secretions. Recommendations for Tdap vaccine in adults under development.
Pneumonia:			
Multidrug-resistant bacterial (see multidrug-resistant organisms)			
Pneumococcal pneumonia	S		Use Droplet Precautions if evidence of transmission within a patient care unit or facility
Pressure ulcer (decubitus ulcer, pressure sore) infected:			
Major	C	DI	If no dressing or containment of drainage; until drainage stops or can be contained by dressing
Minor or limited	S		If dressing covers and contains drainage
Rubella (German measles)	D	U 7 days after onset of rash	Susceptible HCP should not enter room if immune caregivers are available. No recommendation for wearing face protection (e.g., a surgical mask) if immune. Pregnant women who are not immune should not care for these patients. Administer vaccine within three days of exposure to non-pregnant susceptible individuals. Place exposed susceptible patients on Droplet Precautions; exclude susceptible healthcare personnel from duty from day 5 after first exposure to day 21 after last exposure, regardless of post-exposure vaccine.
Scabies	C	U 24 hrs	
Staphylococcal disease (S aureus):			
Skin, wound, or burn:			
Major	C	DI	No dressing or dressing does not contain drainage adequately
Minor or limited	S		Dressing covers and contains drainage adequately
Enterocolitis	S		
Multidrug-resistant (see multidrug-resistant organisms)			
Pneumonia	S		
Scalded skin syndrome	C	DI	
Toxic shock syndrome	S		
Streptococcal disease:			
Group A Setretococcus:			
Skin, wound, or burn:			
Major	C, D	U 24 hrs	No dressing or dressing does not contain drainage adequately
Minor or limited	S		Dressing covers and contains drainage adequately
Endometritis (puerperal sepsis)	S		
Pneumonia	D	U 24 hrs	

Table 5.2 Continued

INFECTION/CONDITION	PRECAUTIONS		
	Type*	Duration†	Comments
Streptococcal diseases Continued…			
Serious invasive disease	D	U 24 hrs	Outbreaks of serious invasive disease have occurred secondary to transmission among patients and healthcare personnel. Contact Precautions for draining wound as above; follow rec. for antimicrobial prophylaxis in selected conditions.
Not group A or B unless covered elsewhere	S		
Tuberculosis (M. tuberculosis):			
Extrapulmonary, draining lesion	A, C		Discontinue precautions only when patient is improving clinically, and drainage has ceased or there are three consecutive negative cultures of continued drainage. Examine for evidence of active pulmonary tuberculosis.
Extrapulmonary, no draining lesion, meningitis	S		Examine for evidence of pulmonary tuberculosis.
Pulmonary or laryngeal disease, confirmed	A		Discontinue precautions only when patient on effective therapy is improving clinically and has three consecutive sputum smears negative for acid-fast bacilli collected on separate days(MMWR 2005; 54: RR-17 http://www.cdc.gov/mmwr/preview/mmwrhtml/rr5417a1.htm?s_cid=rr5417a1_e).
Pulmonary or laryngeal disease, suspected	A		Discontinue precautions only when the likelihood of infectious TB disease is deemed negligible, and either 1) there is another diagnosis that explains the clinical syndrome or 2) the results of three sputum smears for AFB are negative. Each of the three sputum specimens should be collected 8-24 hours apart, and at least one should be an early morning specimen.
Skin-test positive with no evidence of current active disease	S		
Urinary Tract Infection (UTI, including pyelonephritis), with or without urinary catheter	S		
Varicella Zoster	A, C	Until lesions dry and crusted	Susceptible HCP should not enter room if immune caregivers are available; no recommendation for face protection of immune HCP; no recommendation for type of protection, i.e. surgical mask or respirator for susceptible HCP. In immunocompromised host with varicella pneumonia, prolong duration of precautions for duration of illness. Post-exposure prophylaxis: provide post-exposure vaccine ASAP but within 120 hours; for susceptible exposed persons for whom vaccine is contraindicated (immunocompromised persons, pregnant women, newborns whose mother's varicella onset is <5 days before delivery or within 48 hrs after delivery) provide VZIG, when available, within 96 hours; if unavailable, use IVIG, Use Airborne Precautions for exposed susceptible persons and exclude exposed susceptible healthcare workers beginning 8 days after first exposure until 21 days after last exposure or 28 if received VZIG, regardless of postexposure vaccination.
Wound Infections:			
Major	C	DI	No dressing or dressing does not contain drainage adequately
Minor or limited	S		Dressing covers and contains drainage adequately

* Type of Precautions: A, Airborne Precautions; C, Contact; D, Droplet; S, Standard; when A, C, and D are specified, also use S.

† Duration of precautions: CN, until off antimicrobial treatment and culture-negative; DI, duration of illness (with wound lesions, DI means until wounds stop draining); DE, until environment completely decontaminated; U, until time specified in hours (hrs) after initiation of effective therapy; Unknown: criteria for establishing eradication of pathogen has not been determined.

FIGURE 5.1: SAMPLE CONTACT PRECAUTIONS SIGN

CONTACT PRECAUTIONS

Visitors must report to Nursing Station before entering.

☑ Perform hand hygiene before entering and before leaving room

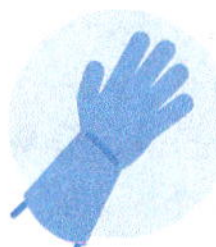

☑ Wear gloves when entering room or cubicle, and when touching resident's intact skin, surfaces, or articles in close proximity

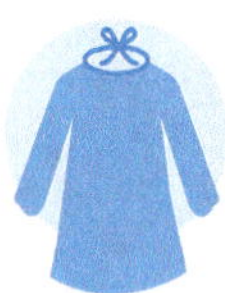

☑ Wear gown when entering room or cubicle and whenever anticipating that clothing will touch resident items or potentially contaminated environmental surfaces

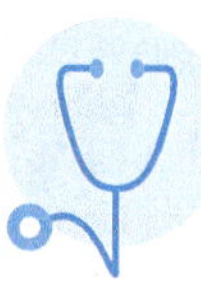

☑ Use resident-dedicated or single-use disposable shared equipment or clean and disinfect shared equipment (BP cuff, thermometers) between residents

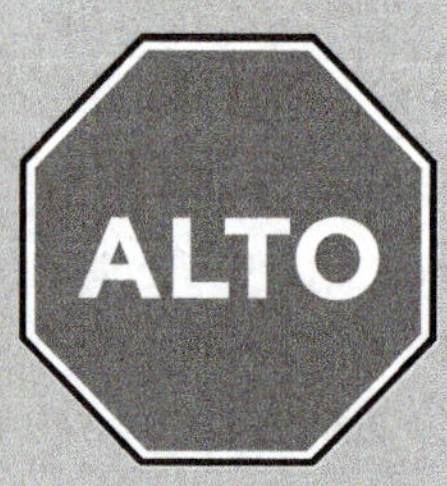

Precauciones Ambientales

Los vistantes deben presentarse primero al puesto de enfermeria antes de entrar.

- *Lávese las manos con agua y jabón.*
- *Póngase guantes al entrar al cuarto.*

Disclaimer: This isolation sign is provided as visual example of what a facility could use and may be modified as necessary to meet a specific LTCF's needs. Any isolation signs used must be compliance with CMS F tag 241 section 483.15(a), state requirements, and specific facility policy.

Also available on the CD-ROM.

FIGURE 5.2: SAMPLE CONTACT (SPECIAL ENTERIC) PRECAUTIONS SIGN FOR USE WITH RESIDENTS WITH *CLOSTRIDIUM DIFFICILE* INFECTIONS

CONTACT PRECAUTIONS

Visitors must report to Nursing Station before entering.

☑ ***SPECIAL ENTERIC***
Perform hand hygiene before entering and before leaving the room. *Must wash with soap and water for 15-20 seconds.*

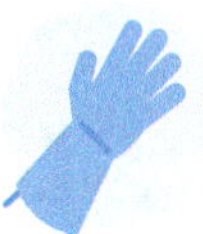

☑ **Wear gloves when entering room or cubicle, and when touching resident's intact skin, surfaces, or articles in close proximity**

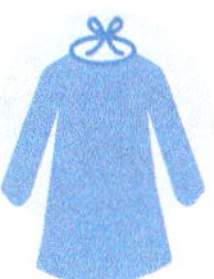

☑ **Wear gown when entering room or cubicle and whenever anticipating that clothing will touch resident items or potentially contaminated environmental surfaces**

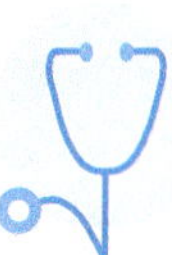

☑ **Use resident-dedicated or single-use disposable shared equipment or clean and disinfect shared equipment (BP cuff, thermometers) between residents**

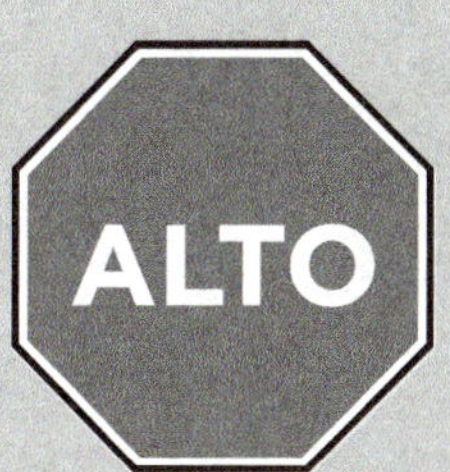

Precauciones Ambientales

Los vistantes deben presentarse primero al puesto de enfermeria antes de entrar.

- *Lávese las manos con agua y jabón.*
- *Póngase guantes al entrar al cuarto.*

Disclaimer: This isolation sign is provided as visual example of what a facility could use and may be modified as necessary to meet a specific LTCF's needs. Any isolation signs used must be compliance with CMS F tag 241 section 483.15(a), state requirements, and specific facility policy.

Also available on the CD-ROM.

FIGURE 5.3: SAMPLE DROPLET PRECAUTIONS SIGN

DROPLET PRECAUTIONS

Visitors must report to Nursing Station before entering.

☑ **Perform hand hygiene before entering and before leaving room**

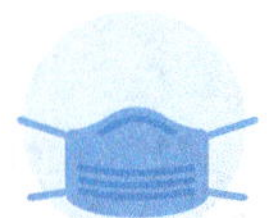

☑ **Wear mask when entering room**

(!) Visitors and health care workers

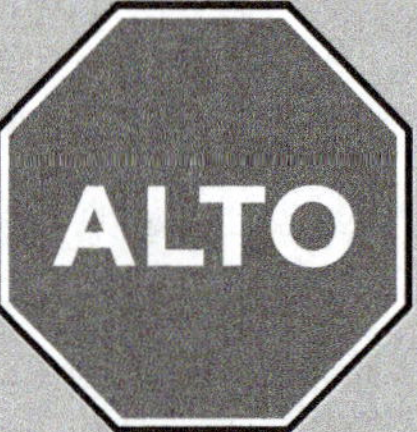

Precauciones de Gotas Diminutas

Los vistantes deben presentarse primero al puesto de enfermeria antes de entrar.

- *Lávese las manos.*
- *Póngase mascara al entrar al cuarto.*

Disclaimer: This isolation sign is provided as visual example of what a facility could use and may be modified as necessary to meet a specific LTCF's needs. Any isolation signs used must be compliance with CMS F tag 241 section 483.15(a), state requirements, and specific facility policy.

Also available on the CD-ROM.

FIGURE 5.4: SAMPLE AIRBORNE ISOLATION SIGN

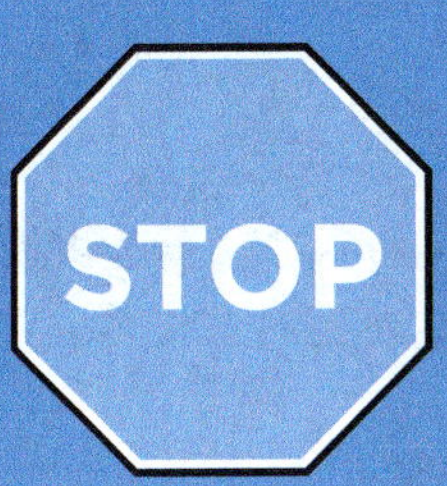

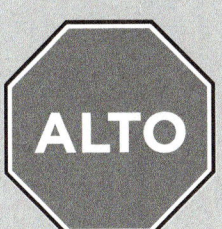

STOP

AIRBORNE PRECAUTIONS

Visitors must report to Nursing Station before entering.

☑ **Perform hand hygiene before entering and before leaving room**

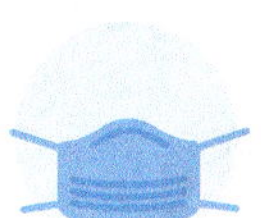

☑ **Wear N95 respirator when entering room**

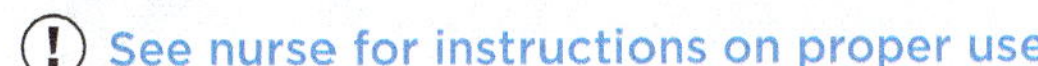

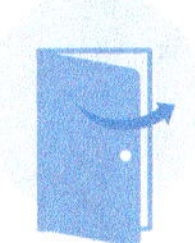

See nurse for instructions on proper use

☑ **Keep door closed**

☑ **Dietary may not enter**

ALTO

Precauciones Ambientales

Los vistantes deben presentarse primero al puesto de enfermeria antes de entrar.

- *Lávese las manos.*
- *Póngase mascara N95 confiltro al entrar al cuarto.*
- *Mantenga la puerta cerrada.*
- *No debe entrar el dietista.*

Disclaimer: This isolation sign is provided as visual example of what a facility could use and may be modified as necessary to meet a specific LTCF's needs. Any isolation signs used must be compliance with CMS F tag 241 section 483.15(a), state requirements, and specific facility policy.

Also available on the CD-ROM.

FIGURE 5.5: ILLUSTRATION OF DONNING PPE

SEQUENCE FOR *DONNING* PERSONAL PROTECTIVE EQUIPMENT (PPE)

The type of PPE used will vary based on the level of precautions required; e.g., Standard and Contact, Droplet or Airborne Infection Isolation.

1. Gown

- Fully cover torso from neck to knees, arms to end of wrists, and wrap around the back
- Fasten in back of neck and waist

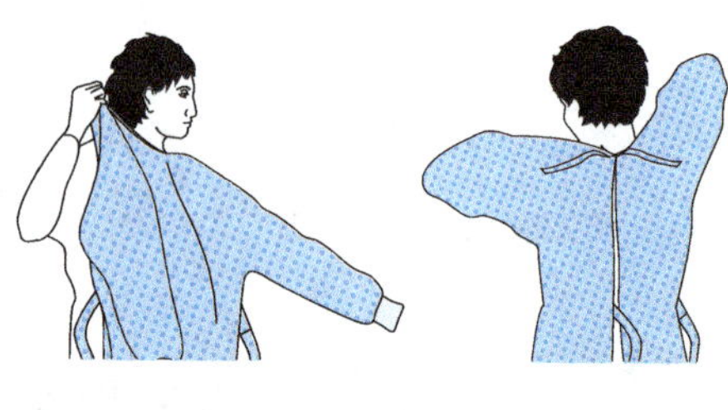

2. Mask or Respirator

- Secure ties or elastic bands at middle of head and neck
- Fit flexible band to nose bridge
- Fit snug to face and below chin
- Fit-check respirator

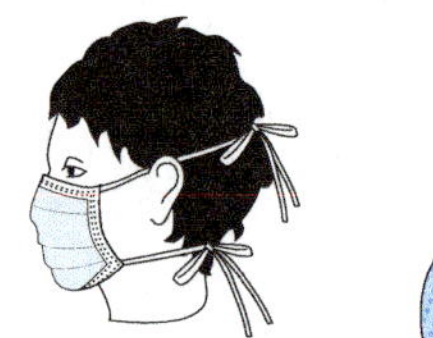

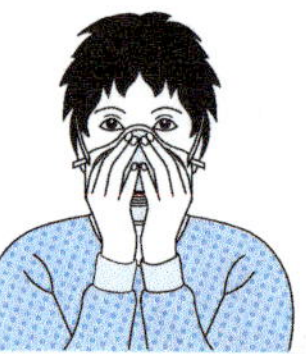

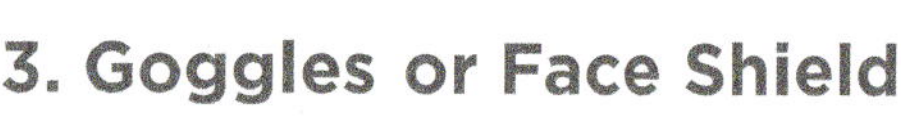

3. Goggles or Face Shield

- Place over face and eyes and adjust to fit

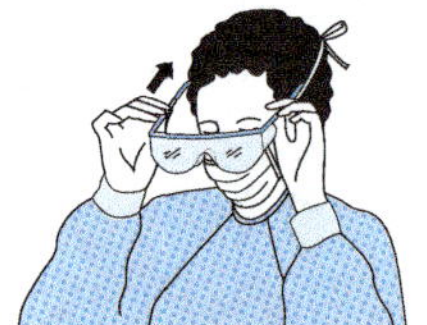

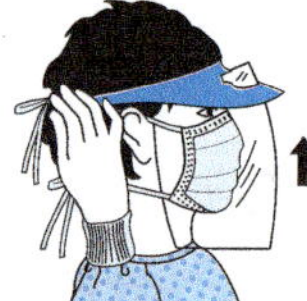

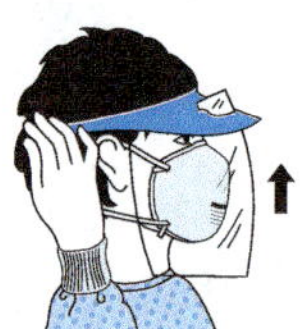

4. Gloves

- Extend to cover wrist of isolation gown

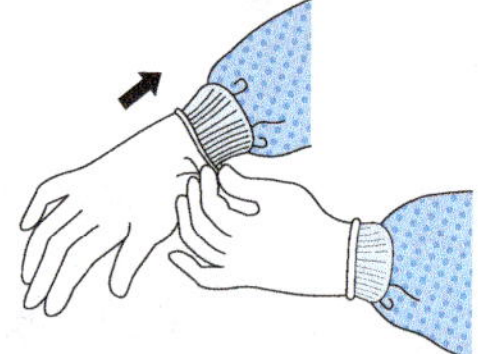

Use Safe Work Practices to Protect Yourself and Limit the Spread of Contamination

- Keep hands away from face
- Limit surfaces touched
- Change gloves when torn or heavily contaminated
- Perform hand hygiene

Adapted from Centers for Disease Control and Prevention. Available at: http://www.cdc.gov/HAI/pdfs/ppe/ppeposter148.pdf

Also available on the CD-ROM.

FIGURE 5.6: ILLUSTRATION OF REMOVING PPE

SEQUENCE FOR *REMOVING* PERSONAL PROTECTIVE EQUIPMENT (PPE)

Except for respirator, remove PPE at doorway or in anteroom. Remove respirator after leaving patient room and closing door.

1. Gloves

- Outside of gloves is contaminated!
- Grasp outside of glove with opposite gloved hand; peel off
- Hold removed glove in gloved hand
- Slide fingers of ungloved hand under remaining glove at wrist
- Peel glove off over first glove
- Discard gloves in waste container

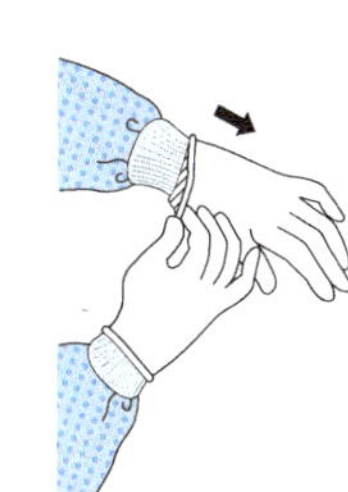
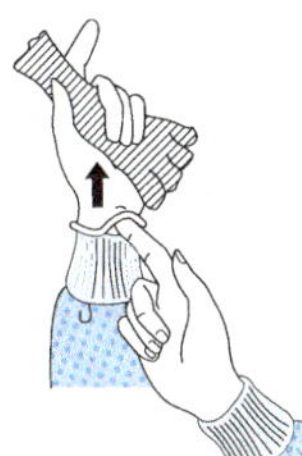
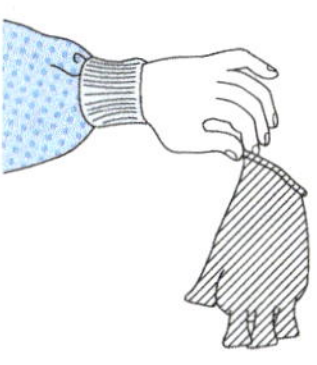

2. Goggles or Face Shield

- Outside of goggles or face shield is contaminated!
- To remove, handle by head band or ear pieces
- Place in designated receptacle for reprocessing or in waste container

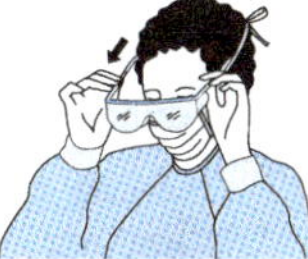
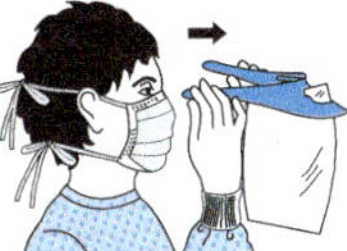
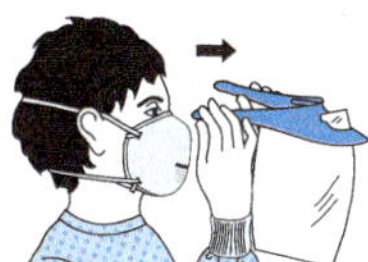

3. Gown

- Gown front and sleeves are contaminated!
- Unfasten ties
- Pull away from neck and shoulders, touching inside of gown only
- Turn gown inside out
- Fold or roll into a bundle and discard

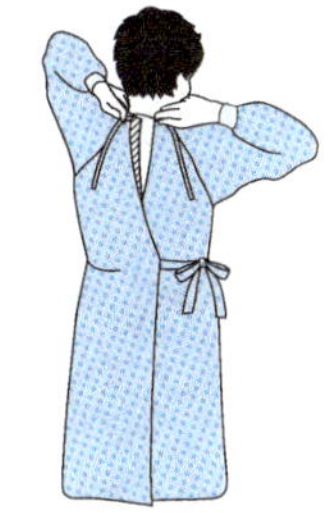
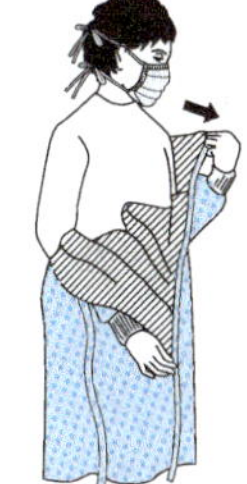
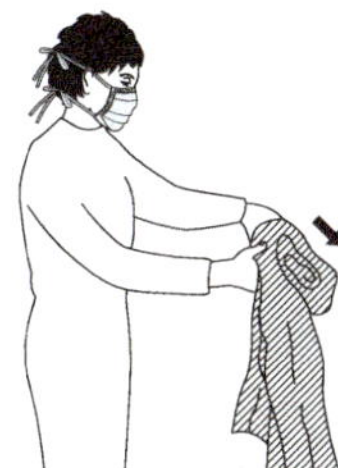

2. Mask or Respirator

- Front of mask/respirator is contaminated— DO NOT TOUCH!
- Grasp bottom, then top ties or elastics and remove
- Discard in waste container

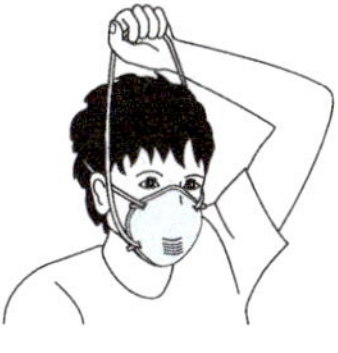
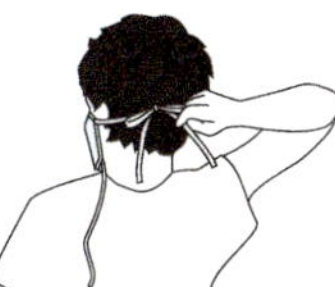
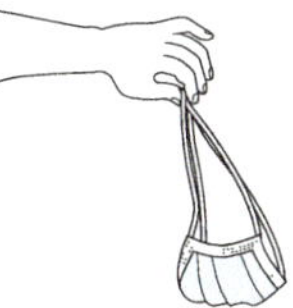

Perform hand hygiene immediately after removing all PPE

Adapted from Centers for Disease Control and Prevention. Available at: http://www.cdc.gov/HAI/pdfs/ppe/ppeposter148.pdf

Also available on the CD-ROM.

TABLE 5.4: SAMPLE INFECTION PREVENTION AND CONTROL IMPROVEMENT AUDIT TOOL

ROOM # ____________ CASE ____ DATE ____/____/____

INDICATOR: TRANSMISSION-BASED PRECAUTIONS	
Completed	Action
☐ Yes ☐ No	Symptoms documented
☐ Yes ☐ No	Preliminary precautions implemented
☐ Yes ☐ No	Condition communicated to resident, family, and team
☐ Yes ☐ No	MD/APN notified
☐ Yes ☐ No	Appropriate diagnostic tests ordered and obtained
☐ Yes ☐ No	Diagnosis of infection on chart
☐ Yes ☐ No	Appropriate precautions and treatment ordered
☐ Yes ☐ No	Room given proper signage for isolation technique
☐ Yes ☐ No	Condition communicated CNA Assignment and IDT
☐ Yes ☐ No	Precautions addressed on Care Plan
☐ Yes ☐ No	Dedicated equipment available in room
☐ Yes ☐ No	PPE properly stored
☐ Yes ☐ No	Hand hygiene observed
☐ Yes ☐ No	Proper use of PPE observed
☐ Yes ☐ No	Appropriate handling of linen observed
☐ Yes ☐ No	Appropriate handling of trash observed

Comments/Action Taken: ____

____

____

Signature of Person Completing Audit: ______________________________________

Also available on the CD-ROM.

REFERENCES

1. Siegel JD, Rhinehart E, Jackson M, Chiarello L, and the Healthcare Infection Control Practices Advisory Committee. *Guideline for isolation precautions: Prevention of transmission of infectious agents in healthcare settings,* June 2007. CDC website. 2007. Available at: http://www.cdc.gov/hicpac/pdf/isolation/Isolation2007.pdf.

2. Nicole LE. Preventing infections in non-hospital settings: Long-term care. *Emerg Infect Dis* 2001; 7(2): 205-207.

3. Saint S, Higgins LA, Nallamothu BK, Chenoweth C. Do physicians examine patients in contact isolation less frequently? A brief report. *Am J Infect Control* 2003; 31(6): 354-356.

4. Abad C, Fearday A, Safdar N. Adverse effects of isolation in hospitalized patients: a systematic review. *J Hosp Infect* 2010 Oct; 76(2): 97-102.

5. Centers for Medicare and Medicaid Services (CMS). *CMS Manual System Pub. 100-07 State Operations Provider Certification. Revisions to Appendix PP – Interpretive Guidelines for Long-term Care Facilities, Tag F441.* CMS website. 2009. Available at: https://www.cms.gov/Regulations-and-Guidance/Guidance/Transmittals/downloads/r51soma.pdf.

6. Siegel JD, Rhinehart E, Jackson M. Management of multidrug-resistant organisms in healthcare setting, 2006. *Am J Infect Control* 2007; 35(10 Suppl 2): S165-S193.

7. Cahill C, Chen S, Rosenberg J, Harriman K. *Enhanced standard precautions for California long-term care facilities,* 2010. California Department of Public Health website. 2010. Available at: http://cdph.ca.gov/programs/hai/Documents/AFL10-27AttachmentIncluded.pdf.

8. Simor AE, Bradley SF, Strausbaugh LJ, Crossley K, Nicolle LE. Clostridium difficile in long-term care facilities for the elderly. *Infect Control Hosp Epidemiol* 2002; 23(11): 696-703.

9. California Department of Public Health (CDPH). *Recommendations for the prevention and control of influenza – California long-term care facilities.* CDPH website. 2011. Available at: http://www.cdph.ca.gov/programs/hai/Documents/Influenza-Recommendations-LTCF-v.12-11.pdf.

10. Centers for Disease Control and Prevention (CDC). *Section 3: Ancillary Respirator Information.* CDC website. 2013. Available at: http://www.cdc.gov/niosh/npptl.

11. Jensen PA, Lambert LA, Iademarco MF, Rizdon R. Guidelines for preventing the transmission of *Mycobacterium tuberculosis* in health-care settings, 2005. *MMWR Recomm Rep* 2005; 54(RR-17): 1-141.

12. Boyce JM, Pittet D; Healthcare Infection Control Practices Advisory Committee; HICPAC/SHEA/APIC/IDSA Hand Hygiene Task Force. Guideline for hand-hygiene in health-care settings: Recommendations of Healthcare Infection Control Practices Advisory Committee and the HICPAC/SHEA/APIC/IDSA Hand Hygiene Task Force. Society for Healthcare Epidemiology of America/Association for Professionals in Infection Control/Infectious Diseases Society of America. *MMWR Recomm Rep* 2002; 51(No.RR-16): 1-45.

13. Dubberke ER, Gerding DN. *Rationale for hand hygiene recommendations after caring for a patient with Clostridium difficile infection.* SHEA website. 2011. Available at: http://www.shea-online.org/Portals/0/CDI%20hand%20hygiene%20update.pdf.

14. Cohen SH, Gerding DN, Johnson S, Kelly CP, Loo VG, McDonald LC, et al. Clinical practice guidelines for Clostridium difficile infection in adults: 2010 update by the Society for Healthcare Epidemiology of America (SHEA) and the infectious diseases society of America (IDSA). *Infect Control Hosp Epidemiol* 2010; 31(5): 431-455.

15. Crobach MJ, Dekkers OM, Wilcox MH, Kuijper EJ. European Society of Clinical Microbiology and Infectious Diseases (ESCMID): data review and recommendations for diagnosing Clostridium difficile-infection (CDI). *Clin Microbiol Infect* 2009; 15(12): 1053-1066.

ADDITIONAL RESOURCES

1. Brinsko V. Nutrition services. In: Carrico R, ed. *APIC Text of Infection Control and Epidemiology,* 3rd ed. Washington, DC: Association for Professionals in Infection Control and Epidemiology, Inc., 2009: 18-1–18-8.

2. Catalano G, Houston SH, Catalano MC, Butera AS, Jennings SM, Hakala SM, et al. Anxiety and depression in hospitalized patients in resistant organism isolation. *South Med J* 2003; 96(2): 141-145.

3. Gasink LB, Singer K, Fishman NO, Holmes WC, Weiner MG, Bilker WB, et al. Contact isolation for infection control in hospitalized patients: is patient satisfaction affected? *Infect Control Hosp Epidemiol* 2008; 29(3): 275-278.

4. Ontario Agency for Health Protection and Promotion, Provincial Infectious Diseases Advisory Committee. *Routine Practices and Additional Precautions in All Health Care Settings,* 3rd edition. Toronto, ON: Queen's Printer for Ontario, 2012.

5. Rosenbaum P, Zeller J, Frank J. Long-term care. In: Carrico R, ed. *APIC Text of Infection Control and Epidemiology,* 3rd ed. Washington, DC: Association for Professionals in Infection Control and Epidemiology, Inc., 2009: 52-1–52-18.

6. Stelfox HT, Bates DW, Redelmeier DA. Safety of patients isolated for infection control. *JAMA* 2003; 290(14): 1899-1905.

CHAPTER 6

Nursing Care to Prevent Infections

Marilyn Hanchett, RN, MA, CPHQ, CIC

KEY CONCEPTS

- The nursing assessment is the cornerstone of resident care and critical to infection prevention efforts.
- Infection prevention risks must be incorporated into nursing assessments and interventions to maximize resident safety.
- A team approach to the delegation and supervision of resident care activities is critical to promoting a culture of safety and preventing infections.

In the ongoing challenges related to aging and comorbid conditions, nursing care of the long-term care resident focuses on promoting independence, maintaining physical status, and ensuring good health and emotional and psychosocial well-being. Although virtually all nursing activities include some component of infection prevention-related safety, this chapter addresses the most common and high-risk assessment factors necessary for infection prevention in this increasingly vulnerable population.

NURSING ASSESSMENT

The admission and ongoing nursing assessments, conducted by a registered nurse, are determined by organizational policy and completed according to specific forms. No matter which documents are used by the organization and/or required by the payer, the assessment must include a focus on those aspects of resident health that may predispose them to otherwise preventable infections. This is especially important since RNs often spend a greater proportion of their work time on indirect resident tasks and other duties that remove them from situations in which ongoing assessments can be readily performed.[1]

However, there are significant challenges to an effective assessment process. To be optimally effective, the assessment must target both known and potential risks among its designated population. The obstacles to achieving this in long-term care include:

- The resident assessment criteria vary widely in their inclusion of infection risks and related comorbid conditions, including but not limited to dementia, diabetes, renal failure, congestive heart failure, and stroke.[2]
- Symptoms may be subtle and not conform to the expected inflammation/infection response. Nonspecific symptoms such as lethargy, change in level of consciousness, weakness, shortness of breath, and lack of fever may be common among elderly residents.[3]
- The facility's understanding of infection risks is heavily influenced by the scope and intensity of its surveillance program, which is often limited.
- The variation across long-term care facilities (LTCFs) in application of surveillance definitions, the collection and aggregation of data, and the methods used for reporting make comparative analyses extremely challenging.

In spite of these challenges, nursing assessment remains the cornerstone of the care management process. The objectives of the assessment process, as it relates to infection prevention, are:

1. Early recognition of factors that may predispose to infection
2. Rapid intervention when infectious symptoms are identified
3. Planning for treatment and prevention of potential cross transmission when the resident's care does not require hospitalization
4. Prompt transfer to the acute care facility when care requirements exceed the diagnostic, medical, or nursing capacity of the LTCF

When the resident returns to the LTCF from a hospital, the assessment process will also incorporate early detection of factors that may lead to readmission to acute care, often within 7 to 30 days.[4] The BRI Scale (Figure 6.1) summarizes the variety of risk criteria that should be incorporated into both the initial and ongoing resident assessments. A general physical assessment for potential or actual infections emphasizes four broad categories: upper and lower respiratory tract infections, gastrointestinal infections, skin and wound infections, and urinary tract infections.[5]

Respiratory Assessment

Upper respiratory infections (URIs) are the most common communicable illness and can spread rapidly within any institution.[6] LTCF residents may be especially susceptible due to advanced age and multiple and chronic impairments, as well as diminished host resistance and other age-related immunological changes.[5] The design of the LTCF, the sharing of bedrooms, ventilation systems, and the layout of common areas can also impact the spread of respiratory infection by droplet, contact, droplet nuclei, and airborne routes.[7] A comprehensive assessment should include analysis of all of these factors.

FIGURE 6.1: BRI SCALE

Infection Risk Scale

PLEASE COMPLETE THIS ASSESSMENT

- On Admission
- With MDS Schedule (where applicable)
- For any significant change in resident condition

RESIDENT INFORMATION:

First name: ______________________

Last name: ______________________

Birthdate/ID: ______________________

	DATE	DATE	DATE	DATE
	__/__/__	__/__/__	__/__/__	__/__/__
	ENTER SCORE: 0 = NO 1 = YES			
Current Active Infection, Ventilator, Dialysis, Immune System Compromise (HIV, Splenectomy, Chemotherapy, Chronic steroid use) *(Automatic High Risk: 18)*				
History of infection/antibiotic use during the last 6 months				
History of hospitalization during the last 6 months				
History of colonization/past infection with MDRO (MRSA, VRE, C-diff)				
MRSA nasal colonization				
Dependent for Personal Care				
Significant, Unplanned Wt. Loss (5%)				
PEG tube/J tube, surgical implant past 12 months				
Swallowing issues/Aspiration Risk				
Diagnosis of Diabetes				
Diagnosis of Urinary Retention				
Diagnosis of Neuropathy				
Diagnosis of Peripheral Vascular Disease				
Open Wounds				
Oxygen/Nebulizer Use				
Vascular Access (PICC, Port, Peripheral IV)				
Urinary Catheter				
Male Gender (MRSA Colonization)				
Refuses Immunization				
TOTAL (MAXIMUM 18)				
✓ Low risk (L) = **0-4** ✓ Moderate risk (M) = **5-9** ✓ High risk (H) = **10-18** *Care suggestions on page 2*				
ADDRESSED ON CARE PLAN AND WITH CARE TEAM				
INITIALS				

Figure 6.1 Continued

Assessment Results

Low Risk = 0–4

- ☐ Care Plan ____________________
- ☐ Staff and Resident Education
- ☐ Hand Hygiene
- ☐ Standard Precautions

Moderate Risk = 5–9

- ☐ Care Plan ____________________
- ☐ Staff and Resident Education
- ☐ Hand Hygiene
- ☐ Standard Precautions
- ☐ Quarterly Assessment and Documentation

High Risk = 10–18

- ☐ Care Plan ____________________
- ☐ Staff and Resident Education
- ☐ Hand Hygiene
- ☐ Standard Precautions
- ☐ Daily Assessment and Documentation

Notes ____________________

Signature ____________________ Date ____________________

Notes ____________________

Signature ____________________ Date ____________________

Notes ____________________

Signature ____________________ Date ____________________

Notes ____________________

Signature ____________________ Date ____________________

Also available on the CD-ROM.

Overutilization of antibiotics for viral URIs remains a serious concern, especially as resistance to common medications escalates worldwide. One study that included residents with more than 700 episodes of acute bronchitis, common cold, influenza-like illness, pharyngitis, sinusitis, and pneumonia reported that antibiotics were prescribed unjustifiably in 20 percent of all cases and more than 66 percent in cases of acute bronchitis.[8] A medication history, to the extent that such information can be obtained, is useful in assessing the resident's past experiences and treatment expectations when managing viral respiratory infections.

Chronic obstructive pulmonary disease (COPD) is common among the elderly and is currently the fourth leading cause of death. One study reported a 23 percent annual hospital readmission rate among LTCF residents.[4] A history of cigarette use is major risk factor for the development of COPD and must be included in the nursing assessment. Assessment of chronic cough, sputum production, oxygen use, and the frequency of exacerbations are necessary to manage symptoms and avoid more serious infection complications. The resident's participation or potential participation in smoking cessation and pulmonary rehabilitation programs must be evaluated. Due to frequency of exacerbations in COPD, the nursing assessment must include the resident's use of long- and short-acting bronchodilators, inhaled steroids, and other drugs to improve lung function. Oxygen therapy may be necessary and can improve quality of life when hypoxia is persistent.[9] Although COPD is not infectious, it is a serious progressive illness that can predispose the resident to other infection risks and, for that reason, should be incorporated into the nursing assessment. Additional information on respiratory treatments is presented in Chapter 7.

Assessment of lower respiratory tract function is also important. According to the Centers for Disease Control and Prevention (CDC), pneumonia kills more people globally each year than any other infectious disease; individuals over age 65 are particularly vulnerable. In the United States, the most common bacterial cause of pneumonia is *Streptococcus pneumoniae* (pneumococcus), and the most common viral causes are influenza, parainfluenza, and respiratory syncytial viruses.[10]

LTCF-acquired pneumonia is among the leading causes of mortality, morbidity, and transfers to acute care facilities. However, hospitalization may not be routinely necessary, depending on the severity of the infection. In cases of pneumonia, LTCF residents may be at greater risk for functional decline, delirium, and pressure ulcers when hospitalized.[11] The nursing assessment in such cases must present all relevant risks factors to the physician before a final decision regarding hospital transfer is made.

Auscultation of the lung fields is included in the assessment. All lung sounds should increase in pitch with inspiration and decrease with expiration. If these sounds are approximately equal, obstruction may be present. Inspiratory crackles (rales) are common in the elderly and do not immediately indicate disease. Inspiratory wheezing suggests obstruction in the trachea whereas expiratory wheezing suggests obstruction in the chest. Consolidation in the lungs, which often leads to infection, will alter breath sounds over any portion of the lung field. A loud stridor on inspiration indicates a medical emergency. The assessment should reflect the resident's baseline lung sounds to help differentiate changes that may be detected and the possibility of any developing infection.[12]

Vaccination can help prevent pneumonia and the resident's immunization profile must be included as part of the nursing assessment. The following types of vaccinations should be included:

- Pneumococcal
- *Haemophilus influenzae* type b (Hib)
- Pertussis (whooping cough)
- Varicella (chickenpox)
- Measles
- Influenza (flu) vaccine

Gastrointestinal Assessment

LTCF residents may experience gastrointestinal changes due to a wide variety of reasons, including medications, limited mobility, decreased fluids, inadequate dietary fiber, poor dentition, and gastroesophageal reflux disease (GERD). Most changes are not an indication of infection. However, the nursing assessment must monitor any changes and promptly identify infection risks.

A common controversy focuses on the risks associated with the often prolonged use of proton pump inhibitors (PPIs), the class of drugs used to decrease gastric acidity and manage symptoms in GERD and *Helicobacter pylori*, the pathogenic agent for peptic ulcer disease. Studies have shown that the risks associated with PPI use are low. The U.S. Food and Drug Administration (FDA) suggests PPIs may be associated with *Clostridium difficile*-associated disease. Although decreased vitamin B12 levels have been reported in the elderly, PPIs have not been linked to cases of *C. difficile* infection (CDI).[13]

Inflammatory (Crohn's disease, ulcerative colitis) and noninflammatory conditions (diverticulosis, noninfectious colitis) are inflammatory rather than infectious conditions. These bowel conditions are not contagious. However, residents who have challenges with toileting may present hygienic and environmental issues related to their daily nursing needs. Standard Precautions, thorough cleaning/disinfection, and the use of facility-approved disinfectants will provide adequate decontamination when such risks are identified in the assessment process.

Bowel changes are not an immediate indicator of infection. Bowel cleansing for diagnostic procedures, tube feedings, medications, and changes in diet can trigger diarrhea. Nursing assessment of diarrhea presents a common challenge among LTCF residents.

Diarrheal illness may also be caused by viruses, bacteria, or parasites. While the modes of transmission are usually fecal-oral and foodborne, person-to-person spread may occur in some cases. Norovirus has become the most common foodborne infection in the United States. *Escherichia coli* and *Salmonella* bacterial gastroenteritis are frequently seen in older adults; parasitic gastrointestinal infections are less common. For a complete review of pathogenic viruses, bacteria and parasites, refer to the *APIC Text.*[14]

CDI is emerging as the most common cause of acute diarrheal illness in LTCFs; outbreaks have been and continue to be reported.[15] In addition, a more virulent strain of CDI has been identified that is more resistant to treatment with fluoroquinolones; metronidazole and vancomycin are now preferred. Overutilization of antibiotics is widely identified as a major contributor to CDI in all healthcare settings.[16]

CDI presents numerous nursing challenges to both the assessment and delivery of care. Residents who are treated in acute care settings may experience a recurrence after discharge to LTCF.[17] The use of a private room and separate bathroom, part of the rigorous Contact Precautions used in acute settings, may not be feasible in LTCFs. Resident cohorting, limiting bathroom use, requiring the use of a bedside commode, using sporicidal cleaning and disinfecting practices, as well as stringent hand hygiene and use of gowns and gloves, must be incorporated into resident management strategies. For additional information on CDI, see the APIC's *Guide to Preventing* Clostridium difficile *Infections.*

The nursing assessment must also identify potential risks for ostomates. Some studies have reported a higher risk of complications among elderly ostomates.[18] Residents with new ostomies may be at higher risk for peristomal complications. Pouching systems that do not fit exactly, leak, or are misapplied can lead to pressure ulcers around the stoma and/or excoriation with repeated exposure to intestinal effluent. *Candida* infections have been reported in these types of situations.[19] Peristomal irritation can lead to other types of infections as well and can aggravate preexisting skin problems in the elderly.[20]

Skin and Wound Assessment

The effect of aging is usually most prominently observed in the skin. The epidermis thins, supporting subcutaneous fat decreases, the elasticity of connective tissue declines, and remaining melanocytes increase, appearing as lentigo or "age spots." The peripheral vasculature becomes more fragile and susceptible to bruising. Growths, such as skin tags, are common in the elderly. The cumulative effect of these changes is that the elderly are at risk for skin injury, and when damaged, tissues usually heal more slowly than in younger individuals. Infection is a risk in any skin impairment. For a detailed review of skin and wound issues, see Chapter 7. A thorough assessment of the resident's skin, including sensitivities, abrasions, wounds, bruises, limitation in self-care, and preferred products must be carefully documented.

In addition to the skin and wound issues addressed in Chapter 7, the nursing assessment should also include, minimally, the resident's health history in the following high-risk areas that may contribute to an integumentary compromise.

- **History of varicella exposure, previous occurrence of zoster, and related immunizations:** The skin lesions and painful neurological involvement that characterize acute attacks intensifies the severity of zoster among older adults. Adults without varicella immunity are susceptible to infection. Antiretroviral therapy will be prescribed. For residents with disseminated cases and/or super infection of lesions, antibiotics will also be included in the treatment plan.[21]
- **History of sun exposure and skin cancer risk:** Prolonged exposure to ultraviolet light can lead basal cell or squamous cell carcinoma. Often these cancers are identified before age 65, but they also occur later in life. The skin changes may develop slowly and can be mistaken for other conditions and/or localized infection. A dermatology consultation may be required.
- **History of amputation and stump integrity:** The socket of the prosthesis, which cradles warm, damp skin, creates an environment for skin breakdown and infection. A localized bacterial infection may progress to cellulitis or produce an abscess. Decreased or absent sensation in the affected extremity will impede resident awareness of early signs of complications, including onset of inflammation and/or infection. Although mobility is the key to regaining postoperative independence, conclusive evidence and the multiple outcome measures applied reflect the need for further research in both the prognosis for mobility among LTCF residents as well as the risks for infection.
- **History of neurological impairment and loss of sensation:** Impaired mobility, which may result from trauma, stroke, degenerative conditions, and/or neuropathy, can predispose the resident to numerous health problems. Unrelieved pressure or damage to the skin can set the stage for infection. Residents may be unable to sense excessive pressure or irritation caused by poorly fitting footgear and/or inadequately secured braces or other assistive devices.

Infestation, Not Infection

Parasitic infestation of lice and scabies has been reported in LTCFs. These parasites cause small red bumps on the skin that initially may mimic other types of skin irritation or rashes. Papules or blisters will develop and the scratching that results from intense itching may cause these lesions to bleed and become infected. Paradoxically, these symptoms may be less pronounced in the elderly, leading to transmission within LTCFs where residents have frequent close contact. Residents should receive a skin scraping for positive diagnosis of scabies prior to initiating treatment. Antiparasitic topical treatments will eliminate the infestation, along with thorough environmental cleaning. Residents identified with or being treated for parasitic infestations do not require disposable dinnerware or utensils, and their clothing and bedding will be satisfactorily decontaminated with routine facility laundering. Prompt identification and rapid intervention are essential to preventing widespread outbreaks within LTCFs.

Urinary Tract Assessment and Prevention of Catheter-associated Urinary Tract Infections

It is estimated that an average of 1.6 to 3.8 infections per resident occur annually in LTCF residents.[22] Urinary tract infections (UTIs) are one of the most common endemic infections. Indwelling urethral catheters in LTCFs have a prevalence rate of 7 to 10 percent but may be higher in residents who are unable to ambulate.[23] Catheter-associated urinary tract infections (CAUTIs) can lead to many complications including cystitis, gram-negative bacteremia, and pyelonephritis. Complications from CAUTIs are pain and discomfort, and lead to hospitalization and increased cost and mortality. Each year, more than 13,000 deaths are associated with UTIs.[24]

The nursing assessment should include risk criteria specific to the development of urinary infections. Postoperative residents who are admitted to LTCFs with an indwelling catheter after major surgery are at higher risk for hospital readmission than those who do not use urinary catheters for extended periods of time.[25] Mobility status is also an important criterion. For residents who require wheelchairs, prostheses, or other mobility aids, maintaining or improving mobility reduced the risk of hospitalization for urinary infection by 38 to 80 percent.[2]

Use of the appropriate descriptors for urinary infections is important both in the assessment as well as ongoing documentation of health status. The following key terminology is essential to accurate documentation:

- **Primary urinary tract infections** are defined in two broad categories described as symptomatic urinary tract infection (SUTI) criteria or asymptomatic bacteremic UTI (ABUTI).
  - *Symptomatic urinary tract infection (SUTI)* – A resident with signs and symptoms of infection and a positive urine culture.
  - *Asymptomatic bacteremic urinary tract infection (ABUTI)* – Isolation of identified measurable amount of bacteria in a urine specimen collected from a resident without signs or symptoms.
- **Catheter-associated urinary tract infection (CAUTI)** is a UTI where an indwelling catheter has been in place for more than two calendar days when all elements of the UTI infection criteria were first present together with the day of placement being day 1, and an indwelling urinary catheter was in place on the date of the event or the day before.[26]
- **Pyuria** is urine containing increased numbers of polymorphonuclear leukocytes reflecting an inflammatory response. Laboratory ranges vary, but pyuria is often defined as greater than 10 leucocytes per microliter (μL) or cubic millimeter (mm3). Pyuria is often seen in elderly residents with sepsis or pneumonia.
- **Urosepsis** is a nonspecific term referring to bacteremia associated with an infection of the urinary tract; it is not considered the same as sepsis.
- **Uropathogens** include pathogenic organisms found in the urinary tract. *E. coli* causes bacterial infections in about 40 percent of residents with indwelling urinary catheters The second most common pathogen is gram-negative, aerobic *Klebsiella* sp., particularly *K. pneumonia*. Most commonly seen in resident with indwelling catheters are *Proteus* species, *Providencia* species, and *Morganella morganii*.[27]

If a urinary catheter is present, the assessment should document the indication(s) for use and the time periods during which it is required. The nursing assessment must also identify any instances of inappropriate use (see Table 6.1). Use of urinary catheters for management of urinary incontinence should not be done in LTCF residents. The facility's Treatment Administration Record (TAR) may be used for monitoring placement. Remind the attending physician of the presence of the catheter and request its removal as soon as possible. Portable bladder scanners can be used to measure urinary retention. This can help to reduce the need for catheterization and also be used to reduce unnecessary procedures.

TABLE 6.1: APPROPRIATE AND INAPPROPRIATE USE OF URINARY CATHETERS

Appropriate Use
• The resident has acute urinary retention or bladder outlet obstruction. • The catheter is necessary to measure urinary output for a specific period of time. • The catheter will assist in healing of open sacral or perineal wounds in incontinent residents. • The resident requires prolonged immobilization and use of a bedpan or urinal is not feasible. • The catheter will improve comfort in end of life care.
Inappropriate Use
• The catheter is used for the convenience of the nursing staff. • The catheter is used in lieu of other bladder management strategies. • The catheter is used for specimen collection when the resident can voluntarily void. • The catheter is left in place when removal is indicated.

The literature reference, as well as medical and nursing protocols reference, contains extensive and detailed information regarding the safe and effective management of indwelling urinary catheters. Basic infection prevention interventions include all of the measures listed in Table 6.2. Individual LTCFs may have additional safety measures.

Residents who have end-stage renal disease will not require a urinary catheter; dialysis will be required. For more information on dialysis, see Chapter 7. Residents with end-stage renal disease may require a suprapubic catheter for peritoneal dialysis. Staff who have specialized training in these procedures are necessary to minimize the risk of infection. Peritonitis remains a common reason for hospital readmission, and gram-positive organisms are often identified. Extremely old age with or without severe functional impairment increased the risk of a poor outcome.[28] Better outcomes have been associated with higher activities of daily living (ADL) scores, expected return to the community at the time of admission, and epoetin (recombinant human erythropoietin) treatment to correct renal anemia.[29]

TABLE 6.2: NURSING CARE TO PREVENT INFECTIONS WITH INDWELLING URINARY CATHETERS

1. Only personnel who have been trained in correct technique to insert catheters should perform a catheter insertion. If it is anticipated the resident may present difficulties in the insertion procedure (e.g., the resident having contractures and/or may be difficult to position or may be confused and try to grab equipment), an assistant may be needed to assist the nurse performing the procedure.
2. Always use Standard Precautions.
3. Hand hygiene should be done before gloving and again when gloves are removed.
4. Aseptic technique and sterile supplies must be used for catheter insertion.
5. To lessen the trauma of catheterization, use the smallest size catheter necessary to allow the free flow of urine.
6. For maximum safe catheter maintenance, maintain a closed sterile urinary draining system.
7. Maintain an unobstructed urine flow. Keep the catheter and tubing free from kinking and secure the tubing per institutional protocol.
8. Keep the collecting bag **below the level of the bladder** at all times. Do not place the bag on the floor.
9. Empty the collecting bag regularly using a separate, clean collecting container marked with the resident's name.
10. Changing indwelling catheters or drainage bags at routine intervals is not recommended.[28] It is suggested to change catheters and drainage bags based on clinical indications such as infection, obstruction, or when the closed system is compromised.
11. Do not clean the periurethral area with antiseptics to prevent CAUTI while the catheter is in place. Routine hygiene of soap and water for daily bathing and showering is appropriate. Perform perineal care after each bowel movement.
12. Unless obstruction is suspected, bladder irrigation is not recommended.
13. When a CAUTI is strongly suspected, remove the old catheter (chronic indwelling catheter in place for more than 14 days) before obtaining a laboratory specimen. This is done to prevent the influence of the possible presence of biofilm. Specimens obtained from drainage bags should never be submitted for analysis.
14. Specimens – Consult the facility-contracted microbiology laboratory for the correct procedure for holding specimens for pickup. It is recommended specimens be cultured within 2 hours, but if this is not possible, the use of refrigeration or chemical preservatives will be required. Follow all requirements for biohazard labeling and preparation prior to transport.
15. Empty the collecting bag regularly using a separate, clean collecting container marked with the resident's name.
16. Urine dipstick tests are convenient to rule out the presence of infection. Using a dipstick, immerse it in fresh urine and remove immediately, hold horizontally to compare to the chart and read.
    - Nitrates – Most urinary pathogens reduce nitrates to nitrites; however, false negatives can occur. Normal urine does not contain nitrites.
    - Leukocyte esterase – This is a reaction produced by neutrophils. A positive test suggests pyuria associated with urinary tract infection.

ADDITIONAL HIGH RISK ASSESSMENT CATEGORIES

Diabetes

Type 1 diabetes has numerous, serious long- and short-term consequences, including infection when inadequately managed. The LTCF resident may present with a history of stroke, visual impairment, amputation, or other significant health problem. However, type 2 diabetes may begin in later life, necessitating blood glucose monitoring, dietary adjustments, altered activity regimens, and other lifestyle modifications that may be especially challenging in older age.

In addition to the risks associated with cardiovascular disease, vision loss, neurological damage, and kidney failure, residents with diabetes are also at risk for wound infection and delayed wound healing. Diabetic residents with pressure ulcers need to be considered as high risk for infection. Residents with surgical incisions may also require additional assessment and monitoring, especially if blood sugars cannot be maintained within normal limits. Medication management, nutrition, glycemic control, management of hypertension, and dyslipidemia are not only required for management of diabetes but also as part of an overall health maintenance and infection prevention plan.[30]

Sexual Health and HIV

Aging does not necessarily lead to a decline in sexuality. However, aging does increase the potential barriers to ongoing sexual activity, including lack of a healthy partner; illness; and/or disability, hormonal fluctuations, and depression.[31] The prevalence of sexual transmitted disease (STD) among older adults has not been widely studied but is thought to be low. While there is some limited evidence of an increase in STDs in people older than 50, there are few longitudinal studies that fully verify this trend, and the incidence of STDs remains much lower than among younger age groups. Routine STD screening for LTCF residents is not generally recommended.[32]

Individuals with human immunodeficiency virus (HIV) are now living into older age due in large part to early diagnosis, prompt initiation of antiretroviral therapy following diagnosis, and restoration and maintenance of a normal CD4 count.[33] The number of older individuals with HIV in the United States is rapidly increasing. Screening for HIV infection should be integrated into the assessment process. For HIV positive residents, additional assessment should address co-infections, comorbid health problems, social isolation, risk of polypharmacy, and, when appropriate, end of life care.[34]

Alcohol and Other Substance Abuse

LTCF residents may develop substance abuse behaviors late in life or may be coping with the health consequences of chronic abuse. Unfortunately, these problems often go unrecognized until a serious consequence (e.g., a fall with or without injury, drug reaction, hostile behavior) reveals the underlying problem.

Alcohol abuse and alcoholism are common but often undetected among LTCF residents. The negative impact of alcohol abuse is often increased among the elderly. This includes an increased risk predisposing the individual to a variety of infections.[35] Similarly, substance abuse maybe unrecognized in the LTCF population. Although the use of illegal "street drugs" is thought to be rare, there is growing evidence of the misuse and abuse of prescription medications. At least one in four older adults use psychoactive drugs with abuse potential, and that use is expected to increase as the population ages. The nonmedical use of prescription drugs among adults older than 50 years is believed to be rapidly increasing.[36] The nursing assessment must take the potential for substance abuse into consideration, especially because these drugs can alter immune response and predispose to opportunistic infections.

Depression

Depression is commonly diagnosed in LTCF residents, especially those older than 65 years. But not all residents receive treatment because (1) depressive symptoms in the elderly may present differently than in younger individuals and (2) depression is often associated with one or more health conditions, often masking its impact or leading clinicians to consider it as an expected part of the overall diagnosis. The incidence of depressive symptoms has been linked with a decline in coping skills and trajectories in later life.[37]

Many immunity-inflammation mediated disorders are comorbid with depression, including diabetes, Crohn's disease, HIV, multiple sclerosis, and cardiac disease. When these conditions are noted on the health history and reported during the assessment, the possibility of depression should also be considered.

Depression does not cause infection but can exacerbate negative behaviors that may predispose to infection. Poor nutrition, immobility, self-neglect, nonadherence to care routines, and avoidance of personal hygiene are just a few common examples of depression-associated behaviors that can increase the resident's risk. The nursing care approach must blend management of depressive symptoms with appropriate infection prevention strategies.

ADDITIONAL INTERVENTIONS TO PREVENT INFECTIONS

Hand Hygiene

Hand hygiene is the mainstay of all infection prevention programs. The availability of both soap and water as well as an alcohol-based hand rub is recommended. In addition to educating facility employees about the need for and correct procedures for hand hygiene, the resident and any family and/or visitors should also be instructed. Residents may need reminders and/or direct assistance with cleaning their hands. For detailed information on hand hygiene, see Chapter 5 on Isolation Precautions.

Nutrition and Hydration

The impact of nutritional status through life is well documented; its relationship to morbidity and mortality among the elderly has also been extensively investigated. Malnutrition increases the risk of frailty and can influence immune response and susceptibility to infection.[38] Decreased taste sensation, loss of appetite, poor or absent dentition, depression, medications, and dysphagia are among the many issues contributing to malnutrition in LTCF residents where the prevalence of malnutrition has been reported to be as high as 37 percent.[39]

Sarcopenia is the loss of lean muscle mass occurring with advanced age. Experts believe that anabolic resistance to nutrients, insulin, and resistance exercise not only contribute to sarcopenia but almost make it difficult to treat. Light resistance exercise, combined with essential amino acid supplements has been beneficial for some residents.[40] Other strategies such as calorie restriction, testosterone supplements, and myostatin inhibition have also been utilized, but a definitive approach to reduce or prevent age-related muscle wasting has not yet been established.[41]

A lack of knowledge and awareness of nutritional issues among staff adds to the challenges faced by LTCFs. Multiple studies report widespread lack of staff knowledge and barriers to addressing it. For example, in one study, only 38 percent correctly identified residents' needs for increased protein and only 15 percent demonstrated correct knowledge of fluid requirements. Although staff overwhelmingly stated that nutritional assessment were important, just 53 percent reported conducting them.[42] Both initial and ongoing training programs in nutrition and aging are clearly needed.

Tube feedings, administered via a gastrostomy tube, provide an ideal medium for bacterial growth if not adequately maintained. In addition to monitoring the gastrostomy tube for patency and position, the stoma site must also be assessed for signs of localized inflammation or infection. Tube feeding products, containers required for their preparation, administration sets, irrigation syringes, and any infusion pumps must be cleaned/disinfected and replaced per institutional policy and procedure.

> A food and fluid intake tracking tool and dehydration checklists are available on the CD-ROM included with this book.

The onset of dehydration may occur slowly or, in cases associated with acute illness, be rapid and dangerous. As fluid loss increases, multiple symptoms can be assessed. However, these may vary among individuals. Common symptoms may include increased respirations and heart rate, deceased perspiration, and urination. Mental status changes, muscle tingling, weakness, and fatigue are also common. Dehydration can progress rapidly in the frail elderly and can escalate to a medical emergency if undetected.

Hypodermoclysis, the subcutaneous infusion of fluids, is safe and effective in LTCFs. Extensive review of the literature indicates that adverse reactions are more common when nonelectrolyte or hypertonic solutions were infused.[43] Randomized control trials have shown that minor side effects are similar to those seen with intravenous therapy; the risks of both inflammation and infection are low.[44] The injection of hyaluronidase prior to infusion of fluids can increase the speed of absorption, but may not enhance the resident's comfort level. As with intravenous infusions, maintenance of sterile supplies and rigorous aseptic technique is required for resident safety.

Oral Care

The oral cavity is frequently neglected when it comes to preventive care in LTCF residents. Lack of care creates an environment for the growth of pathogenic species, which include *Candida* (primarily albicans), *Streptococcus, Lactobacilli,* and others.[45] These disease-causing organisms have been linked to systemic disease, and poor oral hygiene may predispose debilitated residents to problems such as hyperglycemia, cardiac disease, and cerebrovascular accidents.[46,47] In addition, the oral cavity serves as an important reservoir for the growth of respiratory pathogens in patients who are debilitated, hospitalized, or living in a LTCF. LTCF residents often have poorer oral hygiene than community-dwelling individuals, which may foster oropharyngeal colonization with respiratory pathogens. In one study, inadequate oral care and swallowing difficulty were statistically associated with pneumonia. This suggests that oral hygiene interventions may reduce the rate of oral colonization by respiratory pathogens and, subsequently, the risk for pneumonia in this resident population.[48] Factors that favor the overgrowth of pathogenic species include decreased saliva production with age,[49] medication,[50] chronic disease,[47] debility, and poor oral hygiene. In addition, dental diseases such as caries (cavities) and periodontal disease may debilitate the resident further and produce lowered desire to eat and inadequate nutrition.

Many long-term care residents require assistance with ADLs, including oral care.[49,51] Residents who exhibit resistance to mouth care tend not to receive regular care, and residents with dementia, often dependent on others for mouth care, may react with care-resistant behavior.[46] Lack of time, increased workload, limited staff, and the lack of accountability all contribute to the problem of delivering mouth care.[52] Nurses are in a powerful position to support nursing assistants in providing mouth care by providing adequate supplies and support when residents exhibit resistant behaviors.[46]

Regular mouth care, including professional oral care, is effective in reducing infections by many opportunistic pathogens.[53] Regular preventive care has been shown to reduce *Candida* colonization of the oral mucosa as well as denture surfaces, and an amine fluoride-stannous fluoride combination in a mouth rinse and toothpaste has been shown to decrease the *Candida* counts in LTCF residents, as well.[54,55] Mechanical cleaning is more effective for the removal of *Candida* and other organisms than rinsing with povidone iodine alone.[56,57] Professional oral health care provided by dental hygienists is an effective adjunct to regular care performed by the nursing staff and decreases the total oropharyngeal bacteria.[56,57] See Table 6.3.

The most common dental infections of the oral cavity are caries (cavities), gingivitis, and periodontal disease. Severe caries and periodontal disease are relatively easy to diagnose. Large carious lesions will usually present as a black spot or hole in a tooth, and periodontal disease will present as red, swollen gingiva (gums), and loose teeth. Any pain or swelling in the jaws, especially if accompanied by a fever, should be referred as soon as possible to a licensed dentist. The pain and swelling may represent an infection in the bone or an infection in or death of the pulp of a tooth. Sometimes, an infection will produce purulence (pus) that drains through the tooth socket or through the bone. In these cases, pain and swelling may not be present.

Infections in the mucosa and hard surfaces of the upper and lower dental ridges may also occur. *Candida* species are the most common opportunistic infecting organism in the oral cavity. Candidosis, or "thrush," may present as a white coating. It is most commonly seen on the tongue, but may also be seen throughout the mouth. This coating may be scraped off to show a red, sometimes bleeding, surface below. Candidosis may also present as a white area that cannot be scraped off, or, especially under dentures, as a flame-red area. Chronic candidosis may indicate the resident has an immune deficiency.

Herpes simplex is another common infection of the mouth. The primary infection is usually quite mild in children, but if an adult suffers a primary herpes infection, it can be severe and in some cases may require hospitalization. After the primary infection, the herpes virus remains in the nerve root. At various times, usually at times of stress, the virus will migrate down the nerve and cause a lesion that begins with a tingling sensation in the area. Shortly after, small blisters will form and break open. Secondary herpes lesions usually heal in about a week; however, herpes is contagious and gloves should always be worn and changed. Staff should routinely look inside the residents' mouths, using a light and tongue blade, and note when something looks different or "just not right."

Hand hygiene should always be performed before and after providing oral care, and gloves should be worn during the procedure. Because a myriad of conditions may look similar in the oral cavity, and the difference between serious and benign is not readily apparent, regular visits by a dental professional are recommended.

INFUSION THERAPY AS PART OF THE NURSING ASSESSMENT[58]

As residents with more medically complex needs are treated at the LTCF, there is a greater probability that infusion therapy may be necessary. As a result, a variety of invasive devices are increasingly utilized in

TABLE 6.3: SUPPLIES FOR ORAL CARE

Supplies	Use
Foam swabs	Especially for residents who cannot assist with their oral care, foam dental swabs can be used to perform debridement of food. With extremely resistant residents, dental foam swabs may be the only care that can be provided.
Dental floss	Unwaxed dental floss cleans best, but may be difficult to use. Waxed ribbon floss slides more easily between the teeth. Woven floss with fluoride is also available. For residents who have trouble with floss, or for residents who cannot assist, consider flossers that hold the floss and make flossing easier.
Toothbrush	Toothbrushes should have soft bristles. Specialty toothbrushes with extra-large handles are available. The brushing action should rotate from the gingiva to the top of the tooth. Consider an electric toothbrush. Electric toothbrushes clean the teeth very well and can be moved slowly across the tooth surfaces. This allows for a better cleaning with less effort on the part of the resident or staff. Each resident needs to have a personal (their use only) toothbrush.
Toothpaste	If toothpaste is used, it should be used sparingly, especially with residents who cannot assist with their care. Use fluoride toothpaste.
Tongue scraper	Tongue scrapers are available in plastic and are easy to use. Scraping the tongue removes additional organisms and food particles from the mouth. Use the tongue scraper gently.
Mouthwash	Use mouthwashes only with those residents who can assist with their oral hygiene and who can expectorate (to avoid aspiration of the liquid). Dilute as necessary with water if the resident complains of a strong taste. For residents who are unable to assist, a foam swab may be moistened with a mild mouthwash and used to remove debris from the mouth. For prescribed mouthwashes, such as chlorhexidine gluconate, check with the prescribing clinician or the pharmacy before diluting.
Hydrogen peroxide	While prescribed on occasion, hydrogen peroxide should be used only when prescribed and then for the shortest time possible. Hydrogen peroxide promotes the overgrowth of *Candida* species by reducing the number of other organisms in the mouth.
Salt water	As with mouthwash, use only with those residents who can assist with their oral hygiene and who can expectorate (to avoid aspiration of the liquid). Alkaline saltwater rinses (addition of a quarter of a teaspoon of baking soda to 100 mL of saline) can refresh a resident's mouth and is used for soreness as well.

LTCF settings. The nursing assessment must include a thorough documentation of the type of catheter, the procedures used to maintain it, as well as resident response to treatment. See Chapter 7 for an in depth discussion about infusion therapy in LTCFs.

Intravenous peripheral catheters and peripherally inserted central catheters (PICCs) are among those most commonly seen.[59] Implanted ports for residents requiring long-term therapy are also used. Although intravenous catheter infection rates are not among the major categories of infection reported in LTCFs (noninfectious complications may be identified more often), the risk potential of these devices warrants careful monitoring when therapies must be delivered via either of the peripheral or central vasculature.

This is especially important because contamination of the intravenous system can occur in several ways.

1. Migration of skin organisms at the insertion site into the cutaneous catheter tract and along the surface of the catheter with colonization of the catheter tip; this is the most common route of infection for short-term catheters;
2. Direct contamination of the catheter or catheter hub by contact with hands or contaminated fluids or devices;
3. Less commonly, catheters might become hematogenously seeded from another focus of infection; and
4. Rarely, contaminated infusate may lead to sepsis.

Mural thrombus, a stationary blood clot along the blood vessel wall, has been recognized as an infection risk factor, especially in central catheters. The risk of thrombus increases with catheter tip dislodgement or migration, as well as hypercoagulability. However, neither antibiotic nor anticoagulant prophylaxis is recommended by the CDC. Selection of the appropriate size catheter, confirmation of correct placement, stabilization using a sutureless securement device, and regular flushing are routine measures for decreasing the risk of thrombus.

Peripheral Catheters

Prevention of infections, either localized at the insertion site or generalized in a systemic bacteremia, can be optimized by implementation of the following procedures identified by the CDC:[58]

1. In adults, use an upper extremity site for catheter insertion. Replace a catheter inserted in a lower extremity site to an upper extremity site as soon as possible.
2. Select catheters on the basis of the intended purpose and duration of use, known infectious and noninfectious complications (e.g., phlebitis and infiltration), and experience of individual catheter operators.
3. Prepare clean skin with an antiseptic (70 percent alcohol, tincture of iodine, or alcoholic chlorhexidine gluconate solution) before peripheral venous catheter insertion. Antiseptics should be applied and allowed to dry according to the manufacturer's recommendation prior to placing the catheter.
4. Avoid the use of steel needles for the administration of fluids and medication that might cause tissue necrosis if extravasation occurs.
5. Evaluate the catheter insertion site daily by palpation through the dressing to discern tenderness and by inspection if a transparent dressing is in use. Gauze and opaque dressings should not be removed if the resident has no clinical signs of infection. If the resident has local tenderness or other signs of possible central line-associated blood stream infection, an opaque dressing should be removed and the site inspected visually.
6. Remove peripheral venous catheters if the resident develops signs of phlebitis (warmth, tenderness, erythema, or palpable venous cord), infection, or a malfunctioning catheter.
7. There is no need to replace peripheral catheters more frequently than every 72 to 96 hours to reduce the risk of infection and phlebitis in adults.

PICCs

A central catheter can be peripherally inserted using the brachial, basilic, or cephalic vein. The catheter is advanced until the tip is adjacent to the superior vena cava. Peripheral insertion is generally considered more secure for long-term therapies administered in nonhospital settings. Studies have shown that infection rates are lower with PICCs used exclusively in outpatient settings (0.4 per 1,000 catheter days) than in acute care (2-5 per 1,000 catheter days).[60] However, as with any long-term intravenous device, phlebitis, occlusion, thrombus, and infection remain a risk.

PICC catheters may be coated or impregnated with several types of anti-infective chemicals: silver, antimicrobials, or chlorhexidine gluconate. A resident admitted from an acute care setting with a previously inserted PICC may have such a catheter. The long-term efficacy of such products is not well documented and is thought to decrease over time. In addition, the presence of anti-infective coatings may induce a false sense of security regarding the actual safety risk to the resident.[61] Stringent infection prevention measures are needed for both coated and uncoated products.

PICC contamination may be extra or intraluminal. Extraluminal pathogens typically are associated with the resident's micro flora where staphylococci may be identified. Intraluminal contamination is introduced during manipulation of the intravenous system. There are many opportunities for unintentional intraluminal contamination to occur. Poor hand hygiene, contaminated gloves, breaks in aseptic technique, and failure to disinfect access surfaces are common examples of how pathogens can be introduced into an otherwise sterile system.

The solution, amount, and frequency of PICC flushing remains controversial. Heparin solutions and normal saline are commonly used, although other products have been used in experimental studies.[62,63] It is important to know that none of these experimental catheter locking solutions have been approved by the FDA. The LTCF's flushing protocol must be documented and followed carefully. Hand hygiene and disinfection of the access port/needleless connector are required when manipulating the system. Connectors are other adjunct supplies must be changed per protocol.

Upper extremity thrombus, a risk factor of infection, is a common complication of extended PICC placement. However, duration of device use is not the sole risk factor. Studies have reported additional risk factors such as basilic vein placement, renal failure, infusion of total parenteral nutrition, or antibiotics (especially vancomycin) increased thrombus risk.[64]

As with peripheral catheters, the insertion site must be protected when the resident wishes to bathe. Commercially prepared sleeves are useful for this purpose. If the dressing becomes wet or loose, it must be promptly replaced.

Because of their length and frequent movement of the extremities, PICCs are at risk for migration and/or dislodgement. This unintended motion can lead to adverse outcomes. Sutures and tape have been traditionally used for stabilization, but today commercially engineered adhesive anchors or specially designed securement dressings provide enhanced protection.

Implanted Infusion Ports

Introduced in the 1980s, implanted ports rapidly gained widespread acceptance. Initially used for chemotherapy, ports are now utilized for any long-term therapy and when the need for repeated blood sampling would be injurious to the peripheral vasculature.

The port is surgically implanted in subcutaneous tissue, usually in the chest, but arm and abdominal placement may also be used. The tip of the port terminates in a major vessel, often the subclavian. After the surgical site has healed, the nurse uses a special noncoring sterile needle to access the septum of the port, which is just beneath the skin. The same aseptic procedures used with intravenous therapies are required, including a sterile dressing once the needle is in place. Catheter-related thrombus and occlusion are reported with implanted ports, but infections also occur.[27,65] When therapy is completed, the needle is removed, all administration sets appropriately discarded, and the site does not require additional dressing. Implanted ports that are not used regularly must be periodically flushed to maintain patency and prevent occlusion-related infections.

CATHETER SITE DRESSING REGIMENS (ALL TYPES OF CATHETERS)

The insertion site for an intravenous catheter should be protected. Sterile gauze or a sterile, transparent, semipermeable dressing should be used to cover the catheter site. A basic adhesive bandage rarely provides sufficient protection, especially if the administration of medication of fluids will requires several hours.

Additional measures to prevent infection include:

1. If the resident is diaphoretic or if the site is bleeding or oozing, use a gauze dressing until this is resolved.
2. Replace catheter site dressing if the dressing becomes damp, loosened, or visibly soiled.
3. Do not use topical antibiotic ointment or creams on insertion sites, except for dialysis catheters, because of their potential to promote fungal infections and antimicrobial resistance.
4. Do not submerge the catheter or catheter site in water. Showering should be permitted if precautions can be taken to reduce the likelihood of introducing organisms into the catheter (e.g., if the catheter and connecting device are protected with an impermeable cover during the shower).
5. Monitor the catheter site visually when changing the dressing or by palpation through an intact dressing on a regular basis, depending on the clinical situation of the individual resident. If residents have tenderness at the insertion site, fever without obvious source, or other manifestations suggesting local or bloodstream infection, the dressing should be removed to allow thorough examination of the site.
6. Encourage residents or their families to report any changes in their catheter site or any new discomfort to the nurse.

Replacement of Administration Sets and Safety Components

Intravenous tubing and related products can harbor pathogens that can be introduced when the administration set is accessed. Preventative care can minimize the risk associated with the use of these products.

1. In residents not receiving blood, blood products, or fat emulsions, replace administration sets that

are continuously used, including secondary sets and add-on devices, no more frequently than at 96-hour intervals but at least every 7 days.

2. Replace tubing used to administer blood, blood products, or fat emulsions (those combined with amino acids and glucose in a three-in-one admixture or infused separately) within 24 hours of initiating the infusion.
3. Change the needleless components at least as frequently as the administration set. There is no benefit to changing these more frequently than every 72 hours.
4. Change needleless connectors no more frequently than every 72 hours or according to manufacturers' recommendations for the purpose of reducing infection rates.
5. Ensure that all components of the system are compatible to minimize leaks and breaks in the system.
6. Minimize contamination risk by scrubbing the access port with an appropriate antiseptic (chlorhexidine, povidone iodine, an iodophor, or 70 percent alcohol) and accessing the port only with sterile devices.

DELEGATION AND SUPERVISION BY NURSES

Task delegation and the need for supervision of staff exist in multiple areas throughout the LTCF. While this process is by no means restricted to any one discipline, the number of unlicensed staff providing resident care, as well the occasional presence of volunteers, students, and visitors, make these responsibilities a crucial component of professional nursing practice in LTCFs.

Delegation and supervision, roles in the prevention of infection in LTCFs that are not well documented, are nonetheless essential part of the overall process of care delivery and coordination. It is, however, not enough for the nurse to ensure that assigned tasks have been performed correctly. The nurse must also monitor the environment to maximize those factors that support the success of a team approach. This is essential for transforming LTCF organizational culture from a traditional approach of blame and punishment to a proactive position of resident safety.[66]

For example, the nurse may provide inservice education to a group of nurse assistants on the correct use of gloves when Contact Precautions are required. The nurse must not only follow up to check that all the requisite steps in gloving process are being done correctly, but also to ensure that the assistants understand why the various steps are important, how consistency of their performance impacts the risk of cross contamination, encourage peer-to-peer support for the procedure, and to ensure that adequate supplies are in place when and where they are needed. Opportunities for questions, additional learning, and adjustment of any incorrect procedural steps are available in a positive, team-oriented manner. The focus is not just on the gloving technique, but on the resident, whose safety and health status are supported by the use of Contact Precautions.

This is a small but dramatic shift in the nurses' approach to team management. Although there is a compelling need for the development of nurse-sensitive measures for the prevention of infections in long-term care, existing studies indicate that teamwork, nurse leadership, and effective communication are essential to a culture of safety in LTCFs. Additionally, expanding the use of information technology will provide additional support for the delegation and supervision processes. The transition away from a hierarchical team model to a circular system that simultaneously and actively engages all members is a crucial transition in achieving better resident and organizational outcomes.[67]

REFERENCES

1. Dellefield ME, Harrington C, Kelly A. Observing how RNs use clinical time in a nursing home: a pilot study. *Geriatr Nurs* 2012 Jul-Aug; 33(4): 256-263.
2. Rogers MA, Fries BE, Kaufman SR, Mody L, McMahon LF Jr, Saint S. Mobility and other predictors of hospitalization for urinary tract infection: a retrospective cohort study. *BMC Geriatr* 2008 Nov 25; 8: 31.
3. Ashcraft AS, Champion JD. Nursing home resident symptomatology triggering transfer: avoiding unnecessary hospitalizations. *Nurs Res Pract* 2012; 2012: 495103.
4. Ouslander JG, Diaz S, Hain D, Tappen R. Frequency and diagnoses associated with 7- and 30-day readmission of skilled nursing facility patients to a nonteaching community hospital. *J Am Med Dir Assoc* 2011 Mar; 12(3): 195-203.
5. Bentley DW, Bradley S, High K, Schoenbaum S, Taler G, Yoshikawa TT. Practice guideline for evaluation of fever and infection in long-term care facilities. *J Am Geriatr Soc* 2001 Feb; 49(2): 210-222.
6. File, TM. The epidemiology of respiratory tract infections. *Semin Respir Infect* 2000 Sep; 15(3): 184-194.
7. Garibladi RA. Residential care and the elderly: the burden of infection. *J Hosp Infect* 1999 Dec; 43 Suppl: S9-S18.
8. Vergidis P, Hamer DH, Meydani SN, Dallal GE, Barlam TF. Patters of antimicrobial use for respiratory tract infections in older residents of long-term care facilities. *J Am Geriatr Soc* 2011 Jun; 59(6): 1093-1098.
9. Urbano FL, Pascual RM. Contemporary issues in the care of patients with chronic obstructive pulmonary disease. *J Manag Care Pharm* 2005; Jun: 11(5 Suppl A): S2-S13.
10. Centers for Disease Control and Prevention (CDC). *Pneumonia Can Be Prevented – Vaccines Can Help.* CDC website. 2012. Available at: http://www.cdc.gov/features/pneumonia/.
11. Dosa D. Should I hospitalize my resident with nursing home-acquired pneumonia? *J Am Med Dir Assoc* 2005 Sep-Oct; 6(5): 327-333.
12. Williams ME. The basic geriatric examination. Medscape Family Medicine Website. Available at: http://www.medscape.com/viewarticle/712242_5.
13. Thomson AB, Sauve MD, Kassam N, Kamitakahara H. Safety of the long-term use of proton pump inhibitors. *World J Gastroenterol* 2010 May 21; 16(19): 2323-2330.
14. Carrico R, ed. *APIC Text of Infection Control and Epidemiology,* 3rd ed. Washington, DC: Association for Professionals in Infection Control and Epidemiology, 2009.
15. Simor AE, Bradley SF, Strausbaugh LJ, Crossley K, Nicolle LE, SHEA Long-Term-Care Committee. Clostridium difficile in long-term-care facilities for the elderly. *Infect Control Hosp Epidemiol* 2002 Nov; 23(11): 696-703.
16. Makris AT, Gelone S. Clostridium difficile in the long-term care setting. *J Am Med Dir Assoc* 2007 Jun; 8(5): 290-299.
17. Murphy CR, Avery TR, Dubberke ER, Huang SS. Frequent hospital readmissions for Clostridium difficile infection and the impact on estimates of hospital-associated C. difficile burden. *Infect Control Hosp Epidemiol* 2012 Jan; 33(1): 20-28.
18. Hellman J, Lago CP. Dermatologic complications in colostomy and ileostomy patients. *Int J Dermatol* 1990 Mar; 29(2): 129-133.
19. Ratcliff CR, Scarano KA, Donovan AM, Colwell JC. Descriptive study of peristomal complications. *J Wound Ostomy Continence Nurs* 2005 Jan-Feb; 32(1): 33-37.
20. Nybaek H, Jemec GB. Skin problems in stoma patients. *J Eur Acad Dermatol Venereol* 2010; 24(3): 249-257.
21. O'Donnell JA, Hofmann MT. Skin and soft tissues. Management of four common infections in the nursing home patient. *Geriatrics* 2001 Oct; 56(10): 33-38,41.
22. Wickham RS. Advances in venous access devices and nursing management strategies. *Nurs Clin North Am* 1990 Jun; 25(2): 345-364.
23. Magaziner J, Tenney JH, DeForge B, Heble JR, Muncie HL Jr, Warren JW. Prevalence and characteristics of nursing home-acquired infections in the aged. *J Am Geriatr Sci* 1991 Nov; 39(11): 1071-1078.
24. Maki DG, Kluger DM, Crnich CJ. The risk of bloodstream infection in adults with different intravascular devices: a systematic review of 200 publish prospective studies. *Mayo Clin Proc* 2006 Sep; 81(9): 1159-1171.
25. Wald HL, Epstein AM, Radcliff TA, Kramer AM. Extended use of urinary catheters in older surgical patients: a patient safety problem? *Infect Control Hosp Epidemiol* 2008 Feb; 29(2): 116-124.
26. Centers for Disease Control and Prevention (CDC). *HAI Definition and CAUTI Surveillance Training.* CDC Website. Available at: http://www.cdc.gov/nhsn/acute-care-hospital/CAUTI/index.html.
27. Ide Y, Mikami K, Murata K. Long-term outcomes and complications of upper arm central venous access ports. *Gan To Kagaku Ryoho* 2013 Mar; 40(3): 331-335.
28. Anderson JE. Ten years' experience with CAPD in a nursing home setting. *Perit Dial Int* 1997 May-Jun; 17(3): 255-261.
29. Collins AJ. Anaemia management prior to dialysis: cardiovascular and cost-benefit observations. *Nephrol Dial Transplant* 2003; 18 Suppl 2: ii2-ii6.
30. Hoogwerf BJ. Postoperative management of the diabetic patient. *Med Clin North Am* 2001 Sept; 85(5): 1213-1228.
31. Inelmen EM, Sergi G, Girardi A, Coin A, Toffanello ED, Cardin F, et al. The importance of sexual health in the elderly: breaking down barriers and taboos. *Aging Clin Exp Res* 2012 Jun; 24(3 Suppl): 31-34.
32. Poynten IM, Grulich AE, Templeton DJ. Sexually transmitted infections in older populations. *Curr Opin Infect Dis* 2013 Feb; 26(1): 80-85.
33. May MT, Ingle SM. Life expectancy of HIV-positive adults: a review. *Sex Health* 2011 Dec; 8(4): 526-533.
34. Greene M, Justice AC, Lampiris HW, Valcour V. Management of human immunodeficiency virus infection in advanced age. *JAMA* 2013 Apr 3; 309(13): 1397-1405.
35. Rigler SK. *Alcoholism in the elderly.* Am Fam Physician 2000 Mar 15; 61(6): 1710-1716, 1882-1884, 1887-1888 passim.

REFERENCES

36. Simoni-Wastila L, Yang HK. Psychoactive drug abuse in older adults. *Am J Geriatr Pharmacother* 2006 Dec; 4(4): 380-394.

37. Brennan PL, Holland JM, Schutte KK, Moos RH. Coping trajectories in later life: a 20-year predictive study. *Aging Ment Health* 2012; 16(3): 305-316.

38. Fukagawa NK. Protein and amino acid supplementation in older humans. *Amino Acids* 2013; 44(6): 1493-1509.

39. Guigoz Y, Lauque S, Vellas BJ. Identifying the elderly at risk for malnutrition. The Mini Nutritional Assessment. *Clin Geriatr Med* 2002; 18(4): 737-757.

40. Fry CS, Rasmussen BB. Skeletal muscle protein balance and metabolism in the elderly. *Curr Aging Sci* 2011; 4(3): 260-268.

41. Sakuma K, Yamaguchi A. Molecular mechanisms in aging and current strategies to counteract sarcopenia. *Curr Aging Sci* 2010 Jul; 3(2): 90-101.

42. Beattie E, O'Reilly M, Strange E, Franklin S, Isenring E. How much do residential aged care staff members know about the nutritional need of residents? *Int J Older People Nurs* 2013 Feb 11. [epub ahead of print].

43. Rochon PA, Gill SS, Litner J, Fischbach M, Goodison AJ, Gordon M. A systematic review of the evidence for hypodermoclysis to treat dehydration in older people. *J Gerontol A Biol Sci Med Sci* 1997 May; 52(3): M169-176.

44. Arinzon Z, Feldman J, Fidelman Z, Gepstein R, Berner YN. Hypodermoclysis (subcutaneous infusion) effective mode of treatment of dehydration in long-term care patients. *Arch Gerontol Geriatr* 2004 Mar-Apr; 38(2): 167-173.

45. Budtz-Jergensen E, Mojon P, Bannon-Clement JM, Baehni P. Oral candidosis in long-term hospital care: comparison of edentulous and dentate subjects. *Oral Dis* 1996 Dec; 2(4): 285-290.

46. Jablonski RA, Kolanowski A, Therrien B, Mahoney EK, Kassab C, Leslie DL. Reducing care-resistant behaviors during oral hygiene in persons with dementia. *BMC Oral Health* 2011 Nov 19; 11: 30.

47. Haumschild MS, Haumschild RJ. The importance of oral health in long-term care. *J Am Med Dir Assoc* 2009 Nov; 10(9): 667-671.

48. Raghavendran K, Mylotte JM, Scannapieco FA. Nursing home-associated pneumonia, hospital-acquired pneumonia and ventilator-associated pneumonia: the contribution of dental biofilms and periodontal inflammation. *Periodontol* 2000 2007; 44: 164-177.

49. Almstahl A, Kareem KL, Carlen A, Wardh I, Lingstrom P, Wikstrom M. A prospective study on oral microbial flora and related variables in dentate dependent elderly residents. *Gerodontology* 2012 Jun; 29(2): e1011-8.

50. ADA Division of Communication. For the dental patient: How medications can affect your oral health. *J Am Dent Assoc* 2005 Jun; 136(6): 831.

51. Jablonski RA, Kolanowski AM, Litaker M. Profile of nursing home residents with dementia who require assistance with mouth care. *Geriatr Nurs* 2011 Nov-Dec; 32(6): 439-446.

52. Dharamsi S, Jivani K, Dean C, Wyatt. Oral care for frail elders: knowledge, attitudes, and practices of long-term care staff. *J Dent Educ* 2009 May; 73(5): 581-588.

53. Kokubu K, Senpuku H, Tada A, Saotome Y, Uematsu H. Impact of routine oral care on opportunistic pathogens in the institutionalized elderly. *J Med Dent Sci* 2008 Mar; 55(1): 7-13.

54. Budtz-Jergensen E, Mojon P, Rentsch A, Deslauriers N. Effects of an oral health program on the occurrence of oral candidosis in a long-term care facility. *Community Dent Oral Epidemiol* 2000 Apr; 28(2): 141-149.

55. Meurman JH, Parnanen P, Kari K, Samaranayake L. Effect of amine fluoride-stannous fluoride preparations on oral yeasts in the elderly: a randomized placebo-controlled trial. *Gerodontology* 2009 Sep; 26(3): 202-209.

56. Adachi M, Ishihara K, Abe S, Okuda K. Professional oral health care by dental hygienists reduced respiratory infections in elderly persons requiring nursing care. *Int J Dent Hyg* 2007 May; 5(2): 69-74.

57. Ishikawa A, Yoneyama T, Hirota K, Miyake Y, Miyatake K. Professional oral health care reduces the number of oropharyngeal bacteria. *J Dent Res* 2008 Jun; 87(6): 594-598.

58. The Centers for Disease Control and Prevention (CDC). *2011 Guidelines for the Prevention of Intravascular Catheter – Related Infections.* CDC website. 2011. Available at: http://www.cdc.gov/hicpac/pdf/guidelines/bsi-guidelines-2011.pdf.

59. Tsan L, Davis C, Langberg R, Hojlo C, Pierce J, Miller M, et al. Prevalence of nursing home-associated infections in the Department of Veterans Affairs nursing home units. *Am J Infect Control* 2008 Apr; 36(3): 173-179.

60. Safdar N, Maki DG. Risk of catheter-related bloodstream infection with peripherally inserted central venous catheters used in hospitalized patients. *Chest* 2005 Aug; 128(2): 489-495.

61. Chopra V, Anand S, Krein SL, Chenowith C, Saint S. Bloodstream infection, venous thrombosis, and peripherally inserted central catheters: reappraising the evidence. *Am J Med* 2012; 125(8): 733-741.

62. Casey AL, Elliott TS. Prevention of central venous catheter-related infection: update. *Br J Nurs* 2010 Jan 28-Feb 10; 19(2): 78,80,82.

63. Cicalini S, Palmieri F, Petrosillo N. Clinical review: new technologies for prevention of intravascular catheter-related infections. *Crit Care* 2004 Jun; 8(3): 157-162.

64. Marnejon T, Angelo D, Abu Abdou A, Gemmel D. Risk factors for upper extremity venous thrombosis associated with peripherally inserted central venous catheters. *J Vasc Access* 2012 Apr-Jun; 13(2): 231-238.

65. Goltz JP, Noack C, Petritsch B, Kirchner J, Hahn D, Kickuth R. Totally implantable venous power ports of the forearm and chest: initial clinical experience with port devices approved for high-pressure injections. *Br J Radiol* 2012 Nov; 85(1019): e966-972.

66. Scott-Cawiezell J, Vogelsmeier A, McKenney C, Rantz M, Hicks L, Zellmer D. Moving from a culture of blame to a culture of safety in the nursing home setting. *Nurs Forum* 2006 Jul-Sep; 41(3): 133-140.

67. Scott-Cawiezell J, Vogelsmeier A. Nursing home safety: a review of the literature. *Annu Rev Nurs Res* 2006; 24: 179-215.

CHAPTER 7

Residents with Advanced Medical Needs

Steven J. Schweon, RN, MPH, MSN, CIC, HEM

KEY CONCEPTS

- The long-term care-based infection preventionist needs a basic understanding of certain advanced medical conditions of residents, the therapies or devices to treat those conditions, and associated infection risks.
- Infection prevention measures are particularly critical for residents with end-stage renal disease who are in need of dialysis treatments.
- Infection preventionists should understand the different types of infusion therapies and monitor residents receiving infusion therapy as part of the facility surveillance program.
- The infection preventionist needs to monitor resident populations with chronic wounds—particularly pressure ulcers—to ensure implementation of wound care strategies to prevent infection and skin breakdown and to heal existing wounds.

This chapter addresses infection risks associated with different types of advanced therapies and discusses strategies for delivering safe care during these therapies by implementing infection prevention best practices. This includes the use and care of positive airway pressure machines, dialysis, infusion therapy, and advanced wound care. For information regarding infection prevention for common categories of nursing care, please refer to Chapter 6.

OBSTRUCTIVE SLEEP APNEA

Obstructive sleep apnea (OSA) is a respiratory disorder in which a resident frequently stops breathing during sleep. OSA is caused by inadequate motor tone of the tongue and/or airway dilator muscles. OSA has been associated with cardiac, neurological, and endocrine disorders, in addition to perioperative complications.[1] Obesity is another risk factor identified in residents with OSA. Residents with OSA may experience depression, anxiety, and fatigue along with strained interpersonal relationships. The infection preventionist (IP) needs to have a basic understanding of OSA, its associated risk factors, and how it is treated, in order to identify the best approach for cleaning and disinfecting the equipment that is used in its management.

The only initial sign of OSA may be snoring. Other signs and symptoms include witnessed apnea events, excessive daytime sleepiness, difficulty concentrating, mood changes, and gasping or choking during sleep. Diagnosis usually occurs during overnight polysomnography testing that will assess the sleep, respiratory, and cardiac disorders.

The definitive treatment for OSA is positive airway pressure (PAP) delivered as continuous positive airway pressure (CPAP), bilateral positive airway pressure (BPAP), or auto positive airway pressure (APAP) modes during sleep.[2] CPAP is the most commonly used method in long-term care facilities (LTCFs). The resident wears a PAP device during sleep, which acts to prevent the pharynx and tongue from collapsing. These devices are oral, nasal, or oronasal in nature. The sleep lab technical team determines the optimal amount of pressure that is needed for each individual. The pressure settings may need to be adjusted over time, and additional dental and surgical modalities may need to be initiated. Residents who use a PAP device usually have improved sleep quality, decreased daytime fatigue, and improved concentration.

Although CPAP treatments can greatly improve a resident's quality of life, there are factors to take into consideration, particularly in regard to use and care of the equipment. The resident may have difficulty tolerating the treatment if the CPAP mask is tight, leaks, blows air into the eyes, or dries out the nose. Dried nasal passages can lead to increased mucous production in the sinuses, rhinitis, and epistaxis. In addition, wearing a mask can lead to skin irritation or breakdown and aggravate allergies. CPAP may need to be temporarily stopped if the resident has a sinus or an upper respiratory tract bacterial/viral infection. A properly fitting mask and humidification will promote comfort and increase compliance. There are many different mask options to assist with promoting resident comfort.

The mask and CPAP device are intended for single-resident use only. The resident's use of the CPAP mask should also be part of the individual's care plan. The mask and tubing are contaminated with microorganisms after every use and could be transmitted to other residents on the hands and uniforms of caregivers. A daily cleaning and disinfection schedule should be developed with input from the resident, if feasible. Consult the manufacturer of the CPAP device for both the use of the appropriate mask, device, and tubing and for the recommended cleaning and disinfection process. This will ensure that the products used for cleaning and disinfection are compatible with the device and its components. Caution must be used to ensure the settings are not accidently altered during the cleaning process.

The CPAP machine should not be stored on the floor. Water from the humidifier may tip into the machine during movement, resulting in potential damage. The manufacturer may recommend using distilled water in the machine; however, the water in the humidifier is a breeding ground for microorganisms such as *Pseudomonas aeruginosa.* Change the water and clean and disinfect the humidity reservoir per the manufacturer's instructions. The filters should also be changed according to manufacturer's recommendations. Assign responsibility on the Treatment Administration Record (TAR) to ensure daily assessment of the system, water and filter changes, and cleaning and disinfection.

END-STAGE RENAL DISEASE

Dialysis—the mechanical removal of excess fluid, electrolytes, metabolic waste, and toxins that would be normally cleared by the kidneys—has been the foundation and initial choice of treating end-stage renal disease (ESRD). The process uses osmosis, diffusion, and ultrafiltration to reduce the body's metabolic waste. Dialysis cannot cure kidney failure; lifelong treatment is needed to maintain normal fluid and electrolyte balance.

Infection is a leading cause of morbidity and is second only to cardiovascular disease as the leading cause of death in the chronic uremic patient on hemodialysis. Infections are a major cause of hospitalizations and carry a greater mortality risk than the general population.[3] The long-term care facility (LTCF) IP needs to have a basic understanding of dialysis to develop policies and procedures that protect this susceptible population from infection.

ESRD residents are at greater infection risk due to the following factors:

- Need for short-term and long-term vascular access resulting in endogenous bacteria potentially invading the bloodstream
- Multiple, frequent encounters with the healthcare environment, such as the hospital or dialysis center
- Frequent exposure to other residents and healthcare personnel (HCP) that may result in person-to-person infectious agent transmission
- Exogenous pathogen exposure from contaminated sources such as HCP hands, equipment, or supplies
- Comorbidities such as diabetes

The number of individuals with ESRD is expected to increase by 2020.[3] The elderly are a substantial and growing population with ESRD.[4] Chronic kidney disease risk factors include diabetes, hypertension, cardiovascular disease, higher body mass index, and advancing age.[5] Identifying residents at risk for potential ESRD can lead to more aggressive management of these comorbid diseases and risk factors. This in turn may lead to improved disease management and lessen the need for dialysis.

The benefits of dialysis include extending life and improving quality of life. These benefits are more uncertain in the elderly.[6] After initiating dialysis, mortality in the first year exceeds 35 percent among patients 70 years of age and older, and exceeds 50 percent among patients 80 years of age and older.[7] ESRD treatment options include:

- In-center hemodialysis: free-standing dialysis center for hemodialysis treatments
- Home hemodialysis: hemodialysis in the patient's home
- Nocturnal hemodialysis: sleeping at the dialysis center overnight and undergoing hemodialysis
- Daily short dialysis: 5 to 6 days of receiving hemodialysis with shortened treatment time
- Peritoneal dialysis:
  - **Continuous ambulatory peritoneal dialysis (CAPD):** a continuous process using the peritoneum as an artificial kidney
  - **Continuous cyclic peritoneal dialysis (CCPD):** peritoneal dialysis done at night while connected to a machine
- Renal transplant
- No treatment: palliative/comfort care

The Centers for Disease Control and Prevention (CDC) have issued recommendations for preventing infection transmission among chronic hemodialysis patients.[8] The IP must review these recommendations and implement pertinent findings into the organization's infection prevention program.

Dialysis may be started in situations with limited life expectancy to alleviate symptoms like shortness of breath and to improve functional status—the ability to perform activities of daily living such as walking, bathing, or using the toilet. One study noted that after 1 year of initiating dialysis, one of eight nursing home residents had a functional capacity that was maintained at the predialysis level, suggesting functional decline in most residents with ESRD continues despite dialysis.[6] The authors suggest the functional decline in this population is due to:

- A high disability prevalence at baseline
- Coexisting morbidities, such as cerebral vascular accident (CVA), dementia
- Hospitalization
- Physical risks associated with dialysis
- Psychosocial burden
- Kidney failure reflecting multiorgan dysfunction

Vascular Access for Short-term and Long-term Dialysis

Residents who require short-term dialysis will need placement of a temporary dialysis access catheter in the jugular, subclavian, or femoral vein. Residents who require long-term dialysis treatment require permanent, long-term vascular access. This is done via arteriovenous (AV) fistulas or grafts, which are created by surgically connecting an artery and a vein, resulting in a permanent anastomosis under the skin.

AV fistulas are the preferred vascular access route for long-term dialysis patients because they last the longest, have the best performance, and are less prone to infection and clotting. The fistula allows adequate, proper blood flow during dialysis, leading to stronger veins and easing repeated needle insertions. The surgery can be performed as an outpatient procedure. The fistula is usually placed in the nondominant arm and may be visible. The upper arm may be used for placement if the forearm access fails or if the arteries and veins are small and unsuitable for creating the fistula.

Fistulas take a few months to heal and function properly. No phlebotomy or blood pressures are to be performed on the affected arm. Temporary dialysis access is required as it takes several months for the fistula to properly develop. Not all patients may be eligible for a fistula. Stenosis or narrowing of the blood vessel is the most common problem, resulting in decreased blood flow and clotting. The vascular surgeon may opt to send the resident to interventional radiology for probable fibrinolysis and percutaneous transluminal angioplasty or to the operating room for a surgical thrombectomy and revision of the impaired vasculature.

An arteriovenous graft (AVG) is similar to an AV fistula. Instead of a direct artery to vein connection, the AVG is created by indirectly connecting an artery to a vein by synthetic vessel tubing, which supports blood flow. Grafts are used when patients have veins that will not develop into a suitable fistula. The graft is surgically implanted under the skin in the arm, as an outpatient procedure. Following surgery, there may be pain and swelling over the graft for 3 to 4 weeks. Keeping the arm elevated will promote comfort. After the edema abates, the graft can be used for needle insertion during the dialysis treatment. With the graft, there is increased risk of infection and clotting.

Nursing care of the AV fistula and graft to prevent infection includes:

- Following postoperative surgical instructions for wound healing
- Washing over the access site daily with soap and water and again before dialysis
- Ensuring the hemodialysis staff use rigorous aseptic techniques to clean and disinfect the skin before access
- Monitoring the resident and surgical site for potential infection and signs and symptoms include redness, tenderness, purulence, and fever

Additional nursing care considerations for ESRD residents will be required. Consult with the dialysis provider to clarify resident-specific recommendations.

Temporary Dialysis

Central venous catheters (CVC) are inserted and used when there is an emergent dialysis treatment need and while waiting for the AV fistula or graft to mature. Insertion sites include the internal jugular, subclavian, and femoral veins. Placement can be performed as an outpatient procedure. The CDC guidelines for preventing catheter-related infections have evidenced-based recommendations for both catheter insertion and maintenance.[9] Strategies address:

- Hand hygiene and aseptic technique
- Maximal sterile barrier precautions
- Skin preparations
- Catheter site dressing regimens

Tunneled Catheters

A tunneled CVC is inserted surgically. There are two types of CVCs: cuffed or noncuffed. Tunneled noncuff catheters are for emergencies and may be used for up to 3 weeks. Tunneled cuff catheters can be used for temporary access (beyond 3 weeks) while waiting for the AVF or AVG to mature. After placement, dialysis can be performed immediately. Temporary catheters exit from the insertion site. The exit site is treated and dressed using strict aseptic technique. Temporary dialysis catheters have high complication rates, including infection at the exit site and bacteremia. To prevent infection, nursing care of the temporary dialysis catheter should include:

- Following postprocedure instructions for wound healing
- Performing hand hygiene prior to any type of nursing care
- Having the dialysis nurse perform the skin disinfection and dressing change
- Not submerging the catheter or the catheter site in water; showering is acceptable if the catheter and the insertion site can be protected with a tested, impermeable cover
- Keeping the catheter caps on at all times; only the dialysis staff should remove and access
- Notifying the dialysis center immediately if:
  - The cap falls off
  - The catheter develops hole or leak
- Ensuring the hemodialysis staff use rigorous aseptic techniques to clean and disinfect the skin before access

Accessing the vascular system through the AVF, AVG, and the CVC significantly contributes to the risk of infection. The CVC poses the greatest risk with the chance for infection rising the longer the catheter is present or being used. Bacteremia may lead to endocarditis or osteomyelitis, requiring hospitalization. Antimicrobial catheter lock solutions may be used to prevent catheter-associated blood stream infection, but this use has not been approved by the U.S. Food and Drug Administration. Use of the antimicrobial lock solutions may result in toxicity, allergic reactions, hemorrhage, and bacterial resistance.

Dialysis-associated CVC infections result from pathogen transmission from the skin outside the catheter or from catheter intraluminal migration. Less frequent sources include contaminated infusate solution, bacterial seeding from a distant infection site, and dialysate back-flow. AVFs have the lowest infection risk when compared to AVGs and CVCs.

Staphylococcus aureus and coagulase-negative *Staphylococcus* are the most common pathogens responsible for access-related blood stream infections. The risk of methicillin-resistant *Staphylococcus aureus* invasive infection is more than 100 times greater in dialysis patients in comparison to the general population.[3] Gram-negative and polymicrobial organisms also contribute to bloodstream infections. The development of biofilm on indwelling catheters greatly contributes to the infection risk. Early fistula placement, adhering to recommended AVF and AVG infection prevention maintenance practices, and minimizing catheter use will assist with reducing vascular access-associated infections.

The Centers for Medicare & Medicaid Services (CMS) recognizes the importance of proper vascular access to maintaining the resident's overall health, including infection prevention. The Conditions for Coverage are minimum health and safety standards for improving care. LTCFs must meet the following two standards for Medicare and Medicaid reimbursement for hemodialysis residents:[10]

> The interdisciplinary team must provide vascular access monitoring and appropriate, timely referrals to achieve and sustain vascular access. The hemodialysis patient must be evaluated for the appropriate vascular access type, taking into consideration co-morbid conditions, other risk factors, and whether the patient is a potential candidate for arteriovenous fistula placement.
>
> If the patient's vascular access is not an arteriovenous fistula, the record should indicate why the patient was determined to not be a candidate for a fistula.

Dialysis treatments are usually scheduled 3 days a week for 3 to 4 hours at a time. A resident's temperature should be measured and recorded at least before and after each dialysis treatment. Any temperature greater than 100°F (37.8°C), chills, or other unexplained symptoms occurring after onset of hemodialysis should be evaluated for relationship to water treatment, dialysis equipment, and dialysis and reprocessing procedures.[11]

Antimicrobial resistance is common in residents with ESRD due to numerous infection episodes that may have resulted in a prolonged antibiotic(s) treatment course.

Additionally, numerous hospitalizations and surgical procedures may have led to multidrug-resistant organism (MDRO) colonization and potential infection with MRSA, vancomycin-resistant enterococci (VRE), and other multidrug-resistant gram-negative organisms such as *Acinetobacter baumannii* and *Escherichia coli.* Antibiotic exposure also puts these residents at greater risk for *Clostridium difficile* infection.

Suspected remote, nondialysis-associated infections should be quickly identified and properly treated. Culture reports will assist with appropriate antibiotic therapy and prevent bacterial seeding to the dialysis access site.

Peritoneal dialysis (PD) uses the peritoneal membrane for waste removal. A surgically placed catheter is inserted into the abdominal cavity for dialysate infusion. This approach takes several hours a day, 7 days a week. Infection complications include peritonitis, tunnel infection, exit site infection, and death. Deep cuff infections may require catheter removal. To prevent infection, HCP caring for the PD catheter must use meticulous sterile technique, including performing hand hygiene prior to access and wearing a mask when connecting the catheter to the tubing.

An additional infection risk is exposure to the Hepatitis B virus (HBV), Hepatitis C virus (HCV), and the human immunodeficiency virus (HIV) from other patients' blood during the dialysis treatment. HBV and HCV outbreaks have been reported in dialysis facilities.[3] Exposure occurs when there is a breakdown in sterile technique and other infection prevention precautions that may lead to contaminated equipment. The use of erythropoietin has reduced the need for blood transfusions and potential exposure to contaminated products. HBV transmission in hemodialysis facilities has been decreasing due to implementing infection prevention practices and vaccinating patients and staff with the HBV vaccine.

The CDC recommends HBV vaccination for hemodialysis patients and those with renal disease that may result in dialysis, although the vaccine response is less robust when compared to the general population.[3,12] A higher vaccine dose is given and serology testing is done after the series has been completed to confirm immunity. Ensure the resident is vaccinated, either through the LTCF or the hemodialysis facility. Unfortunately, there is no HCV vaccine available at the time of this manual's publication. All HCP should use Standard Precautions when coming into contact with body fluids. Additionally, safe injection practices should be the standard of care for all residents, regardless of their hepatitis or HIV status. Clean and disinfect the resident's environment and medical equipment on a regular schedule using EPA-registered, facility-approved, cleaner and disinfectant.

Dialysis centers should perform HBV and HCV resident testing on a schedule. The IP must be able to interpret hepatitis serology laboratory reports (see Table 7.1). Because HCV is increasing in the community, screening for long-term care residents may be required. See Figure 7.1 for the recommended testing process for HCV.

In addition to the infection risks already discussed, residents with chronic kidney disease are susceptible to influenza and pneumococcal disease and associated secondary complications. LTCFs should offer the seasonal and pandemic (if available) influenza vaccine per facility policy, as well as the one dose pneumococcal polysaccharide vaccine to ESRD residents. Provide a booster dose if more than 5 years have lapsed since initial administration of the vaccine. Additionally, offer the influenza and HBV vaccine to all the facility's HCP as an adjunct resident safety measure.

Educate the resident and their family on the importance of infection prevention strategies, including maintaining the hemodialysis catheter, hand hygiene, and vaccination. Document the teaching and the response. Additionally, educate the front-line staff on the importance of infection prevention in this vulnerable population. Carefully monitor for possible signs of infection including fever, chills, rigors, drainage from the catheter exit site, redness/tenderness around the catheter exit site, and a general feeling of weakness/not feeling well. The CDC has additional dialysis safety educational materials available for the IP, HCP, and residents.[13]

The resident may have to travel to a dialysis unit or the procedure may be performed within the facility. The dialysis staff must report any resident infections to the LTCF nursing staff. The IP should visit the dialysis unit,

TABLE 7.1: INTERPRETING HEPATITIS B SEROLOGY RESULTS

Test	Result	Interpretation
HBsAg anti-HBc anti-HBs	negative negative negative	Susceptible
HBsAg anti-HBc anti-HBs	negative positive positive	Immune due to natural infection
HBsAg anti-HBc anti-HBs	negative negative positive	Immune due to hepatitis B vaccination
HBsAg anti-HBc IgM anti-HBc anti-HBs	positive positive positive negative	Acutely infected
HBsAg anti-HBc IgM anti-HBc anti-HBs	positive positive negative negative	Chronically infected
HBsAg anti-HBc anti-HBs	negative positive negative	Interpretation unclear; four possibilities: • Resolved infection (most common) • False-positive anti-HBc, thus susceptible • "Low level" chronic infection • Resolving acute infection

Adapted from: A Comprehensive Immunization Strategy to Eliminate Transmission of Hepatitis B Virus Infection in the United States; Recommendations of the Advisory Committee on Immunization Practices, Part I: Immunization of Infacts, Children, and Adolescents, MMWR 2006;54(No. RR-16) Courtesy of Centers for Disease Control and Prevention. Available at: http://www.cdc.gov/hepatitis/hbv/pdfs/serologicchartv8.pdf.

become familiar with the staff, and review the dialysis policy and procedure manual. Additionally, the dialysis unit should submit a scheduled report to the Infection Prevention and Control Committee. The report should include identified infections, water testing results, and any problems with the dialysis units.

INFUSION THERAPY

Infusion therapy is the administration of fluids and medications through a catheter into a vein. In recent years, infusion therapy has shifted from being managed entirely in the acute care hospital setting to the long-term care environment. Hospitals are now discharging sicker patients who require infusion therapy to LTCFs. LTCFs may also receive patients who are not sick enough to qualify for hospitalization and do not have the option to receive infusion therapy at home. Residents with acute and chronic diseases such as cardiac disease, diabetes, or cancer may also receive infusion therapy in the LTCF to prevent unnecessary hospitalization and assist with maintaining health and promoting longevity.

There are several factors that are driving this infusion therapy practice change from acute care to long-term care. These factors include prospective payment reimbursement changes, managed care mandates and restrictions, and patients/family members desiring a quicker hospital discharge. The LTCF's stable, home-like environment and high quality of care make it a safer setting for residents with cognitive and functional challenges. This change also results in reduced healthcare costs and hospital admissions, increased LTCF admissions, and a greater continuity of care.

Historically, LTCF have been unable to provide infusion therapy beyond peripheral IVs due to lack of expertise in advanced infusion therapy and a lack of onsite radiology/laboratory services. Additionally, physicians may not have been available onsite to assess the resident in the event of complications. With the shift in providing infusion therapy in LTCFs rather than hospitals, many LTCFs now have trained, competent staff using evidenced-based policies and procedures to safely administer total parenteral nutrition (TPN), pain management, antimicrobials (e.g., antibiotics, antiviral, and antifungal medications), chemotherapy, inotropics, transfusion therapy, and end-of-life medications through midline and central venous catheters. The resident population of LTCFs is more susceptible to infection due to declining immune function that is part of the normal aging process. Infection risk increases in LTCF populations with debilitated and chronically ill residents of all ages.

FIGURE 7.1: RECOMMENDED TESTING SEQUENCE FOR IDENTIFYING CURRENT HEPATITIS C (HCV) INFECTION

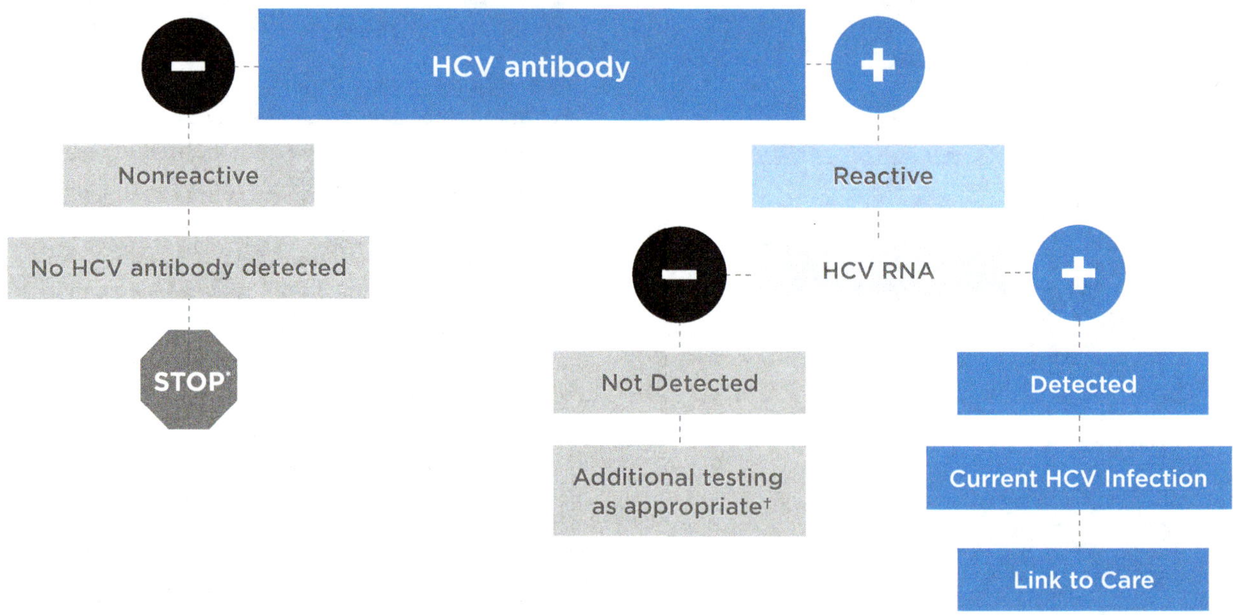

* For persons who might have been exposed to HCV within the past 6 months, testing for HCV RNA or follow-up testing for HCV antibody is recommended. For persons who are immunocompromised, testing for HCV RNA can be considered.

† To differentiate past, resolved HCV infection from biologic false positivity for HCV antibody, testing with another HCV antibody assay can be considered. Repeat HCV RNA testing if the person tested is suspected to have had HCV exposure within the past 6 months or has clinical evidence of HCV disease, or if there is concern regarding the handling or storage of the test specimen.

Source: CDC. *Testing for HCV infection: An update of guidance for clinicians and laboratorians.* MMWR 2013;62(18). Courtesy of Centers for Disease Control and Prevention. Available at: http://www.cdc.gov/hepatitis/hcv/PDFs/hcv_flow.pdf

For residents who receive infusion therapy, the catheter type, duration of use, access frequency, and catheter care are all additional factors that can contribute to infection. The IP should be knowledgeable about the aging process, physical assessment, and infection prevention interventions to promote safe work practices and optimal outcomes while administering infusion therapy. The IP should use evidenced-based guidelines and recommendations from the CDC[9] and the Infusion Nurses Society[14] to develop policies and procedures that minimize the risk of catheter-related infections and other complications from infusion therapy. The IP should also include monitoring of residents who are receiving infusion therapy as part of the infection prevention and control surveillance plan.

Infusion therapy is an invasive procedure and informed consent is required prior to proceeding. The advantages and risks of the insertion procedure and ongoing therapy need to be fully understood at the onset. The resident should have an active role with all decision making, when possible. However, the resident's cognitive function may be impaired due to:

- Medications and polypharmacy
- Sensory defects, such as hearing deficit
- Chronic medical conditions like cerebral vascular accident (CVA) or Alzheimer's disease
- Acute medical condition such as infection
- Hypoxemia
- Dehydration
- Electrolyte alteration

The LTCF must be aware of the resident's advance directives, existing healthcare proxies, and cognitive status prior to moving forward with an invasive procedure. The resident's family may be a resource to obtain consent when the resident is not considered capable of decision making.

The type of catheter depends on the type and duration of therapy. Options include:

- Peripheral catheter insertion
- Midline catheter insertion
- Peripherally inserted central catheters (PICC)
- Long dwelling implantable ports

An acute infectious process such as pneumonia may hamper cognition due to hypoxia. An infection may also result in pain, which may impair thinking. If infection is suspected, it may be necessary to transport the resident with a suspected infection to another facility for laboratory studies. This may result in a therapeutic intervention delay and may impede recovery. Additionally, hospitalization may be required if the resident is severely compromised.

From the infection prevention and resident safety perspective, determine the ideal location for cannulation. Aging results in less venous elasticity, making vein cannulation more challenging. Assess if the resident has a history of phlebitis. If the resident is receiving physical or occupational therapy involving the arm, an alternative location should be used to minimize catheter movement. Assess if the resident is agitated, confused, or disoriented; there is the potential risk of the resident pulling out the infusion tubing and the catheter. Placing the infusion therapy in the nondominant extremity may foster independence. Additionally, aging results in decreased pain sensation and skin thickness. This may alter the resident's perception of infiltration, tissue damage, and skin tears/ulceration.

Central line insertion requires strict aseptic technique to prevent infection.[9,14] Prior to cannulation, the insertion site is treated with an antimicrobial agent to reduce the potential for infection. Follow the manufacturer's recommendations when applying the antimicrobial agent and be aware that excessive friction during application may damage the resident's skin. Using alcohol may result in skin dryness. Excessive hair over the insertion site should be clipped; shaving with a razor may result in skin breakdown, leading to a portal of entry for microorganisms and potential infection. A stabilization device should be used to secure the catheter and prevent phlebitis after the procedure is completed. Using tape may result in a skin tear. During and after the procedure, the resident may require frequent reassurances and reminders about the need for infusion therapy. The nursing staff should be well educated in the dressing change procedure and may require competency verification to ensure safe practice.

Hand hygiene must be performed prior to administering infusion therapy. Medication labels should be carefully checked for the correct resident's name and expiration date. The medication should be observed for cloudiness, discoloration, particulates, and leakage. Any medication with these changes should not be administered and the pharmacy must be consulted immediately.

Intravenous medications requiring refrigeration should be stored between 36°F and 46° F (2° C and 8° C.) This is different than recommended food storage temperatures, so separate temperature logs should be developed. Only medications should be stored in the medication refrigerator. Staff should check and document the refrigerator temperature at least daily. Deficiencies should be reported to the maintenance department and the pharmacy. Expiration dates should be monitored. The electrical outlet serving the refrigerator should have an alternative, immediate power source such as a generator in the event of a power outage.

Most LTCFs outsource their pharmaceutical and infusion support to a consulting pharmacy or infusion service for medications, supplies, equipment, and technical support. These vendors partner closely with the LTCF to ensure safe resident care. This may include product selection. The IP should review policies and procedures for consistency and to ensure they are aligned with best practices.

Teaching the resident and family about infusion therapy will assist with informed consent, promote health, and prevent adverse outcomes, including infection. Infection prevention topics include:

- Monitoring the infusion site for possible redness, warmth, swelling, edema
- Changing tubing and dressings on a set schedule and recording on the TAR
- Frequently assessing the resident for signs of

possible infection such as fever and notifying a physician if necessary

The resident needs strict monitoring to ensure the treatment is being tolerated and there are no complications. LTCF nursing staff must be educated and able to manage the resident's infusion therapy and prevent infection. Policies, procedures, and competencies ensure staff is practicing safely and promoting infection prevention. The IP should randomly audit infusion therapy care practices to ensure they are consistent with policy.

In certain fragile residents, intravenous access may not be a viable option. Alternative infusion therapies include hypodermoclysis—the infusion of solution into subcutaneous tissue. It is performed when the resident is unable to take fluids intravenously or orally. The IP must be aware of the various infusion options and the potential for infection.

For additional information on infusion therapy, see Chapter 6.

SKIN, SOFT TISSUE, AND WOUND INFECTIONS

The integument is the largest organ in the body. It is the first line of protection against bacterial invasion and it assists with regulating temperature. Skin breakdown caused by trauma allows microorganisms to enter the body and multiply. The entry of microorganisms triggers the immune response. Tissue injury will trigger an inflammatory response. Infection occurs when the host is unable to effectively manage and contain the bacterial invasion. Paradoxically, the inflammatory response stimulates wound vasoconstriction, which results in tissue hypoxia and increased bacterial growth.

Wounds can result from:

- Surgery; infection is classified as a surgical site infection (SSI)
- Impaired blood flow from venous and arterial insufficiency
- Burns
- Injury
- Neuropathy and impaired sensation resulting from diabetes or multiple sclerosis
- Terminal illness, as part of multisystem organ failure (MSOF)
- Pressure, usually over a bony prominence, resulting in a pressure ulcer

A wound is tissue injury caused by trauma such as cutting, piercing, or tearing. Wounds are classified as acute (sudden onset) or chronic (nonhealing). Acute wounds usually close with minimal intervention while chronic wounds require aggressive treatment and care and may be very challenging to manage. This chapter addresses advanced wound care management, specifically in regard to pressure ulcers. For basic skin and wound assessment guidance, please refer to Chapter 6 on Nursing Care.

The IP must have a basic understanding of wound care management, including an understanding of:

- Wound pathophysiology
- Strategies to prevent complications and promote healing
- Treatment modalities including managing the infected wound
- Prevention strategies to prevent skin disruption and compromise
- Chronic wounds as a risk factor for MDRO colonization

Pressure ulcers develop due to immobility through prolonged lying or sitting position and a sedentary lifestyle. The constant pressure deprives the tissues of oxygen and nutrients, resulting in ischemia, cellular death, and tissue necrosis. A shear can cause additional injury. Additional risk factors for pressure ulcer development include:

- Fever
- Anemia
- Infection
- Hypotension
- Malnutrition
- Spinal cord injury (SCI)
- Neurological disease
- Decreased body mass index (BMI)
- Increased metabolic rate
- Skin maceration
- Ischemia
- Advanced age

- Chronic illness such as diabetes or cancer
- Weakness
- Altered mental status
- Skin conditions such as edema or pruritus
- Incontinence
- Vascular disease
- History of pressure ulcers

CMS provides specific regulatory guidance and oversight on the prevention of pressure ulcers in LTCF residents. The CMS State Operations Manual F314 §483.25(c) states:[15]

1. A resident who enters the facility without pressure sores does not develop pressure sores unless the individual's clinical condition demonstrates that they were unavoidable; and
2. A resident having pressure sores receives necessary treatment and services to promote healing, prevent infection, and prevent new sores from developing.

LTCFs are required to have individualized interventions in place for residents at risk of developing pressure ulcers to prevent their formation. For residents with pressure ulcers, CMS requires that facilities have treatment protocols in place based on current standards of practice and in accordance with facility policies and procedures.

Wounds may be found in both hospitalized patients who are transferred to LTCFs and in residents currently living within the facility. Wounds such as the Kennedy terminal ulcer may also develop in late stages of the dying process. Wound care not only increases the potential for human suffering, but also the risk of rehospitalization, the need for advanced clinical therapies including surgery, and the economic burden for healthcare providers. Interventions to prevent skin breakdown, maintain skin integrity, and prevent wound development include:

- Performing meticulous skin care with a pH-balanced skin cleanser instead of soap
- Using a lower pH cleanser, applying a moisture barrier to the skin, and changing pads frequently for residents who are incontinent
- Repositioning every 2 hours and as needed; tissue tolerance testing assists with personalizing repositioning routines and schedules in the chair and bed
- Using a pressure-reducing mattress
- Assessing skin integrity frequently
- Avoiding friction and shearing forces
- Using pressure-relieving cushions
- Providing enteral or parenteral support
- Preventing muscle spasms that can lead to abrasions
- Preventing contractures that impede flexibility and mobility
- Optimizing blood supply and tissue perfusion
- Maintaining glycemic control
- Reducing edema
- Maintaining warmth and preventing chilling of the extremities

Variables that influence wound healing include the size and depth; superficial wounds involving the epidermis and dermis will heal faster than deeper wounds extending to the muscle and bone. Wound healing is also impacted by:

- The resident's age
- Presence of infection
- Circulation
- Medications
- Nutrition
- Activity
- Hydration
- Moisture and fluid balance

Wound colonization is characterized by microorganisms on the wound surface without a host immune response. There are no signs or symptoms of infection. Bacterial colonization is normal in all wounds and may help protect the wound against virulent organisms.

Infection, the presence of microorganisms resulting in disease, is the most common complication of pressure ulcers and may at times be difficult to diagnose.[16] Nursing staff must continually assess the resident for potential infection. Due to immune system decline, an elderly resident may not be able to mount a fever and a robust immune response when encountering infection. The nurse must also inspect the wound for:

- Thick green or yellow drainage
- Purulence

- Foul odor
- Redness and warmth (postoperative inflammation of a surgical incision is expected for several days after the procedure)
- Edema
- Bleeding
- Hardness
- Pain
- Delayed healing
- Wound breakdown

There may be leukocytosis. Infection may also spread to surrounding tissues, potentially resulting in cellulitis and a sinus tract abscess. The resident with diabetes may have elevated blood glucose levels. Residents who are immunocompromised may have a diminished localized and systemic response to infection.

Routine wound cultures may not be routinely obtained unless infection is suspected. Specific surveillance cultures for the presence of a MDRO may be ordered. Aerobic bacteria are found in all pressure ulcers with anaerobes tending to be present in larger wounds. The most common organisms isolated from pressure wounds include *Proteus mirabilis*, Group D Streptococci, *Escherichia coli*, *Staphylococcus* species, *Pseudomonas* species, and *Corynebacterium* organisms.[15] An infectious disease physician will coordinate antibiotic treatment.

Wound cultures may assist with the infection diagnosis. Specimens obtained from viable instead of necrotic tissue are the most beneficial. There are different techniques to obtain cultures:

- The tissue biopsy is the gold standard.[17] This technique is invasive, skill-intensive, and may be unavailable in some settings. Viable wound tissue is removed with a scalpel or punch biopsy instrument. This technique is beyond the nursing scope of practice.
- The needle-aspiration technique obtains fluid from multiple insertions into the tissue surrounding the wound. This technique is also beyond the nursing scope of practice.
- The swab culture technique is widely available, and the wound surface organism is cultured instead of tissue. It may be difficult to recover anaerobic organisms. Cleansing the wound prior to culturing will assist with removing organisms in the wound exudate and nonviable tissue. There are different culture techniques when obtaining the specimen; consider consulting with the wound care specialist for the optimal approach.

The microbiology laboratory isolates, identifies, and quantifies the types and amounts of organisms obtained. The amount of organisms present reflects microorganism replication. Alternatively, semiquantitative cultures reflect colony counts that are reported from 1 to 4+, with 4+ indicating the largest amount. Antimicrobial testing is performed to determine if a particular antibiotic agent is sensitive, intermediate, or resistant to the cultured microorganism. The minimum inhibitory concentration (MIC) is a laboratory measurement that tests for the lowest concentration of the antibiotic agent that will inhibit the growth of the microorganism. An antibiotic with a low MIC can be an indication of a more effective choice. Additionally, clinically, the resident's signs, symptoms, and culture results are all assessed to assist with the infection diagnosis.

Deep tissue infections may require parenteral antibiotic therapy and surgical intervention/debridement. Oral antibiotic therapy may be used for less serious wounds. Topical antibiotics, depending on the type of wound, may also be prescribed. Antibiotic effectiveness will depend on the blood flow to the infected tissue.

Infection may also become more invasive, spreading to the bone, especially when the bone is exposed (osteomyelitis), and to the bloodstream (bacteremia and sepsis), potentially resulting in hospitalization. Underlying muscle and bone may be destroyed. The resident may experience fever, chills, weakness, mental status changes, tachycardia, hypotension, and leukocytosis, which increases the mortality risk.

When performing surveillance, use the 2012 LTCF surveillance definitions for consistency, formerly referred to as the McGeer Criteria.[18] These definitions are for epidemiological use only and were not designed for clinical diagnosis or as minimum criteria for starting antibiotics. The criteria for meeting the clinical diagnosis definition may vary from the epidemiological definition. Appropriate antibiotic therapy in the LTCF depends on:

- Whether the infection is localized or systemic
- Drug allergies
- Metabolic impairments such as decreased renal or liver function
- How effectively the antibiotic penetrates the tissues
- Resident's body weight
- Medication impact upon the hemopoietic system
- Delivery route, such as oral or intravenous

Antibiotic therapy will alter the gastrointestinal flora, which may increase the risk of *C. difficile* infection. The management of the resident with a pelvic, perineal, or rectal wound coupled with *C. difficile* diarrhea can make wound care very challenging.

Antibiotic resistance is an ongoing concern. The culture and sensitivity report will help guide appropriate antibiotic therapy. The microbiology lab should notify the nursing unit of epidemiologically significant organisms such as MRSA. Depending on the LTCF's policy, residents may need Contact Precautions if the culture is positive for MDROs like MRSA, VRE, or a multidrug-resistant gram-negative bacilli. In addition, antibiotic therapy may result in secondary infections such as oral candidiasis, requiring treatment with an antifungal agent.

When developing a treatment strategy, determine the stage of the wound and outline the therapy goals accordingly. A wound care specialist may be consulted and can become an active team member. A surgery consult may also be needed. Devitalized tissue should be debrided.

Sterile technique involves hand hygiene, sterile field, gloves, dressings, and instruments. Clean technique involves hand hygiene, clean field, clean gloves, and sterile instruments. Practice Standard Precautions when providing wound care. Wear the appropriate personal protective equipment, including facial protection and a gown if splashing is anticipated. Avoid cross-contamination of healthy tissue during care. A position statement is available to assist the IP when determining if sterile or clean technique should be performed during treatment; refer to Table 7.2 for additional guidance.[19]

Monitor wound infections closely for potential improvement opportunities. Regardless of the treatment interventions, the IP should have a generalized knowledge of wound healing. The IP needs to review policies to ensure:

- When sterile versus clean technique is used
- Cleaning/disinfecting practices are in place for equipment (e.g., special beds, support mattresses, or whirlpool baths)
- Wound care competencies are offered when appropriate, with emphasis on infection prevention during dressing changes

Cleansing wound solutions are used to decrease the bioburden and contamination and promote wound healing. The solution used depends on the nature of the wound and may include the following:

- Normal saline is used for wound irrigation and as a rinse after other solutions are used.
- Povidone-iodine is useful against microorganisms and should be discontinued when granulation tissue occurs. Iodine toxicity can occur in residents with large, open wounds.
- Acetic acid is effective against *Pseudomonas aeruginosa*.
- Sodium hypochlorite is used to debride necrotic tissue. Zinc oxide should be used around the tissues edges to prevent skin irritation.
- Hydrogen peroxide is not recommended for long-term use due to its toxicity to fibroblasts.

Wound cleanser and normal saline solutions are prepared commercially and are sterile. Date all products being used and follow manufacturer recommendations with expiration dates. For example, a normal saline bottle should be disposed 24 hours after opening.

The purpose of wound debridement is to remove necrotic tissue, eschar, and slough that promote infection and delay healing. Debridement may be done by use of enzymes; mechanical nonselective debridement such as wet-to-dry dressings, whirlpool treatments, and forceful irrigation; or sharp debridement through surgery.

A multitude of semipermeable and occlusive dressings are available for healing. They assist with keeping the wound bed moist and promote healing. The purpose of these dressings is to:

- Reduce the incidence of secondary infection
- Prevent maceration of healthy skin around wound
- Reduce the risk of traumatic removal

TABLE 7.2: SUGGESTED PRECAUTIONS FOR CHRONIC WOUND PROCEDURES

Intervention	Hand-washing	Gloves	Supplies Includes solutions and dressing supplies	Instruments
Wound Cleansing	Yes	Clean*	Normal saline or commercially prepared wound cleanser—sterile; maintain as clean per care setting policy**	Irrigation with sterile device; maintain as clean per care setting policy
Routine dressing change without debridement	Yes	Clean*	Sterile; maintain as clean per care setting policy**	Sterile; maintain as clean per care setting policy**
Dressing change with mechanical, chemical, or enzymatic debridement	Yes	Clean*	Sterile; maintain as clean per care setting policy**	Sterile; maintain as clean per care setting policy**
Dressing change with sharp, conservative bedside debridement	Yes	Sterile*	Sterile	Sterile

* It must be remembered that reimbursement of wound care delivered in the outpatient and home care setting is governed by regulations mandated by the Healthcare Financing Administration (HCFA). HCFA requires use of sterile supplies and equipment, including gloves. Deviations from HCFA regulations in the delivery of wound care could result in submission of fraudulent claims for reimbursement.

** "Maintain clean as per care setting policy" means each care setting must address the parameters for maintenance, such as expiration dates for supplies, consideration of cost, and correct interpretation of the manufacturer's recommendations.

From *APIC-WOCN position statement: Clean versus sterile: Management of chronic wounds.* Available at: http://www.apic.org/Resource/TinyMceFileManager/Position Statements/Clean-Vs-Sterile.pdf.

The different dressing types include:

- Alginates
- Foams
- Gauzes
- Hydrocolloids
- Hydrogels
- Transparent films
- Wound fillers
- Wound pouches

Negative pressure therapy using a vacuum-assisted closure (wound vac) enhances healing by stimulating circulation with leukocytes, reducing the bacterial load and edema, and increasing granulation tissue formation. Other therapies to reduce bacterial bioburden and promote healing include hyperbaric oxygen therapy, silver impregnated dressings, and ultraviolet light (UV). Additional wound healing references are available from http://www.woundheal.org/whs-wound-care-guidelines.

Depending on the type and size of the wound, showering and bathing may be possible. Consult with the wound care specialist for guidance. A plastic cover may need to be used during showering for protection. Bathing in hot water can lead to additional skin dryness and breakdown. Skin lotion should never be applied directly into the wound. During routine care, the nursing staff should have a heightened awareness for additional skin breakdown.

REFERENCES

1. Park JG, Ramar G, Olson E. Updates on definition, consequences, and management of obstructive sleep apnea. *Mayo Clin Proc* 2011; 86(6): 549-555.

2. Simmons S, Pruitt B. Sounding the alarm for patients with obstructive sleep apnea. *Nursing* 2012; 42(4): 34-41.

3. U.S. Department of Health and Human Services (HHS). *National action plan to prevent healthcare-associated infections: Roadmap to elimination.* HHS website. (n.d.). Available at: http://www.hhs.gov/ash/initiatives/hai/esrd.html.

4. Kurella M, Covinsky KE, Collins AJ, Chertow GM. Octogenarians and nonagenarians starting dialysis in the United States. *Ann Intern Med* 2007; 146: 177-183.

5. United States Renal Data System (USRDS). *2012 annual data report. CKD in the general population.* USRDS website. 2012. Available at: http://www.usrds.org/2012/pdf/v1_ch1_12.pdf.

6. Tamura MK, Covinsky KE, Chertow GM, Yaffe K, Landefeld CS, McCulloch CE. Functional status of elderly adults before and after initiation of dialysis. *N Engl J Med* 2009; 361(16): 1539-1547.

7. Collins AJ, Kasiske B, Herzog C, Chavers B, Foley R, Gilbertson D, et al. Excerpts from the United States Renal Data System 2004 annual data report: atlas of end-stage renal disease in the United States. *Am J Kidney Dis* 2005; 45: Suppl 1: A5-A7, S1-S280.

8. Centers for Disease Control and Prevention (CDC). Recommendations for preventing transmission of infections among chronic hemodialysis patients. *MMWR Recomm Rep* 2001; 50(RR05): 1-43.

9. O'Grady N, Alexander M, Burns LA, Dellinger EP, Garland J, Heard SO, et al. *Guidelines for the prevention of intravascular catheter-related infections, 2011.* CDC website. 2011. Available at: http://www.cdc.gov/hicpac/pdf/guidelines/bsi-guidelines-2011.pdf.

10. Centers for Medicare & Medicaid Services (CMS), HHS. Medicare and Medicaid programs; conditions for coverage for end-stage renal disease facilities; final rule. *Fed Regist* 2008; 73(73): 20369-20484.

11. Garcia-Houchins S. Dialysis. In: Carrico R, ed. *APIC Text of Infection Control and Epidemiology,* 3rd ed. Washington, DC: Association for Professionals in Infection Control and Epidemiology, Inc., 2009: 48-1–48-17.

12. Immunization Action Coalition (IAC). *Summary of recommendations for adult immunization.* IAC website. 2012. Available at: http://www.immunize.org/catg.d/p2011.pdf.

13. Centers for Disease Control and Prevention (CDC). *Dialysis safety.* CDC website. 2013. Available at: http://www.cdc.gov/dialysis/.

14. Alexander M, Corrigan A, Gorski L, Hankins J, Perucca R. *Infusion nursing,* 3rd ed. St. Louis: Elsevier, 2010: 571-582.

15. Centers for Medicare & Medicaid Services (CMS). *State operations manual. Appendix PP – Guidance to surveyors for long term care facilities.* CMS website. 2011. Available at: http://www.cms.gov/Regulations-and-Guidance/Guidance/Manuals/downloads/som107ap_pp_guidelines_ltcf.pdf.

16. Salcido R, Lorenzo CT. *Pressure ulcers and wound care.* Medscape website. 2012. Available at: http://emedicine.medscape.com/article/319284-overview.

17. Baranoski S, Ayello EA. *Wound care essentials. Practice principles,* 2nd ed. Philadelphia: Lippincott Williams & Wilkins, 2008: 93-114.

18. Stone ND, Ashraf MS, Caler J, Crnich CJ, Crossley K, Drinka PJ, et al. Surveillance definitions in long-term care facilities: Revisiting the McGeer Criteria. *Infect Control Hosp Epidemiol* 2012; 33(10): 965-977.

19. Wooten MK, Hawkins, K, WOCN Council, APIC 2000 Guidelines Committee. *WOCN position statement: Clean versus sterile: Management of chronic wounds.* WOCN website. 2005. Available at: http://c.ymcdn.com/sites/www.wocn.org/resource/resmgr/docs/clvst.pdf.

CHAPTER 8

Seasonal Influenza

James F. Marx, PhD, RN, CIC

KEY CONCEPTS

- A long-term care facility's infection prevention program must include a seasonal influenza plan with a vaccination program for residents and staff as well as specific measures to prevent influenza transmission.
- The infection preventionist should be familiar with the steps to take during an influenza outbreak.
- The long-term care infection preventionist must comply with national reporting requirements for immunization rates in healthcare personnel and residents.[1]

Seasonal influenza, also called "the flu," is caused by a virus that infects the respiratory tract. Unlike other viral respiratory infections, like the common cold, influenza can cause severe illness and life-threatening complications in many people. In the United States, on average 5 to 20 percent of the population gets influenza and more than 200,000 people are hospitalized from seasonal influenza-related complications.[2] Influenza seasons are unpredictable and can sometimes be severe. Estimates of annual influenza-associated deaths in the United States range from a low of about 3,000 to a high of about 49,000 people.[3] The elderly, young children, pregnant women, and people with certain health conditions are at high risk for serious influenza complications. The best way to prevent influenza is by getting vaccinated each year.[3] Influenza vaccines protect against the most likely forecasted strains of the virus that change every year. Everyone 6 months and older should get vaccinated annually unless medically contraindicated.[3] Full immunity is developed about 2 weeks after vaccination.

Preventing transmission of influenza viruses within long-term care facilities (LTCFs) requires a multifaceted approach that includes the following:

1. Vaccination
2. Laboratory confirmation
3. Infection prevention measures
4. Antiviral treatment and chemoprophylaxis

INCUBATION, TRANSMISSION, AND COMMUNICABILITY

Adults can be infectious for about 1 day before symptoms develop and up to 7 days after becoming sick.[1,3] Children can pass on the virus for more than 7 days. Symptoms start 1 to 4 days after the virus enters the respiratory tract. Influenza virus can be passed on to someone else before the person knows they are sick. Some people can be infected with the virus and have no symptoms. During this time, those persons may still spread the virus to others (Figure 8.1).[1,3]

People with influenza can spread it to others up to 6 feet away. Influenza viruses are spread mainly by droplets made when people with flu cough, sneeze, or talk. These droplets can land in the mouths or noses of people who are nearby or possibly be inhaled into the lungs. Less often, a person might also get influenza by touching a surface or object that has the virus on it and then touching their own mouth, nose, or eyes.[3]

SYMPTOMS

Influenza symptoms can be mild to severe and at times can lead to death. Influenza is different from a cold, although the two illnesses may have similar symptoms. Influenza symptoms usually appear suddenly; some or all of the following may be present:[3]

- Chills, fever, or feeling feverish (it is important to note that not all flu cases will be accompanied by fever)
- Cough
- Sore throat
- Runny or stuffy nose
- Muscle or body aches (sometimes called myalgia)
- Headaches
- Fatigue, vomiting, and diarrhea (more common in children than adults)

Types of Influenza Viruses[4]

There are three types of influenza viruses: A, B, and C. Human influenza A and B viruses cause seasonal epidemics of disease almost every winter in the U.S.

- Influenza A viruses are divided into subtypes based on two proteins on the surface of the virus: the hemagglutinin (H) and the neuraminidase (N). There are 17 different hemagglutinin subtypes and 10 different neuraminidase subtypes. Influenza A viruses can be further broken down into different strains.
- Influenza B viruses are not divided into subtypes, but can be further broken down into different strains.
- Influenza type C infections cause a mild respiratory illness and are not thought to cause epidemics. The seasonal flu vaccine does not protect against influenza C viruses.

FIGURE 8.1: INFLUENZA VIRUS INFECTION TIMELINE

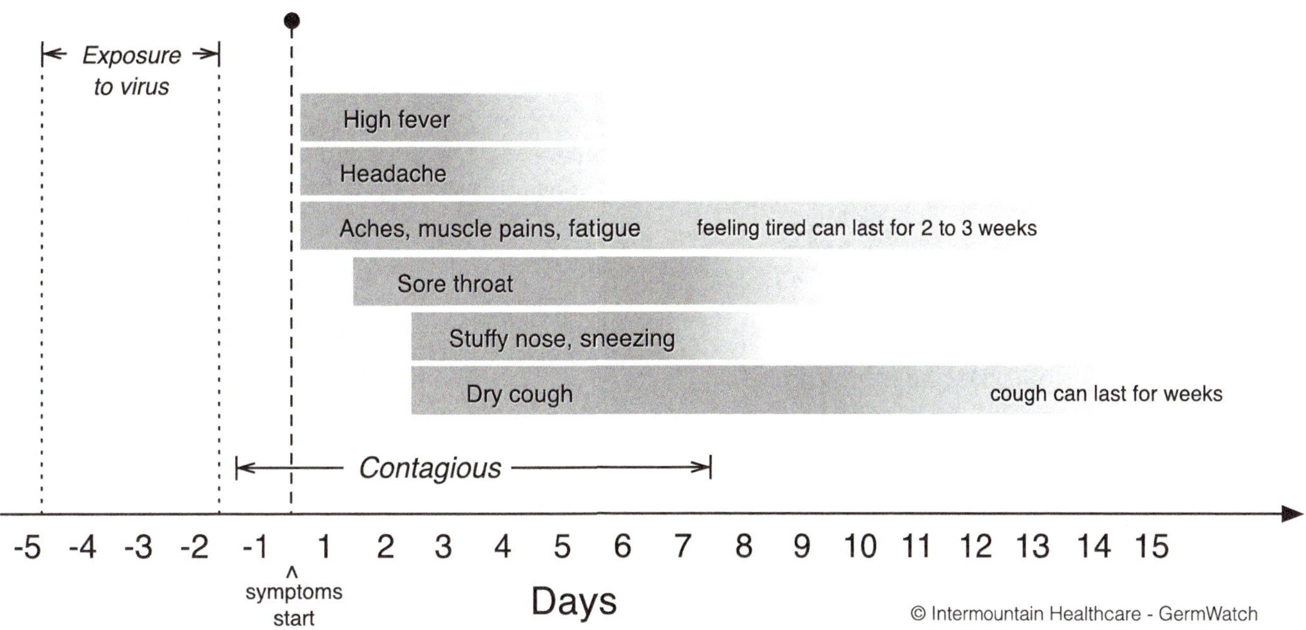

Courtesy of Intermountain Healthcare. Influenza timeline. Intermountain Healthcare website. 2013. Available at: http://intermountainhealthcare.org/health-resources/germwatch/germschool/Pages/influenza.aspx. Used with permission.

ANNUAL INFLUENZA VACCINATION PROGRAM

Immunization programs in LTCF have existed for years. Since 2005, administration of vaccination for both influenza and pneumococcus has existed through the Minimum Data Set (MDS).[5] The long-term care MDS is a standardized, federal documentation requirement for all residents in Medicare and Medicaid-certified LTCFs regardless of the resident's source of payment. However, documentation alone has been insufficient to maximize resident or healthcare personnel (HCP) participation. The Centers for Medicare & Medicaid Services (CMS) data reflect variations in levels of immunization among short- and long-stay long-term care residents.

In an effort to improve vaccination levels, the long-term care component of the *National Action Plan to Prevent Healthcare Associated Infections: Roadmap to Elimination* (often referred to as the HHS National Action Plan) includes resident and HCP influenza vaccinations as two of its five priority areas.[6] The plan proposes metrics and measures that reflect both the National Quality Strategy and are consistent with the aims of Better Care and Healthy People/Healthy Communities and Affordable Care. The vaccination goals are consistent with the national 90 percent compliance targets identified in the Healthy People 2020 objectives.

Residents

Since October 2005, CMS has required LTCFs participating in Medicare and Medicaid programs to offer all residents influenza and pneumococcal vaccines and to document the results of vaccination efforts. According to these requirements, each resident is to be vaccinated unless medically contraindicated or the vaccine is not available because of shortage. However, residents or their legal representative can decline the vaccination. This information should be reported as part of the CMS MDS, which tracks LTCF health parameters.[3]

How Influenza Viruses are Named[4]

The Centers for Disease Control and Prevention (CDC) follows an internationally accepted naming convention for influenza viruses. This convention was accepted by the World Health Organization (WHO) in 1979 and published in February 1980 in the *Bulletin of the World Health Organization*. The approach uses the following components:

1. The antigenic type (e.g., A, B, C)
2. The host of origin (e.g., swine, equine, chicken, etc.; for human-origin viruses, no host of origin designation is given)
3. Geographical origin (e.g., Denver, Taiwan, etc.)
4. Strain number (e.g., 15, 7, etc.)
5. Year the virus was isolated (e.g., 57, 2009, etc.)
6. For influenza A viruses, the hemagglutinin and neuraminidase antigen description in parentheses: (H1N1), (H5N1)

For example:

- A/duck/Alberta/35/76 (H1N1) for a virus from duck origin
- A/Perth/16/2009 (H3N2) for a virus from human origin

Vaccination should begin as soon as vaccine is available. Signed consent is not a federal requirement, but it is usually a state requirement.[3] The LTCF should communicate the benefits of vaccination and provide educational materials, including the current influenza Vaccine Information Statement, to all residents and their families. Facilities should offer vaccination to new residents as soon as possible after admission. The HHS National Action Plan proposed the goal of 85 percent coverage within 5 years for seasonal influenza vaccination among eligible residents during the recent or most current influenza season.[6] An 85 percent resident participation goal as part of the LTCF seasonal influenza plan should be established and results reported.

Staff

HCP who get vaccinated help to reduce the transmission of influenza, decrease staff illness and absenteeism, and lower influenza-related illness and death, especially among people at increased risk for severe influenza illness.[3] Influenza outbreaks in hospitals and LTCFs have been attributed to low influenza vaccination coverage among HCP. National Health Interview Survey (NHIS) data from the 2007 to 2008 influenza season reported only 36.2 percent of HCP in LTCF received the vaccine or approximately half the immunization rate of hospital-based HCP.[7] Most recent data obtained by the CDC during the 2010 to 2011 influenza season showed that HCP vaccination in LTCFs had increased to 64.4 percent but still lagged behind the 71.1 percent in acute care.[8] The Healthy People 2020 goal is to vaccinate 90 percent or more of HCP.[9] With that goal in mind, the HHS National Action Plan proposed a goal of 70 percent HCP vaccination by 2015.[6]

The annual staff vaccination program begins in late summer. The program should include the following:

- Order vaccine administration supplies and begin vaccination as soon as vaccine is available.[3]
- Set a goal to vaccinate at least 90 percent of all direct and nondirect caregivers and include compliance rates as part of the regular infection prevention metrics for discussion with the Infection Prevention and Control Committee.
- Consider a program that makes annual influenza vaccination a condition of employment.[10]
- As an alternative, require staff who decline vaccination to wear a mask while on duty for duration of the influenza season.[10]
- Continue vaccinating new staff through the end of the influenza season.

See the LTC influenza checklist for a complete list of program activities (Table 8.1) and on the CD-ROM.

INFLUENZA DEFINITIONS AND SURVEILLANCE

LTCFs should use a standard definition of infection for influenza-like illness (ILI) to conduct surveillance and

TABLE 8.1: LTCF ANNUAL INFLUENZA PROGRAM CHECKLIST

LATE SUMMER/EARLY FALL (AUGUST-SEPTEMBER)

- ☐ Check with pharmacy to confirm availability of vaccine; ensure sufficient quantity has been ordered
- ☐ Check with pharmacy to confirm the availability of antiviral medications for influenza
- ☐ Review most recent influenza information from the CDC, as well the local and/or state health department
- ☐ Develop and launch an information and "flu shot" awareness campaign for LTCF residents, visitors, and employees
- ☐ Verify that physician orders for vaccine are or will be completed by specific date
- ☐ Verify that supplies needed for vaccine administration are or will be available by specific date

PRESENT INFLUENZA EDUCATION FOR RESIDENTS, VISITORS, AND EMPLOYEES (REPEAT AS NEEDED)

- ☐ Provide education related to influenza symptoms, prevalence in the community, and risks to those unvaccinated
- ☐ Provide education related to vaccine use and safety
- ☐ Review the illness reporting process for both residents and staff; review when symptomatic staff should not report for work and/or require medical clearance before resuming duties
- ☐ Review hand hygiene and respiratory etiquette procedures

COORDINATE LTCF PREVENTION ACTIVITIES WITH THE HEALTH DEPARTMENT

- ☐ Obtain and review the case definition and outbreak reporting criteria required by the state
- ☐ Identify the contact person(s) at the local and/or state health department
- ☐ Identify what information is needed and the required time frames for reporting influenza to the local and/or state health department
- ☐ Participate in health department updates, meetings, and training related to seasonal influenza

IN RESPONSE TO A SINGLE, CONFIRMED CASE

- ☐ Activate LTCF policy and procedure for individual resident isolation and restriction of group activity
- ☐ Follow up with the physician to determine the need for antiviral medication
- ☐ Reinforce need for hand hygiene and isolation precautions with everyone visiting or assisting the resident
- ☐ Confirm the immunization status of any roommates; relocate roommates if necessary and monitor closely for signs and symptoms
- ☐ Reinforce the need for rigorous influenza management and prevention practices by all employees

IN RESPONSE TO MULTIPLE CASES (OUTBREAK SITUATION)

- ☐ Activate the LTCF's outbreak notification system, including the administrator, director of nursing, and medical director
- ☐ Notify the local and/or state health department according to state requirements for influenza
- ☐ Stop all new resident admissions and limit facility visiting to the extent possible
- ☐ Post signage alerting families and visitors of the risk of influenza transmission; provide ongoing information and education to families and visitors as needed
- ☐ Review the need with the medical director and/or other facility leaders for an antiviral prophylaxis program in the LTCF
- ☐ Verify the immunization state of all unaffected residents and employees
- ☐ Encourage staff caring for infected residents to retain these assignments; avoid to the extent possible reassigning employees who have been exposed to care for other, healthy residents
- ☐ Ensure HCP utilize appropriate PPE and perform hand hygiene frequently

Also available on the CD-ROM.

should consider laboratory testing to rule out influenza. The 2012 surveillance definitions for LTCFs (previously referred to as the McGeer criteria) provide an updated case definition for ILI:[11]

Both Criteria 1 and 2 must be present:

1. Fever
2. At least three of the following influenza-like illness subcriteria:
    a. Chills
    b. New headache or eye pain
    c. Myalgia or body aches
    d. Malaise or loss of appetite
    e. Sore throat
    f. New or increased dry cough

The updated definition for ILI also notes the following: "If criteria for influenza-like illness and another upper or lower RTI [respiratory tract infection] are met at the same time, only the diagnosis of influenza-like illness should be recorded. Because of increasing uncertainty surrounding the timing of the start of influenza season, the peak of influenza activity, and the length of the season, "seasonality" is no longer a criterion to define influenza-like illness."[11]

INFLUENZA OUTBREAK INVESTIGATION AND CONTROL

If a cluster of acute respiratory illness is reported, this suggests an influenza outbreak is occurring. It is of critical importance to establish the diagnosis through laboratory testing. If there is one laboratory-confirmed influenza case in a resident or HCP, the IP must begin an outbreak investigation.[3,11] When ILI case detection exceeds the expected rated for the LTCF, and/or when any resident or HCP tests positive for influenza, further investigation and possible outbreak management may be required. If the investigation suggests an outbreak, notify the LTCF leadership and interdisciplinary team and check with the state or local health department for outbreak reporting requirements. To conduct an outbreak investigation, the IP should do the following.

Establish the Existence of an Outbreak[12]

Review current literature, particularly from the CDC and state and local health departments, to be aware of other influenza or influenza-like outbreaks locally, nationally, and internationally. Look for reports of specific flu strain outbreaks or anomalies of which to be aware. Create a line list of residents and staff who exhibit influenza-like symptoms (see example line list on the CD-ROM). Be sure to include the date of symptom onset. Compare data to historical facility rates and any current reports from state and local health departments.

Verify the Diagnosis[12]

It is important to verify diagnosis of the specific type of influenza using diagnostic testing. Collect specimens from three to four residents and/or staff with ILI as soon as possible after the onset of symptoms. Several commercial rapid diagnostic tests are available that can detect influenza viruses within 15 minutes. However, these rapid tests are used primarily for screening purposes and differ in the types of influenza viruses they can detect and strains they can distinguish. A positive test will confirm the influenza diagnosis; however, a negative test does not exclude an influenza diagnosis. For this reason, laboratory-based testing provides the most reliable diagnostic method for confirming an influenza diagnosis.

Define and Identify Cases[12]

Complete the case finding line list using the ILI definition and include results from any laboratory testing performed. To differentiate data and better track events in real time, it may be helpful to classify cases as confirmed, probable, or possible. Collaborate, if possible, with affiliated system IPs or with state or local department of health for assistance with defining outbreak status.

Describe and Orient the Data in Terms of Time, Place, and Person[12]

Based on the incubation period and communicability, determine how cases are associated by person, place, or time. Identify resident location or staff assignment patterns.

It may be helpful to create a map or diagram of the facility to pinpoint where potentially infectious HCP cases have been compared to where resident cases are located.

Develop, Evaluate, and Refine Hypotheses[12]

The outbreak data collected can be used to develop a hypothesis regarding the origin of the outbreak, the type of influenza involved, and patterns of transmission. The hypothesis should be evaluated and refined as more data is collected during the outbreak investigation process. Further outbreak management is dependent on consensus among LTCF leadership. This is an important step to help the IP and interdisciplinary team identify any anomalies in data such as unexpected presentations of symptoms, transmission rates, test results, or mortality that may indicate an unexpected strain of influenza (e.g., H1N1).

Implement Initial Control Measures[12]

The IP should initiate infection prevention and control measures as soon as an outbreak is suspected. Some of the more restrictive measures listed here may only be initiated once an influenza outbreak is confirmed.

- **Respiratory hygiene and cough etiquette.**[13] The following measures to contain respiratory secretions are recommended for all individuals with signs and symptoms of a respiratory infection:
  - Cover the mouth and nose with a tissue when coughing or sneezing.
  - Use in the nearest waste receptacle to dispose of the tissue after use.
  - If tissue is not available, cough or sneeze into the upper sleeve or elbow, not the hands.
  - Perform hand hygiene (e.g., hand washing with nonantimicrobial soap and water, alcohol-based hand rub) after having contact with respiratory secretions and contaminated objects/materials.
- **Availability of supplies.** LTCF should ensure the availability of materials for adhering to respiratory hygiene and/cough etiquette in waiting areas for residents and visitors. The CDC website provides posters and fliers that may be placed in waiting areas and around the facility. Facilities should also provide the following:
  - Tissues and no-touch receptacles for used tissue disposal
  - Conveniently located dispensers of alcohol-based hand rub where sinks are not available
  - Supplies for hand washing (i.e., soap, disposable towels) where sinks are available[3]
  - Surgical masks for use by symptomatic residents or visitors
- **Transmission-based Precautions.** Implement Standard and Droplet Precautions for any resident with suspected or confirmed influenza for 7 days after illness onset or until 24 hours after the resolution of fever and respiratory symptoms, whichever is longer.[3] Droplet Precautions should be started on a symptomatic resident, regardless of the rapid influenza test results. Precautions include[13]:
  - **Personal protective equipment (PPE):** HCP should wear a surgical mask when entering a resident's room with suspected or confirmed influenza; remove and dispose of mask in a waste container when leaving the room and perform hand hygiene. Do not reuse masks.
  - **Hand hygiene:** Perform hand hygiene before and after resident contact; after contact with potential infectious material or contaminated surfaces; and before putting on and after removal of PPE, including gloves. Hand hygiene can be accomplished by washing with soap and water for at least 15 seconds or by using an alcohol-based hand rub. Soap and water should be used is if hands are visibly soiled.
- **Placement of residents:** A private room for a symptomatic resident is preferred, but if a private room is not available, place symptomatic residents with one another (cohorting). If the symptomatic resident is in a semiprivate room, maintain a spatial separation of at least 3 feet between residents and draw a curtain between resident beds.[13]
- **Movement of residents.** Facilities should limit movement of symptomatic residents. If residents are ill on specific units, do not move residents to other units. Keep ill residents and exposed roommate(s) in their room, restrict them from group activities, and serve meals in their room. If other residents become symptomatic, cancel group activities and serve all meals in the residents' rooms. If residents need to leave their room, have them wear a mask, if possible. Offer tissues and reinforce hand hygiene. Discourage any reuse of tissues by residents.

- **Admissions.** It may be necessary to limit new and returning residents during a suspected or confirmed outbreak. If admissions are necessary, ensure new or returning residents do not have acute respiratory illness or can be accommodated in Droplet Precautions. Admit asymptomatic new or returning residents to unaffected units, if possible. Assign staff to work on only one unit, if possible. Restrict staff movement from areas of the facility having outbreaks to areas without symptomatic residents. Assist residents with hand hygiene, especially before leaving and entering rooms and after contact with respiratory secretions and contaminated tissues.[2] Temporary suspension of group activities and/or congregate dining may be necessary during confirmed outbreak situations.
- **Chemoprophylaxis and treatment.** According to CDC recommendations, "all long-term care facility residents who have confirmed or suspected influenza should receive antiviral treatment... Antiviral treatment works best when started within the first 2 days of symptoms. However, these medications can still help when given after 48 hours to those that are very sick, such as those who are hospitalized, or those who have progressive illness."[3] Antiviral medication should be started as soon as possible for residents with suspected or confirmed influenza who are at higher risk for influenza complications on the basis of their age or underlying medical conditions. Clinical judgment is an important component of resident treatment decisions. Therefore, it is essential that the facility's medical director lead outbreak investigation and response.
- **Cleaning and disinfection.** Use routine cleaning and disinfecting strategies during influenza season. An Environmental Protection Agency-registered hospital-grade disinfectant must have an influenza or virucidal statement on the label. Focus on cleaning frequently touched surfaces in common areas and resident rooms more frequently than usual. Special handling of soiled linens and dietary trays is not necessary.[2]
- **Symptomatic staff.** Staff who become symptomatic should not work until they have been afebrile for at least 24 hours.[3] Monitor staff absenteeism due to respiratory symptoms and exclude those with influenza-like symptoms from work. Consider antiviral prophylaxis for all vaccinated and unvaccinated staff.[3]
- **Visitors.** Visitors should be limited to people who are necessary for the resident's emotional well-being and care. Visitors should be screened for symptoms of acute respiratory illness prior to entering the LTCF. Visitors who have been in contact with an infected resident are a possible source of influenza for other residents, visitors, and staff. Facilities should provide signage for visitor instruction before they enter residents' rooms on hand hygiene and use of PPE according to current facility policy. Facilities should instruct visitors of infected residents to limit their movement within the facility.

Communicate Findings[12]

All LTCF staff need to be regularly updated regarding seasonal influenza trends, facility response, emerging threats, and outbreak management, as needed. Check with the state regarding public reporting requirements for influenza. Be sure to include documentation of outbreak management and response in committee minutes, reports, or other communication systems used by the LTCF.

REFERENCES

1. Centers for Disease Control and Prevention (CDC). *Seasonal influenza (flu): How flu spreads.* CDC website. 2012. Available at: http://www.cdc.gov/flu/about/disease/spread.htm.

2. State of California Department of Public Health. *Recommendations for the prevention and control of influenza California long-term care facilities.* CDPH website. 2011. Available at: http://www.cdph.ca.gov/programs/hai/Documents/Influenza-Recommendations-LTCF-v.12-11.pdf.

3. Centers for Disease Control and Prevention (CDC). *Seasonal influenza (flu): Interim guidance for influenza outbreak management in long-term care facilities.* CDC website. 2011. Available at: http://www.cdc.gov/flu/professionals/infectioncontrol/ltc-facility-guidance.htm.

4. Centers for Disease Control and Prevention (CDC). *Seasonal influenza (flu): Types of influenza viruses.* CDC website. 2012. Available at: http://www.cdc.gov/flu/about/viruses/types.htm.

5. Research Data Assistance Center. Long term care minimum data set 3.0. ResDAC website. 2011. Available at: http://www.resdac.org/cms-data/files/mds-3.0.

6. U.S. Department of Health and Human Services (HHS). *National Action Plan to Prevent Healthcare-Associated Infections: Roadmap to Elimination Part 6: Long-Term Care Facilities.* HHS website. 2013. Available at: http://www.hhs.gov/ash/initiatives/hai/actionplan/hai-action-plan-ltcf.pdf.

7. Greby SM, Lu P, Euler G, Williams WW, Singleton JA. *2009 Adult Vaccination Coverage, NHIS.* CDC website. 2011. Available at: http://www.cdc.gov/vaccines/stats-surv/nhis/2009-nhis.htm.

8. Centers for Disease Control and Prevention (CDC). Influenza vaccination coverage among health care personnel—United States, 2010-11 influenza season. *MMWR Recomm Rep* 2011; 60(32): 1073-1077.

9. U.S. Department of Health and Human Services (HHS). *Healthy People 2020.* HHS website. 2013. Available at: http://www.healthypeople.gov/2020/default.aspx.

10. Greene LR, Cox T, Dolan S, Gray P, Khoury R, Kulich P, et al. *APIC position paper: Influenza vaccination should be a condition of employment for healthcare personnel, unless medically contraindicated.* APIC website. 2011. Available at: http://www.apic.org/Resource_/TinyMceFileManager/Advocacy-PDFs/APIC_Influenza_Immunization_of_HCP_12711.PDF.

11. Stone ND, Ashraf MS, Calder J, Crnich CJ, Crossley K, Drinka PJ, et al. Surveillance definitions of infections in long-term care facilities: revisiting the McGeer criteria. *Infect Control Hosp Epidemiol* 2012; 33(10): 965-977.

12. Centers for Disease Control and Prevention (CDC). *Steps of an outbreak investigation.* CDC website. 2004. Available at: http://www.cdc.gov/excite/classroom/outbreak/steps.htm.

13. Siegel JD, Rhinehart E, Jackson M, Chiarello L, and the Healthcare Infection Control Practices Advisory Committee. *Guideline for isolation precautions: Prevention of transmission of infectious agents in healthcare settings.* CDC website. 2007. Available at: http://www.cdc.gov/hicpac/pdf/isolation/Isolation2007.pdf.

CHAPTER 9

Occupational Health

James F. Marx, PhD, RN, CIC

KEY CONCEPTS

- New hires should be screened to protect residents and staff from communicable diseases.
- Employees need training on the proper use of personal protective equipment to prevent transmission of infections.
- The infection preventionist must promote hand hygiene as the cornerstone to all infection prevention and control interventions.
- Facilities must offer employees recommended vaccines to promote a comprehensive, safe work environment.
- Safe injection practice is important to protect resident and healthcare personnel from exposure to infectious disease.

Healthy employees promote healthy residents. Keeping employees and residents safe from infectious disease requires a combination of education, vaccination, and safe work practices. To ensure this, it is important to include healthcare personnel safety as part of the long-term care facility's (LTCF) infection prevention and control program. For the purpose of this chapter, the term healthcare personnel (HCP) is used to describe employees, volunteers, medical providers, and contractors such as phlebotomists, x-ray technicians, physical therapists, and occupational therapists.

The Centers for Medicare & Medicaid Services (CMS) states, "the facility must prohibit employees with a communicable disease or infected skin lesions from direct contact with residents or their food, if direct contact will transmit the disease."[1] HCP should be free of transmissible conditions that could impact resident health.[2] Those who have direct contact with residents can transmit infection between residents, can become infected by the resident, or can be the source of exposure to the resident. Direct contact includes bathing, dressing, transferring, repositioning, and ambulating. Even indirect contact can transmit infection through droplets, air, or contaminated objects.[3] Examples of transmissible infections or conditions are scabies, norovirus, influenza, and tuberculosis (TB). Volunteers and visitors can also transmit infection.

JOB DESCRIPTION RISK ASSESSMENT

Direct care givers have the greatest risk of exposure to infection and pose the greatest risk of infection transmission to residents. Some nondirect care staff, such as food service workers, may also pose a risk of infection transmission (e.g., cooks with gastroenteritis). The LTCF's infection prevention and control plan and risk assessment should take into account the risk of infection associated with different job responsibilities.

The risk assessment should include a review of employee job descriptions and qualifications. A job description that contains an infection risk assessment can identify groups who are at increased risk of exposure to infections or who may be the source of infection. It may also be helpful in prioritizing vaccination efforts and education programs. The following examples are a general guide to an HCP's infection risk:

- **High risk:** frequent contact with resident skin and body fluids
  - Nursing assistants
  - Nurses
  - Occupational and physical therapists
  - Phlebotomists
  - Radiology technicians
  - Transporters
  - Activity aides
  - Laundry workers
  - Environmental services staff
  - Physicians and physician extenders
- **Medium risk:** infrequent contact with resident skin or body fluids
  - Social services
  - Dietary
- **Low risk:** unlikely to have contact with resident skin or body fluids
  - Supply technician
  - Billing clerk
  - Medical records/health information staff

A comprehensive facility risk assessment should consider the resident population's comorbidities and communicable disease risks. For instance, if the facility serves a population known to have chronic bloodborne pathogens such as HIV, a post-exposure plan needs to be in place. Post-exposure follow-up procedures need to address exposures that may occur at any time of the day, night, weekend, and holidays. A letter of agreement between the facility and a local hospital emergency room can help expedite the post-exposure follow-up process. Consider using the hospital's post-exposure follow-up policies as a guide. Review local, state, or federal requirements for implementing an injury and illness prevention program. An evaluation of every exposure provides an opportunity for improvement. Exposures should be presented and discussed in a quality improvement or infection prevention and control committee meeting.

NEW HIRE SCREENING

New hires should be screened for communicable diseases prior to assuming their work assignments.[4] Screening may be done by physical examination, health questionnaire, blood tests, or some combination. CMS does not publish a list of required communicable diseases; therefore, the facility must decide what diseases should be screened based on requirements of federal, state, provincial, or local health departments. Some potential communicable diseases for new hire screening are TB, other vaccine-preventable diseases, respiratory tract infection, gastroenteritis, or scabies. For example, employees may be screened for TB using a skin test or blood test upon hire and annually thereafter.[5] For healthcare staff who have diagnosed communicable diseases that under normal circumstances do not pose a threat of transmission to residents, check with state, provincial, or local health departments for eligibility for employment. This may include sexually transmitted diseases, HIV, and Hepatitis C.

Keep in mind that HCP may work at more than one facility. If so, try to coordinate screening tests and immunization records to reduce the cost of screening. Some states offer online immunization record retrieval—similar to checking for current practice certification or licensure. The CDC website provides a list and links for state immunization programs.

Health questionnaires are used to determine immunization status and to obtain histories of any conditions that might predispose personnel to acquiring or transmitting communicable diseases. However, routine physical exams are usually cost-prohibitive for the LTCF. Physical exams and laboratory testing are typically done only if infection risks have been identified during the screening process.[4]

PREVENTING EXPOSURE

Preventing exposure begins by communicating with the potential resident's transferring facility or by conducting an intake interview. Review the potential resident's past medical and vaccination history, medications, laboratory tests, and radiology reports. Admission decisions should be based on the facility's ability to provide the resident the care needed.[3] Residents colonized or infected with multidrug-resistant organisms (MDROs) must be managed in a skilled nursing facility in a way that avoids or minimizes the risk of transmission to the HCP or other residents. See Chapter 14 for more information on interfacility transfers and transitions.

Early identification of common communicable conditions such as norovirus, scabies, influenza, group A streptococcus, and TB can prevent transmission to staff and other residents.[4] A comprehensive infection prevention and control plan should identify and apply written case definitions consistently. Case definitions should be reviewed and approved by LTCF leadership. Case definitions help to identify true cases and help avoid counting colonization or noninfectious resident conditions. Outbreak definitions should include the number of cases during a specific time period. See Chapter 4 for additional information about outbreak identification.

> ***Sample Case Definitions***
>
> - One laboratory confirmed influenza case in a resident living in the facility for more than 5 days.
> - Three cases of laboratory confirmed *Clostridium difficile* in 1 week among residents living in the facility for more than 3 days and no prior history of *C. difficile*.
> - Ten percent or more of the residents have vomiting or new onset diarrhea.

OCCUPATIONAL HEALTH TRAINING AND EDUCATION

All employees should receive education and training on the use of hand hygiene, environmental hygiene, personal protective equipment (PPE), and Standard and Transmission-based Precautions upon hire and annually thereafter. HCP whose job descriptions are identified as high risk may be required to have additional training and must be offered vaccinations in accordance with state and federal requirements.

Infection preventionists (IPs) will be most successful with staff training programs that use a variety of educational techniques. For example, techniques that engage the employee in hands-on activities may be more useful than lecture or video. Consider using a return demonstration exercise of infection prevention techniques, such as putting on and taking off PPE. See Chapter 13 for more information on staff education and training.

Personal Protective Equipment

PPE can reduce transmission of infection but can also transmit infection if used improperly.[2] For instance, transmission of Hepatitis B may occur if a caregiver's hands become contaminated during a fingerstick blood sugar check, and then the caregiver uses the same gloves to check the blood sugar of another resident. PPE includes employer-provided gloves, protective gowns, face masks, face shields, and eye goggles. Uniforms, such as scrubs, are not considered PPE. It is important to make PPE readily available and to train employees on its proper use. Employees must first understand modes of infection transmission. This may include direct and indirect transmission of MDROs from surfaces, droplet transmission of influenza, and scabies from direct skin contact.

The selection and use of PPE depends on the task being performed. Direct care givers should use Standard Precautions during resident care. Additional precautions may be needed for procedures with high-exposure risk. These procedures generally involve anticipated contact with body fluids, mucus membranes, or nonintact skin. Follow the Centers for Disease Control and Prevention (CDC) recommendations for donning and removing PPE.[3] See Chapter 5 for more information on Standard and Transmission-based Precautions.

PPE must be made available and readily accessible for staff use. Gloves are the most common PPE; however, placing gloves in convenient locations may be a challenge with residents who are cognitively impaired. Unintended access to PPE by cognitively impaired residents can pose a serious safety risk. In addition, the appearance of glove boxes may detract from the "homelike" environment. Finding a balance between resident safety and staff accessibility requires coordination among the interdisciplinary team and agreement with senior leadership.

Hand Hygiene

The cornerstone of infection prevention is hand hygiene. Hand hygiene can be accomplished by using soap and water or alcohol-based hand rub.[6] According to the CDC guidelines for hand hygiene:

> Alcohols are not appropriate for use when hands are visibly dirty or contaminated with proteinaceous materials... Alcohol-based hand rubs are the most efficacious agents for reducing the number of bacteria on the hands of personnel. Antiseptic soaps and detergents are the next most effective, and non-antimicrobial soaps are the least effective... Alcohol-based hand rubs are recommended for routine decontamination of hands for all clinical indications (except when hands are visibly soiled).[6]

HCP can avoid acquiring or transmitting infections or infectious disease by consistently practicing hand hygiene after contact with a resident or resident environment, after glove use, before eating, and when hands are visibly soiled.[6] Hand hygiene should also be performed before resident contact to protect the resident.

Accessibility to hand hygiene stations or dispensers is an important component to hand hygiene compliance.[6] Personal carriage of hand sanitizer has been suggested as one way to increase accessibility and compliance.[7] Point of care (POC) alcohol-based hand rub dispensers is another way to improve hand hygiene compliance. The risks and benefits of POC alcohol-based hand rubs needs to be evaluated based on resident and visitor population because there is risk of ingestion. Be familiar with how to treat residents who may ingest alcohol-based hand rub by following the procedure listed on the Safety Data Sheet for that product. The American with Disabilities Act (ADA) requires dispensers to be no more than 48 inches from the floor.[8] The closer the dispenser is to the situation that requires hand hygiene, the higher the hand hygiene compliance rate.[7] A lack of sinks with soap and paper towels in the typical long-term care setting requires an assessment for placement of alternate methods of hand hygiene.[6]

VACCINATION

Reducing the risk of infection through vaccination has been one of public health's greatest achievements in the past 100 years.[9] Vaccine preventable diseases likely to occur in long-term care facilities are Hepatitis B, influenza, pneumococcal infection, and varicella (residents with herpes zoster or shingles).

Under federal Occupational Safety and Health Administration (OSHA) Section 1910.1030(f)(2)(i), Hepatitis B vaccinations must be offered after education and provided within 10 days of a potential exposure incident.[10] Hepatitis B vaccination for adults is administered in a series of three intramuscular injections. The second dose is given a minimum of 4 weeks after the first, and the third dose is given 5 months after the second dose. It is important to note that there is maximum time period between vaccines. Employees who have ongoing contact with residents or blood and are at risk for injuries with sharps must be tested for antibody to Hepatitis B surface antigen (anti-HBs) 1 to 2 months after the completion of the three-dose vaccination series.[11] Employees who do develop antibodies will have life-long immunity. Employees who do not respond to the primary vaccination series must be revaccinated with a second three-dose vaccine series and retested.[11] Nonresponders must be medically evaluated.

CMS requires influenza and pneumococcal vaccination screening for all new resident admissions.[1] A growing number of healthcare facilities are now requiring HCP annual influenza vaccination. The LTCF IP should be familiar with the APIC position paper on HCP influenza vaccination as a condition of employment.[12]

Other less common vaccine-preventable diseases in long-term care are pertussis, diphtheria, and meningococcal disease. The combined Tdap (tetanus-diphtheria-acellular pertussis) vaccine is recommended for all healthcare personnel. Specialty units with pediatric residents should also consider vaccination for measles, mumps, and rubella. Other recommended vaccines for all adults are shingles, tetanus, typhoid, Hepatitis A, polio, and pneumococcal disease. Refer to the CDC report and recommendations for immunization for a complete list of vaccine-preventable diseases.[11]

Vaccine Information Statements

Vaccine Information Statements (VISs) are information sheets produced by the CDC that explain to vaccine recipients, parents, or legal representatives both the benefits and risks of a vaccine.[13] They are available in many different languages. VISs were written to fulfill the information requirements of the National Childhood Vaccine Injury Act of 1986. U.S. federal law requires that VISs be given to the recipient, including adult recipients, before each vaccine dose is given (National Childhood Vaccine Injury Act of 1986, 42 U.S.C. 300aa-1 to 300aa-34). A VIS for pneumococcal polysaccharide vaccine (PPSV) vaccine for adults is not required; however, providing a copy of this VIS may, in part, fulfill the requirement for informed consent.[13] A written vaccine declaration form can help document refusal and aid in identifying opportunities to increase vaccination rates. A sample influenza declination form can be found at http://www.immunize.org/catg.d/p4068.pdf. More information on VISs can be found on the CDC website or at http://www.immunize.org/.

When administering vaccines to HCP, record the following required information on the HCP's permanent and accessible medical record:

- The edition date of the VIS (found on the back in either the left or right bottom corner)
  - Note: When multiple VISs are given for a combination vaccine, record the individual edition dates.
- The date the VIS is provided (i.e., the date of the visit when the vaccine is administered)
- The name, address, and title of the person who administered the vaccine
- The date the vaccine is administered
- The vaccine manufacturer and lot number

Informed Consent

There is no federal requirement for informed or written consent prior to vaccination.[14] However, some states have informed consent laws. Check the state's medical consent law to determine if there are any specific informed consent requirements relating to immunization and to determine if consent must be oral or written. VISs might be used for informed consent as long as they conform to the appropriate state laws. State-specific immunization laws can be found on the CDC website.

Vaccine Adverse Event Reporting

The Vaccine Adverse Event Reporting System (VAERS) is a national passive reporting system that accepts reports from the public on adverse events associated with vaccines licensed in the United States.[15] Anyone can file a VAERS report, including healthcare providers, manufacturers, vaccine recipients, or vaccine recipients' parents or guardians. The form can be found at http://vaers.hhs.gov/resources/vaers_form.pdf. Healthcare providers are required to report certain adverse events depending on which vaccine is given.[16] The VAERS form requests the following information:

- The type of vaccine received
- The timing of the vaccination
- The onset of the adverse event
- Current illnesses or medication
- Past history of adverse events following vaccination

Demographic information about the recipient VAERS forms can be completed online, or you can complete a paper form and mail or fax it to VAERS.

National Vaccine Injury Compensation Program

One of the barriers to vaccination is the fear of liability. The National Vaccine Injury Compensation Program (VICP) is intended to provide compensation to persons who may have been unavoidably injured by vaccines rather than passing the costs on to vaccine manufacturers and providers.[17] Generally, neither providers nor manufacturers are liable for adverse vaccine reactions (excluding professional negligence). Information about VCIP, including an education sheet, may be found through the U.S. Department of Health and Human Services Health Resources and Services Administration website.

ONGOING HEALTHCARE PERSONNEL SCREENING

Periodic health screenings offer a way to check if HCP has developed any potential communicable disease(s). Some state health departments require annual health screenings for HCP in long-term care. LTCFs frequently screen HCP for TB to ensure that exposure or transmission has not occurred either in the course of their employment or as a result of contact with infected individuals in the community.[11,18,19]

HCP sick policies should be written and enforced in way that encourages HCP to self-monitor and report an infectious illness. Educate employees to report symptoms of infection such as a fever, diarrhea, cough, sore throat, and skin lesions to the IP or employee health nurse. Coordinate efforts with the human resources department to determine the best way to query employees about why they call in sick. Unfortunately, if being away from work will impact the HCP financially, they are less likely to report their illness. Review the facility's sick time policy to see that employees are not penalized for using sick time when necessary. Presenteeism, or coming to work when ill, is an ongoing problem in healthcare.[20] Pressure to work while ill can occur when staffing is an issue or when not working will result in a reduction in pay.

A comprehensive guideline for infection prevention and control in HCP was last published by the CDC in 1998[4] and by Health Canada in 2002.[21] Potential work restrictions are based on consideration of the type of employee illness and the level of resident contact. These factors and their associated restrictions are summarized by the CDC in the Table 9.1.[4]

INJURY AND ILLNESS PREVENTION PROGRAMS

A comprehensive occupational health program in LTCFs will include an Injury and Illness Prevention Program (IIPP) outlined by OSHA (for U.S.-based facilities).[22] States may have additional OSHA requirements.[23] The following OSHA requirements affect LTCFs:

- Musculoskeletal disorders
- Bloodborne pathogens
- TB and other airborne/droplet diseases
- Workplace violence
- Slips, trips, and falls
- Methicillin-resistant *Staphylococcus aureus* (MRSA)
- Chemicals/hazardous drugs

OSHA Form 300 is a log of work-related injuries and illnesses and is required to be posted annually in the facility from February 1 to April 30.[24,25] The listed events include any needlestick injury or cut from a sharp object that is contaminated with another person's blood or other potentially infectious material and latent or active TB infection as evidenced by a positive skin test/blood test or diagnosis by a physician or other licensed healthcare professional after exposure to a known case of active TB. The facility must assign responsibility for this task. The form does not need to be submitted to OSHA unless requested.[25]

Medical files for all HCP on staff must be retained for the duration of employment plus 30 years unless employment is less than 1 year. Employees who leave within 1 year should be provided a copy of their medical record. For more record keeping information, see information on OSHA's website.

OSHA BLOODBORNE PATHOGENS

IPs need to fully understand the various components of bloodborne pathogen standards, including training requirements and documentation. OSHA has published training requirements for bloodborne pathogens.[10] The federal OSHA bloodborne pathogen standard can be found at: https://www.osha.gov/pls/oshaweb/owadisp.show_document?p_table=standards&p_id=10051/. State OSHA requirements may differ.[23] Canadian health and safety resources can be found at: http://www.hrsdc.gc.ca/eng/labour/health_safety/index.shtml.

Key provisions of the bloodborne pathogens standard are:

- Create a bloodborne pathogens exposure control plan (a model plan is available on OSHA's website)
- Update the plan annually
- Common considerations in long-term care
  - Location of sharps disposal containers
    - Must be accessible to the employee at the point of sharps use to avoid transporting sharps a long distance
  - Proper discarding of used razors
    - Nursing assists should not replace the protective plastic cover on a disposable razor to avoid risk of a sharps injury
  - Cleaning and disinfection of common use items:
    - Use an EPA-approved hospital disinfectant with an HIV or Hepatitis B label claim for common use equipment, such as blood glucose meters, and/or any surfaces that are potentially contaminated with blood or other potentially infectious body substances
    - Clean and disinfect equipment according to manufacturer's directions
  - Separate handling and storage of clean and soiled items
  - Labeling and storage of laboratory specimens
    - Specimens should be handled and stored as potential biohazards
  - Use of engineered sharp safety devices is required
    - Have staff practice with the device before using on a resident; solicit input from staff about how the device functions
  - Hepatitis B vaccination
    - Required to be offered after education on bloodborne pathogens and within 10 days of the first potential exposure
  - Post-exposure follow-up within the prescribed time periods
    - Potential HIV exposures should be treated within hours of an exposure incident[24]
  - Availability of PPE (gloves, gowns, facial protection)
    - Consider the location of supplies to encourage use
  - New hire and annual employee education that contains all elements prescribed in the OSHA Standard

SAFE INJECTION PRACTICES

Unsafe injection practices have led to transmission of bloodborne pathogens and other microbial pathogens.

TABLE 9.1: CDC WORK RESTRICTIONS FOR HEALTHCARE PERSONNEL

Summary of suggested work restrictions for healthcare personnel exposed to or infected with infectious diseases of importance in healthcare settings, in the absence of state and local regulations.

Disease/Problem	Work Restriction	Duration	Cat.
Conjunctivitis	Restrict from patient contact and contact with the patient's environment	Until discharge ceases	II
Cytomegalovirus infections	No restriction		II
Diarrheal diseases:			
Acute stage (diarrhea with other symptoms)	Restrict from patient contact, contact with the patient's environment, or food handling	Until symptoms resolve	IB
Convalescent stage, *Salmonella* spp.	Restrict from care of high-risk patients	Until symptoms resolve; consult with local and state health authorities regarding need for negative stool cultures	IB
Enteroviral infections	Restrict from care of infants, neonates, and immunocompromised patients and their environments	Until symptoms resolve	II
Hepatitis A	Restrict from patient contact, contact with patient's environment, and food handling	Until 7 days after onset of jaundice	IB
Hepatitis B:			
Personnel with acute or chronic hepatitis B surface antigemia who do not perform exposure-prone procedures	No restriction*; refer to state regulations; standard precautions should always be observed		II
Personnel with acute or chronic hepatitis B e antigenemia who perform exposure-prone procedures	Do not perform exposure-prone invasive procedures until counsel from an expert review panel has been sought; panel should review and recommend procedures the worker can perform, taking into account specific procedure as well as skill and technique of worker; refer to state regulations	Until hepatitis B e antigen is negative	II
Hepatitis C	No recommendation		
Herpes simplex:			
Genital	No restriction		II
Hands (herpetic whitlow)	Restrict from patient contact and contact with the patient's environment	Until lesions heal	IA
Orofacial	Evaluate for need to restrict from care of high-risk patients		II
Human immunodeficiency virus	Do not perform exposure-prone invasive procedures until counsel from an expert review panel has been sought; panel should review and recommend procedures the worker can perform, taking into account specific procedure as well as skill and technique of the worker; standard precautions should always be observed; refer to state regulations		

Table 9.1 Continued

Disease/Problem	Work Restriction	Duration	Cat.
Measles:			
Active	Exclude from duty	Until 7 days after the rash appears	IA
Postexposure (susceptible personnel)	Exclude from duty	From 5th day after 1st exposure through 21st day after last exposure and/or 4 days after rash appears	IB
Meningococcal infections	Exclude from duty	Until 24 hours after start of effective therapy	IA
Mumps:			
Active	Exclude from duty	Until 9 days after onset of parotitis	IB
Postexposure (susceptible personnel)	Exclude from duty	From 12th day after 1st exposure through 26th day after last exposure or until 9 days after onset of parotitis	II
Pediculosis	Restrict from patient contact	Until treated and observed to be free of adult and immature lice	IB
Pertussis:			
Active	Exclude from duty	From beginning of catarrhal stage through 3rd wk after onset of paroxysms or until 5 days after start of effective antimicrobial therapy	IB
Postexposure (asymptomatic)	No restriction, prophylaxis recommended		II
Postexposure (symptomatic)	Exclude from duty		IB
Rubella:			
Active	Exclude from duty	Until 5 days after rash appears	IA
Postexposure (susceptible personnel)	Exclude from duty	From 7th day after 1st exposure through 21st day after last exposure	IB
Scabies	Restrict from patient contact	Until cleared by medical evaluation	IB
***Staphylococcus aureus* infection:**			
Active, draining skin lesions	Restrict from contact with patients and patient's environment or food handling	Until lesions have resolved	IB
Carrier state			IB
Streptococcal infection, group A	No restriction, unless personnel are epidemiologically linked to transmission of the organism		IB
Tuberculosis:			
Active disease	Exclude from duty	Until proved noninfectious	IA
PPD converter	No restriction		IA
Varicella:			
Active	Exclude from duty	Until all lesions dry and crust	IA
Postexposure (susceptible personnel)	Exclude from duty	From 10th day after 1st exposure through 21st day (28th day if VZIG given) after last exposure	IA

Table 9.1 Continued

Disease/Problem	Work Restriction	Duration	Cat.
Zoster:			
Localized, in healthy person	Cover lesions; restrict from care of high-risk patients†	Until all lesions dry and crust	II
Generalized or localized in immunosuppressed person	Restrict from patient contact	Until all lesions dry and crust	IB
Postexposure (susceptible personnel)	Restrict from patient contact	From 10th day after 1st exposure through 21st day (28th day if VZIG given) after last exposure or, if varicella occurs, until all lesions dry and crust	IA
Viral respiratory infections, acute febrile	Consider excluding from the care of high risk patients‡ or contact with their environment during community outbreak of RSV and influenza	Until acute symptoms resolve	IB

* Unless epidemiologically linked to transmission of infection

† Those susceptible to varicella and who are at increased risk of complications of varicella, such as neonates and immunocompromised persons of any age.

‡ High-risk patients as defined by the ACIP for complications of influenza.

From Centers of Disease Control and Prevention. Guideline for infection control in Health care personnel, 1998. Available at: http://www.cdc.gov/hicpac/pdf/InfectControl98.pdf.

More than 30 outbreaks of viral hepatitis have been reported in the United States since 2000.[26] Identified unsafe practices can be placed into four categories: syringe reuse between patients; contaminated multiuse vials or intravenous solutions; failure to follow basic safe injection practice during preparation and administration of medication; and inadequate disinfection of multiple patient-use glucose testing equipment.[26] Policy and procedures should follow the CDC recommendations for safe injection practices as outlined in the 2007 *Guideline for Isolation Precautions.*[3]

LTCFs should implement the following practices to protect residents:

- Use aseptic technique to avoid contamination of sterile injection equipment.[3]
- Never administer medications from a syringe to multiple residents, even if the needle or cannula on the syringe is changed. Needles, cannulae, and syringes are sterile, single-use items; they should not be reused for another resident or reused to access a medication or solution that might be used for a subsequent resident.[3]
- Use fluid infusion and administration sets (i.e., intravenous bags, tubing, and connectors) for one resident only and dispose appropriately after use. A syringe or needle/cannula is considered contaminated once it has been used to enter or connect to a resident's intravenous infusion bag or administration set.[3]
- Use single-dose vials for injectable medications whenever possible.
- Never administer medications from single-dose vials or ampules to multiple residents or combine leftover contents for later use.[3]
- Use multidose vials properly. If multidose vials must be used, both the needle or cannula and syringe used to access the multidose vial must be sterile.[3]
- Do not keep multidose vials in the immediate resident treatment area and store in accordance with the manufacturer's recommendations; follow the directions on how long a multidose vial can be used, discarding if sterility might have been compromised.[3]
- Do not use bags or bottles of intravenous solution as a common source of supply for multiple residents.[3]
- Follow infection prevention practices for special lumbar puncture procedures:[3]
  - Wear a surgical mask when placing a catheter or injecting material into the spinal canal or subdural space (i.e., during myelograms, lumbar puncture, and spinal or epidural anesthesia).
- Do not share fingerstick devices, also called lancing devices, even with close family and friends; this includes both the lancet (i.e., the sharp instrument that actually punctures the skin) *and* the pen-like device that houses the lancet. Neither should be used for more than one person.

- Do not share blood glucose meters whenever possible. If they must be shared, the device should be cleaned and disinfected *after every use*, per manufacturer's instructions. If the manufacturer does not specify how the device should be cleaned and disinfected, then it should not be shared. Outbreaks of Hepatitis B associated with the misuse of blood glucose testing equipment and supplies have been reported in assisted living facilities.[27]
- Do not share insulin pens between residents. In 2009, the U.S. Food and Drug Administration issued an alert reminding HCP that insulin pens should never be shared due to the risk of transmitting bloodborne diseases such as HIV and Hepatitis C.[28]
- Dedicate multidose insulin vials to a single resident whenever possible. If they must be used for more than one resident, they should not be stored or accessed in the immediate resident treatment area. This is to prevent inadvertent contamination of the vial through direct or indirect contact with potentially contaminated surfaces or equipment that could then lead to infections in subsequent residents.

More information regarding blood glucose monitoring and insulin administration best practices is available on the CDC website.

SHARP SAFETY PROGRAM FOR EMPLOYEES

OSHA addresses sharps handling and employee safety in its Bloodborne Pathogen Standard. The Standard requires use of engineered safety devices as well as documentation of staff exposures; however, compliance in the United States remains less than one hundred percent.[10] For example, only 33 percent of skilled nursing facilities in California reported using a sharp injury log, as required by the state OSHA, and 71 percent reported using engineered safety devices.[29] For a complete list of federal OSHA programs, see the Department of Labor website: http://www.osha.gov/dcsp/osp/index.html. Some states have local programs. The IP must review both the federal and state requirements as applicable and be prepared to implement sharps injury prevention practices in the LTCF.

A sharps safety risk assessment is the first step in developing a prevention program. A sample assessment is available from the CDC at: http://www.cdc.gov/sharpssafety/pdf/sharpsworkbook_2008.pdf. Some key assessment areas, as well as potential training topics include the use of engineered sharps safety devices, sharps disposal at point of use, and safe disposal of razors, syringe/needles, and fingerstick lancets.

> It is important for the IP to remember that ***OSHA requirements are only applicable to LTCF staff*** and do not apply if residents perform unassisted blood glucose testing using their own equipment.

Although glove use during injection of nonvascular spaces (subcutaneous, intramuscular, or intradermal) is not required under the federal bloodborne pathogens standard,[30] glove use may be necessary and HCP performing fingersticks and/or injections must be prepared to use critical thinking to determine the need for protection. Gloves should be worn when the employee anticipates occupational exposure to blood or other potentially infectious material as defined by OSHA.[31] If facility policy requires wearing gloves during injection, then the facility needs to enforce this policy. Check for other state or local requirements regarding the use of gloves during injections.

OSHA TUBERCULOSIS EXPOSURE CONTROL PLAN

HCP exposure to TB is an ongoing challenge in long-term care. Although a TB exposure control plan is not a federal OSHA requirement, it may be required at the state level. The OSHA website includes information and tools for creating and implementing a TB exposure control plan at: http://www.osha.gov/SLTC/etools/hospital/hazards/tb/tb.html.

Key provisions to prevent TB exposure are:

- Create a TB exposure control plan
- Review and update the plan annually
- Common considerations in long-term care:
  - Screen new hire employees and new resident admissions

- » The CDC has a tuberculin skin testing interpretation help sheet at: http://www.cdc.gov/tb/publications/factsheets/testing/skintesting.pdf
- Rescreen employees annually
  - » There is no annual screening recommendation for residents (http://www.cdc.gov/mmwr/preview/mmwrhtml/00001711.htm)
- Train and educate employees upon hiring and annually thereafter
- Determine if the facility meets the requirements for respirator fit testing
  - » Respirators are specially designed face masks with a tight fitting seal that covers the nose and mouth; anyone using a respirator is required to be medically evaluated and fit tested to ensure HCP safety
- Ensure the LTCF has adequate administrative and environmental controls, including airborne precautions capabilities and a respiratory protection program, if it accepts patients with suspected or confirmed infectious TB disease
- If the LTCF does not have capability to care for residents with confirmed infectious TB, ensure the LTCF has:
  - » A written protocol for the early identification of patients with symptoms or signs of TB disease
  - » Procedures for referring these patients to a setting where they can be evaluated and managed; patients with suspected or confirmed infectious TB disease should not stay in LTCFs unless adequate administrative and environmental controls and a respiratory protection program are in place
- Persons with TB disease who are determined to be noninfectious can remain in the LTCF and do not need to be in an Airborne Precautions room[18]

OCCUPATIONAL HEALTH PROGRAM ASSESSMENT

IPs should include at least an annual assessment of occupational health as a component of the infection prevention and control program. Checklists are practical tools to accomplish this and can be customized according to each facility's needs. See Table 9.2 for an example.

TABLE 9.2: SAMPLE OCCUPATIONAL HEALTH PROGRAM ASSESSMENT

For each statement, please select a YES or NO response, as appropriate.	Yes	No
The infection preventionist is responsible for implementing employee health policies. If no, who is responsible? ___	☐	☐
The infection preventionist is responsible for tracking HCP immunizations as part of the infection prevention and control program and reporting findings to an oversight committee (e.g., infection control, quality improvement, nursing practice).	☐	☐
Our facility requires HCP to have immunization or proof of immunity for Hepatitis B.	☐	☐
Our facility requires HCP to have immunization or proof of immunity for varicella (chickenpox).	☐	☐
Our facility requires HCP to have immunization or proof of immunity for measles/mumps/rubella (MMR) and pertussis.	☐	☐
Our facility provides staff with seasonal influenza vaccine at no cost to staff.	☐	☐
Our facility requires a signed declination if the HCP declines influenza vaccination.	☐	☐
Our facility requires HCP who decline influenza vaccinations to wear a mask while at work.	☐	☐
Our facility requires HCP to receive annual influenza vaccine as a condition of employment.	☐	☐
Our facility requires HCP to be screened for tuberculosis (e.g., tuberculin skin testing skin test or blood test) at time of employment.	☐	☐
Our facility requires HCP to be screened for tuberculosis (e.g., tuberculin skin test, blood test, or symptom questionnaire) annually.	☐	☐

Also available on the CD-ROM.

Modified from Centers for Disease Control and Prevention. Long term care baseline prevention practices assessment tool for states establishing HAI prevention collaboratives using ARRA funds. Available at: http://www.cdc.gov/HAI/toolkits/LTC_Assessment_tool_final.pdf.

Also see the "Additional Resources" document on the CD-ROM for a list of URLs and documents for many of the tools and guidelines mentioned in this chapter.

REFERENCES

1. Centers for Medicare & Medicaid Services (CMS). *CMS Manual System, Pub. 100-07 State Operations Provider Certification.* CMS website. 2009. Available at: http://www.cms.gov/Regulations-and-Guidance/Guidance/Transmittals/downloads/R51SOMA.pdf.
2. Smith PW, Bennett G, Bradley S, Drinka P, Lautenbach E, Marx J, et al. SHEA/APIC guideline: Infection prevention and control in the long-term care facility. *Am J Infect Control* 2008; 36: 504-535.
3. Siegel JD, Rhinehart E, Jackson M, Chiarello L, and the Healthcare Infection Control Practices Advisory Committee. *2007 Guideline for Isolation Precautions: Preventing Transmission of Infectious Agents in Healthcare Settings.* CDC website. 2007. Available at: http://www.cdc.gov/hicpac/2007IP/2007isolationPrecautions.html.
4. Bolyard EA, Tablan OC, Williams WW, Pearson ML, Shapiro CN, Deitchman SD. Guideline for infection control in healthcare personnel, 1998. *Am J Infect Control* 1998; 26: 289-354.
5. Mazurek GH, Jereb J, LoBue P, Iademarco MF, Metchock B, Vernon A, et al. Guidelines for using the QuantiFERON-TB Gold test for detecting Mycobacterium tuberculosis infection, United States. *MMWR Recomm Rep* 2005; 55(RR-15): 49-55.
6. Boyce JM, Pittet D; Healthcare Infection Control Practices Advisory Committee; HICPAC/SHEA/APIC/IDSA Hand Hygiene Task Force. Guideline for Hand Hygiene in Health-Care Settings. Recommendations of the Healthcare Infection Control Practices Advisory Committee and the HICPAC/SHEA/APIC/IDSA Hand Hygiene Task Force. *MMWR Recomm Rep* 2002; 51(RR-16): 1-56.
7. Kendall A, Landers T, Kirk J, Young E. Point-of-care hand hygiene: Preventing infection behind the curtain. *Am J Infect Control* 2012; 40: S3-S10.
8. United States Access Board. *American with Disabilities Act, Section 4.2.5.* USAB website. 2002. Available at: http://www.access-board.gov/guidelines-and-standards/buildings-and-sites/about-the-ada-standards/background/adaag#4.2.
9. Centers for Disease Control and Prevention (CDC). Ten great public health achievements – United States, 1900-1999. *MMWR Morb Mortal Wkly Rep* 1999; 48(20): 241-242.
10. Occupational Safety & Health Administration (OSHA). *Bloodborne pathogens.* OSHA website. 1991. Available at: http://www.osha.gov/pls/oshaweb/owadisp.show_document?p_table=standards&p_id=10051.
11. Shefer A, Atkinson W, Friedman C, Kuhar DT, Mootrey G, Bialek SR, et al. Immunization of health-care personnel: recommendations of the Advisory Committee on Immunization Practices (ACIP). *MMWR Recomm Rep* 2011; 60(7): 1-45.
12. Green LR, Cox T, Dolan S, Gray P, Khoury R, Kulich P, et al. *APIC position paper: Influenza vaccination should be a condition of employment for healthcare personnel, unless medically contraindicated.* APIC website. 2011. Available at: http://www.apic.org/Resource_/TinyMceFileManager/Advocacy-PDFs/APIC_Influenza_Immunization_of_HCP_12711.PDF.
13. Centers for Disease Control and Prevention (CDC). *Vaccine information statements.* CDC website. 2013. Available at: http://www.cdc.gov/vaccines/pubs/vis/vis-facts.htm#faq.
14. Kissam S, Gifford DR, Patry G, Bratzler DW. Is signed consent for influenza or pneumococcal polysaccharide vaccination required? *Arch Intern Med* 2004; 164(1): 13-16.
15. Vaccine Adverse Event Reporting System. *Frequently asked questions.* VAERS website. 2012. Available at: http://vaers.hhs.gov/about/faqs.
16. Vaccine Adverse Event Reporting System. *VAERS table of reportable events following vaccination.* VAERS website. 2008. Available at: http://vaers.hhs.gov/resources/VAERS_Table_of_Reportable_Events_Following_Vaccination.pdf.
17. U.S. Department of Health and Human Services (HHS). National Vaccine Injury Compensation Program. HRSA website. (n.d.). Available at: http://www.hrsa.gov/vaccinecompensation/index.html.
18. Jensen PA, Lambert LA, Iademarco MF, Ridzon R; CDC. Guidelines for preventing the transmission of *Mycobacterium tuberculosis* in health-care settings, 2005. *MMWR Recomm Rep* 2005; 54(RR-17): 1-144.
19. Nicolle LE. Preventing infections in non-hospital settings: long-term care. *Emerg Infect Dis* 2001; 7(2): 205-207.
20. Widera E, Chang A, Chen HL. Presenteeism: a public health hazard. *J Gen Intern Med* 2010; 25(11): 1244-1247.
21. Steering Committee on Infection Control Guidelines. Prevention and control of occupational infections in health care. An infection control guide. Canada Communicable Disease Report. *Can Comm Dis Rep* 2002; 28 Suppl 1: 1-264.
22. Occupational Safety & Health Administration (OSHA). *Nursing Homes and Personal Care Facilities.* OSHA website. (n.d.). Available at: http://www.osha.gov/SLTC/nursinghome/index.html.
23. Occupational Safety & Health Administration (OSHA). *State Occupational Safety and Health Plans.* OSHA website. (n.d.). Available at: http://www.osha.gov/dcsp/osp/index.html.
24. Occupational Safety & Health Administration (OSHA). *Recording and reporting occupational injuries and illnesses; Annual summary.* OSHA website. 2001. Available at: http://www.osha.gov/pls/oshaweb/owadisp.show_document?p_table=STANDARDS&p_id=12776.
25. Occupational Safety & Health Administration (OSHA). *Forms for Recording Work-Related Injuries and Illnesses.* OSHA website. 2004. Available at: http://www.osha.gov/recordkeeping/new-osha300form1-1-04.pdf.
26. Dolan SA, Barnes S, Cox TR, Felizardo G, Patrick M, Ward, KS. *APIC Position Paper: Safe injection, infusion and medication vial practices in healthcare.* APIC website. 2009. Available at: http://www.ascquality.org/Library/safeinjectionpracticestoolkit/Safe Injection Infusion and Medication Vial Practices in Healthcare (APIC).pdf.

REFERENCES

27. Thompson ND, Schaefer MK. "Never events": hepatitis B outbreaks and patient notifications resulting from unsafe practices during assisted monitoring of blood glucose, 2009–2010. *J Diabetes Sci Technol* 2011; 5(6): 1396-1402.

28. U.S. Food and Drug Administration (FDA). Information for Healthcare Professionals: Risk of Transmission of Blood-borne Pathogens from Shared Use of Insulin Pens. FDA website. Available at: http://www.fda.gov/Drugs/DrugSafetyPostmarketDrugSafetyInformationforPatientsandProviders/DrugSafetyInformationforHeathcareProfessionals/ucm133352.htm.

29. Gillen M, Davis M, McNary J, Boyd A, Lewis J, Curran C, et al. Sharps injury recordkeeping activities and safety product use in California healthcare facilities. *Am J Infect Control* 2002; 30(5): 269-276.

30. Occupational Safety & Health Administration (OSHA). *Standards interpretations, Standard 1910.1030.* OSHA website. 1992. Available at: http://www.osha.gov/pls/oshaweb/owadisp.show_document?p_table=INTERPRETATIONS&p_id=20819.

31. Occupational Safety & Health Administration (OSHA). *OSHA Fact Sheet, Bloodborne pathogens standard.* OSHA website. 2011. Available at: http://www.osha.gov/OshDoc/data_BloodborneFacts/bbfact01.pdf.

CHAPTER 10

Environment and Equipment

Dolly Greene, RN, CIC
Steven J. Schweon, RN, MPH, MSN, CIC, HEM

KEY CONCEPTS

- Environmental sanitation is an integral part of the responsibilities of the LTCF in providing a safe and sanitary environment for the residents and staff.
- There is increasing evidence indicating that the environment in healthcare facilities can be a reservoir for infectious agents such as bacteria, fungus, and viruses.
- Cleaning and disinfection will provide a safe and sanitary environment for residents and staff.
- Cleaning, disinfecting, and storing equipment and supplies is important in preventing the transmission of potential pathogens within the long-term care facility.
- The infection preventionist serves as an important resource for environmental services by providing appropriate tools, training, education, and audits to monitor and maintain infection prevention and control practices.

In the past, the department responsible for the care and hygiene of the long-term care facility (LTCF) was often referred to as the housekeeping department. As cleaning and sanitation practices are increasingly viewed in the broader context of facility safety and disease prevention, the preferred terminology has changed to environmental services (EVS). The new term reflects the expanding scope of these programs.

As a result of these changing views, environmental hygiene in LTCF has become a priority for infection preventionists (IPs). According to Drs. Weber and Rutala, international experts in environmental infection prevention, "Over the past decade, there has been a growing appreciation that environmental contamination makes an important contribution to hospital-acquired infection with MRSA and VRE. More recently, environmental contamination has been demonstrated to play an important role in acquisition of infection with *C. difficile*, norovirus and *Acinetobacter* species."[1]

Recent studies have demonstrated that several major pathogens are shed by residents and contaminate surfaces at concentrations sufficient for transmission. Some items such as the call bell, bed frame, and over-bed table have been known to harbor pathogenic microorganisms that survive for extended periods of time. Incomplete cleaning and disinfection procedures, combined with the persistence of pathogens in the environment, increase the likelihood that healthcare personnel (HCP) hands will unknowingly become contaminated. Since hand hygiene compliance is a challenge in all types of healthcare facilities, the use of hand washing and alcohol-based hand rubs may not be sufficient to reduce microorganisms and create a safe environment for the residents, staff and visitors.[2]

Environmental risks are further exacerbated by interinstitutional transfers. As residents participate in social activities beyond their facility and/or are transferred between facilities for specific medical needs, the risk of exposure to pathogenic microorganisms in the environment increases. Although this phenomenon has not yet been thoroughly investigated in long-term care settings, the application of disease transfer models indicates that practices initially used for early prevention may require modification once a pathogenic microorganism becomes endemic within the facility.[3]

CLEANING VS. DISINFECTION

The terms "cleaning" and "disinfection" are often used together, and the IP must understand the difference between them.

Cleaning is the physical removal of dirt, body fluids, and other organic matter. Cleaning is accomplished by a combination of detergent, water, and applied friction. Cleaning does not mean that the surface is free of pathogens. It reduces the number of potential pathogens to the point in which their presence is unlikely to cause harm. For that reason, a clean surface cannot be presumed to be disinfected or sterile.

Disinfection destroys the number of potential pathogens on a surface. Although this is most commonly done using Environmental Protection Agency (EPA)-approved chemicals, alternate methods using heat, ultraviolet light, and fogging can also be used in some situations. A surface cannot be disinfected unless it has been cleaned. Organic matter such as blood and body fluids will inactivate disinfectants. Different disinfectants kill specific types of organisms but do not produce sterility no matter their strength or frequency of use.[4,5]

SELECTION OF CLEANING AND DISINFECTING PRODUCTS[3]

In the United States, the EPA registers disinfecting products and indicates their level of effectiveness. Products used in hospitals and other healthcare facilities are commonly referred to as "hospital-grade disinfectants." Products selected for use in LTCF should meet these criteria.[5]

The IP's role in the selection of cleaning and disinfecting products varies by facility. If the IP is not directly involved in the product review and selection process, it is essential that the IP knows not only the types of products used at the LTCF, but also the circumstances for which these products are used. This includes the use of cleaners and disinfectants that are one-step or combination commercial products and the use of diluted bleach (sodium hypochlorite), whether prepared by EVS staff or premixed in a commercial product. Disinfectants should be broad spectrum—meaning, they can eliminate bacteria, viruses, protozoa, fungi, and, in some cases, spores. The IP should check the product information to find out "kill claims" or "label claims" and other key specifications to be sure the product meet the needs of the LTCF. The EPA registration label lists essential information on every approved product. For instructions on how to read an EPA label, see Figure 10.1.

> While emerging environmentally preferable "eco-friendly" products are now available, the criteria that define a "green" cleaner have not yet been established. ***As a general rule, environmentally preferable cleaning products claim to be biodegradable, do not include phosphate or chlorine, and are not manufactured from petrochemicals.*** Until more studies have been done, these types of products are most appropriate for low-risk, community settings.[6]

Another important consideration is the direct contact time required for the disinfectant to be effective. This information is also specified on the label. However, in some cases, the products once applied will dry before the length of time stated on the label. In this case, repeated applications will be necessary. Repeated applications increase EVS work time and add costs to the LTCF. Failing to meet the label requirements for direct contact time has resulted in survey citations. For this reason, IPs should evaluate a range of products available, as newer products now offer shorter required contact times.

The decision to use a particular agent requires careful consideration of other variables as well. For example, a product recommendation should include not only its effectiveness against the potential pathogen identified on the label, but also its safety for residents and staff and potential damage to equipment and/or the environment. Many LTCFs choose to implement a tiered approach to environmental cleaning. Often when the LTCF is struggling with recurrent or persistent types of infections such as *Clostridium difficile*, or has identified an outbreak, changes in both products and cleaning/disinfecting practices may be necessary. However, all chemicals have drawbacks; it is imperative that the IP understand the potential advantages and disadvantages when recommending or evaluating LTCF product use. A summary of this information is presented in Table 10.1.[3,7]

CLEANING PRACTICES AND LTCF RISK FACTORS

The LTCF is a complex environment that contains a diversity of microbial flora, many of which may pose a risk to the residents, staff, and visitors. Residents in LTCFs are particularly susceptible to infection due to their age-related decline in immunologic function. In addition, they may have a variety of conditions that predispose them to infection. (See Chapter 6 on nursing care for a description of common infection risks in the long-term care population.)

Core infection prevention program areas to successfully address these challenges include:

- Hand hygiene (see Chapter 5)
- Use of personal protective equipment (PPE) when indicated (see Chapters 5 and 9)
- Use of Isolation Precautions (see Chapter 5)
- Identification and consistent implementation of standard protocols for environmental hygiene
- A system to regularly monitor the effectiveness of cleaning and disinfecting practices and make sustainable improvements as needed

CLEANING POLICIES, PROCEDURES, AND SCHEDULES

Facility procedures must clearly describe the steps to be taken in order to ensure a safe and hygienic environment. The IP should review the EVS policies and procedures with

FIGURE 10.1: DISINFECTANT PRODUCT LABELS

Understanding the information on a disinfectant product label is essential for effective disease organism removal and the safety of those handling the product. Always read the product label before use. It is a violation of federal law to use a product in a manner inconsistent with its labeling. In order to increase awareness of what a product label contains, this handout will provide you with a step-by-step guide of a disinfectant label.

Only products with EPA registration numbers should be used. This number indicates the product has been reviewed by the EPA and poses minimal risk to animals, people and the environment when used in accordance with their label.

This section will describe the hazards related to humans and animals when using this product. It recommends personal protective gear that should be worn, what effects it will have on the environment and treatment information should it be splashed into the eyes or ingested.

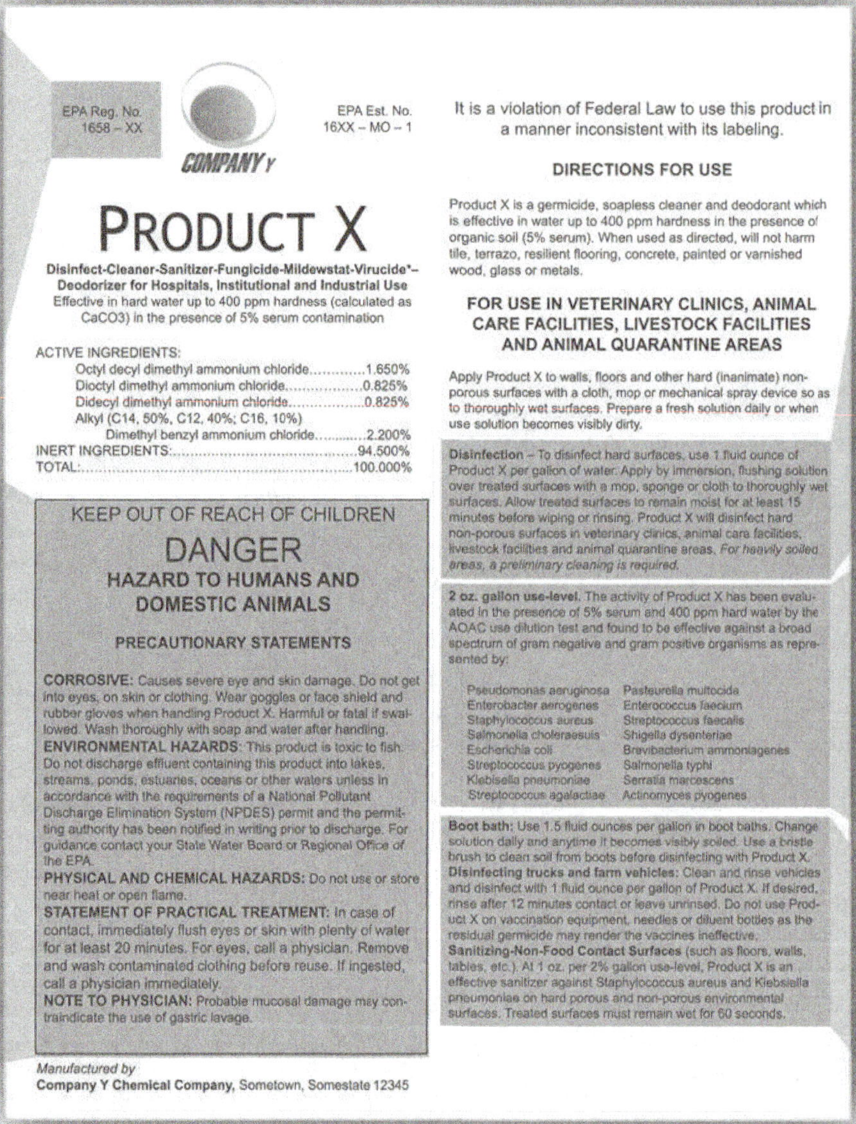

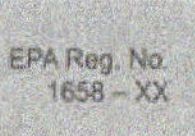

COMPANY Y

EPA Est. No.
16XX – MO – 1

PRODUCT X

Disinfect-Cleaner-Sanitizer-Fungicide-Mildewstat-Virucide*–
Deodorizer for Hospitals, Institutional and Industrial Use
Effective in hard water up to 400 ppm hardness (calculated as CaCO3) in the presence of 5% serum contamination

ACTIVE INGREDIENTS:
Octyl decyl dimethyl ammonium chloride............1.650%
Dioctyl dimethyl ammonium chloride.................0.825%
Didecyl dimethyl ammonium chloride.................0.825%
Alkyl (C14, 50%, C12, 40%; C16, 10%)
Dimethyl benzyl ammonium chloride...........2.200%
INERT INGREDIENTS:.......................................94.500%
TOTAL:...100.000%

KEEP OUT OF REACH OF CHILDREN

DANGER

HAZARD TO HUMANS AND DOMESTIC ANIMALS

PRECAUTIONARY STATEMENTS

CORROSIVE: Causes severe eye and skin damage. Do not get into eyes, on skin or clothing. Wear goggles or face shield and rubber gloves when handling Product X. Harmful or fatal if swallowed. Wash thoroughly with soap and water after handling.
ENVIRONMENTAL HAZARDS: This product is toxic to fish. Do not discharge effluent containing this product into lakes, streams, ponds, estuaries, oceans or other waters unless in accordance with the requirements of a National Pollutant Discharge Elimination System (NPDES) permit and the permitting authority has been notified in writing prior to discharge. For guidance contact your State Water Board or Regional Office of the EPA.
PHYSICAL AND CHEMICAL HAZARDS: Do not use or store near heat or open flame.
STATEMENT OF PRACTICAL TREATMENT: In case of contact, immediately flush eyes or skin with plenty of water for at least 20 minutes. For eyes, call a physician. Remove and wash contaminated clothing before reuse. If ingested, call a physician immediately.
NOTE TO PHYSICIAN: Probable mucosal damage may contraindicate the use of gastric lavage.

Manufactured by
Company Y Chemical Company, Sometown, Somestate 12345

It is a violation of Federal Law to use this product in a manner inconsistent with its labeling.

DIRECTIONS FOR USE

Product X is a germicide, soapless cleaner and deodorant which is effective in water up to 400 ppm hardness in the presence of organic soil (5% serum). When used as directed, will not harm tile, terrazo, resilient flooring, concrete, painted or varnished wood, glass or metals.

FOR USE IN VETERINARY CLINICS, ANIMAL CARE FACILITIES, LIVESTOCK FACILITIES AND ANIMAL QUARANTINE AREAS

Apply Product X to walls, floors and other hard (inanimate) non-porous surfaces with a cloth, mop or mechanical spray device so as to thoroughly wet surfaces. Prepare a fresh solution daily or when use solution becomes visibly dirty.

Disinfection – To disinfect hard surfaces, use 1 fluid ounce of Product X per gallon of water. Apply by immersion, flushing solution over treated surfaces with a mop, sponge or cloth to thoroughly wet surfaces. Allow treated surfaces to remain moist for at least 15 minutes before wiping or rinsing. Product X will disinfect hard non-porous surfaces in veterinary clinics, animal care facilities, livestock facilities and animal quarantine areas. *For heavily soiled areas, a preliminary cleaning is required.*

2 oz. gallon use-level. The activity of Product X has been evaluated in the presence of 5% serum and 400 ppm hard water by the AOAC use dilution test and found to be effective against a broad spectrum of gram negative and gram positive organisms as represented by:

Pseudomonas aeruginosa — Pasteurella multocida
Enterobacter aerogenes — Enterococcus faecium
Staphylococcus aureus — Streptococcus faecalis
Salmonella choleraesuis — Shigella dysenteriae
Escherichia coli — Brevibacterium ammoniagenes
Streptococcus pyogenes — Salmonella typhi
Klebsiella pneumoniae — Serratia marcescens
Streptococcus agalactiae — Actinomyces pyogenes

Boot bath: Use 1.5 fluid ounces per gallon in boot baths. Change solution daily and anytime it becomes visibly soiled. Use a bristle brush to clean soil from boots before disinfecting with Product X.
Disinfecting trucks and farm vehicles: Clean and rinse vehicles and disinfect with 1 fluid ounce per gallon of Product X. If desired, rinse after 12 minutes contact or leave unrinsed. Do not use Product X on vaccination equipment, needles or diluent bottles as the residual germicide may render the vaccines ineffective.
Sanitizing-Non-Food Contact Surfaces (such as floors, walls, tables, etc.). At 1 oz. per 2% gallon use-level, Product X is an effective sanitizer against Staphylococcus aureus and Klebsiella pneumoniae on hard porous and non-porous environmental surfaces. Treated surfaces must remain wet for 60 seconds.

Some products may have multiple uses (i.e., cleaning versus disinfection) and require different dilutions and contact times for such actions.

This section describes what disease organism the product controls, as well as where, how and when to use it.

Specialty applications for the product (i.e., boot baths, vehicle disinfection) will also be listed.

the Center for Food Security & Public Health
IOWA STATE UNIVERSITY®

disinfectant_product_label

Used with permission courtesy of Iowa State University Center for Food Security & Public Health.

TABLE 10.1: SUMMARY OF USES, ADVANTAGES, AND DISADVANTAGES OF SURFACE DISINFECTANTS[3,7]

Use	Advantages	Disadvantages
ALCOHOL		
• Disinfection of small surfaces • Disinfection of oral and rectal thermometers, stethoscopes, external surfaces of some equipment	• Bacteriocidal, tuberculocidal, fungicidal, virucidal • Fast-acting • Easy to use • No toxic residue	• Not EPA registered • Not sporicidal • No detergent or cleaning properties • Affected by organic matter • Flammable • Evaporates rapidly making extended exposure time difficult • May damage instruments (e.g., harden rubber)
CHLORINE		
• Disinfection of environmental surfaces (e.g., countertops, floors) • Disinfectant used in water treatment • 1:10 dilution of 5.25-6.15% sodium hypochlorite recommended for decontaminating blood spills • Other dilutions as appropriate	• EPA registered • Broad spectrum, bactericidal, virucidal, fungicidal, sporicidal, tuberculocidal • No toxic residue • Not affected by water hardness • Inexpensive • Fast acting	• Concentration of 5.25-6.15% can cause ocular irritation or oropharyngeal, esophageal, and gastric burns • Corrosive to metals in high concentrations (>500 ppm) • Inactivated by organic material • Discoloration/"bleaching" of fabrics • Release of toxic chlorine gas if mixed with ammonia or acid • Must be mixed fresh daily; loses concentration over time
HYDROGEN PEROXIDE		
• Disinfects inanimate surfaces (floors, walls, countertops) • Can be used for spot-disinfecting on fabrics • Higher concentrations used for high-level disinfection	• EPA registered • Bactericidal, virucidal, fungicidal, sporicidal • Fast acting (30 second – 1 min bactericidal/virucidal claim, 5 min mycobactericidal claim) • Not affected by organic matter • Stable • Noncorrosive • Non-staining • Lowest EPA toxicity category	• Can be more expensive than other low level disinfectants • May be incompatible with some materials including brass, zinc, copper, and nickel/silver plating • Contact with eyes causes severe damage
IODOPHORS		
• More commonly used as an antiseptic • Used to disinfect blood culture bottles and hydrotherapy tanks	• Bactericidal, mycobactericidal, virucidal	• Not sporicidal • Prolonged contact time needed to kill fungi • Damages silicone catheters • Antiseptic iodophors not suitable as hard-surface disinfectants
QUARTERNARY AMMONIUM COMPOUNDS		
• Cleans/disinfects floors, walls, and furnishings • Can be used to disinfect medical equipment that comes into contact with intact skin	• EPA registered • Bactericidal, fungicidal, virucidal against enveloped viruses • Surface compatible	• Not sporicidal, tuberculocidal, or virucidal against nonenveloped viruses • Poor mycobactericidal activity • High water hardness and cotton/gauze pads reduce microbicidal properties • Documented reports of asthma caused by exposure to benzalkonium chloride • Affected by organic matter

Table 10.1 Continued

Use	Advantages	Disadvantages
PHENOLICS		
• Surface disinfectant (e.g., bedside tables, bedrails, laboratory surfaces) • Noncritical medical device disinfectant	• EPA registered • Tuberculocidal, fungicidal, virucidal, bactericidal • Inexpensive	• Absorbed by porous materials • Irritates tissue • Some phenolics cause depigmentation of skin

facility leadership at least annually to verify that practices are up-to-date. Examples of cleaning practices that must be specified in LTCF EVS policy and procedure include:

- Approved cleaning and disinfecting products, their use(s), and storage
- Procedure and schedules for routine cleaning and trash removal
- EVS staff safety, PPE, eye protection as needed, chemical safety, and safety data sheet (SDS; formerly known as Material Safety Data Sheets or MSDSs)
- Terminal cleaning procedure
- Cleaning in isolation rooms and multidrug-resistant organism (MDRO) awareness
- Floor cleaning and buffing
- Hazardous and nonhazardous spills
- Disposal of biohazard containers, including steps to take if/when sharps are discovered in the regular trash
- Use of wipes, mops, and other cleaning supplies
- Maintenance of the EVS cart
- Routine cleaning of common areas
- Cleaning of glass and windows
- Maintenance of carpets, privacy curtains, mattresses, and other soft surfaces

The EVS supervisor is responsible for maintaining a schedule of cleaning tasks and the employee responsible for them. The IP should perform regular observations and audits of EVS department cleaning procedures and correct use of infection prevention and control practices. Procedures should clearly describe accountability for the following oversight functions:

- Cleaning/disinfecting is an ongoing process in the facility.
- Cleaning/disinfecting procedures incorporate the principles of infection prevention and control.
- Cleaning schedules ensure routine cleaning is consistent.
- Cleaning/disinfecting procedures are aligned with the best practices in patient/resident safety science.

Routine Cleaning Recommendations

- Clean all surfaces such as tabletops, window ledges, bedside tables, counters, sinks, tubs, floors, toilet seats, etc. according to an established EVS schedule. Use the LTCF's approved hospital-grade cleaner/disinfectant according to manufacturer directions. Cleaning must be done before any surface can be disinfected.
- Clean hard surfaces as needed when spills or soiling occurs.
- Vacuum all carpets daily and as needed to maintain a safe, clean, and sanitary environment. Clean carpets as needed.
- Clean walls and blinds according to the LTCF cleaning schedule and whenever dust/soil is visible.
- Wet dust horizontal surfaces regularly by moistening a clean cloth with a small amount of an EPA-registered, hospital-grade detergent/disinfectant to remove organism-laden particles from the surfaces in the resident area.[3,8]
- Clean high-touch surfaces daily and more often as needed during outbreaks. Frequency may need to be increased during cold or flu season.
- Use friction (wiping or scrubbing) in addition to a germicide to remove surface soil from contaminated items prior to disinfection.
- Verify that the EVS staff is using correct dilution of disinfectants/germicides, recommended contact time, and appropriate environmental conditions, as these conditions may greatly affect the adequacy of disinfection. Follow manufacturer's directions for use.
- Disposable cleaning supplies should be discarded prior to cleaning the next room.

Always follow safety precautions regarding cleaning chemical. All chemical products used in the facility must have a SDS on file and readily accessible to staff. Chemicals must be securely stored when not in use. All cleaning supplies should be stored in the original containers when possible, and any new container should be adequately labeled (not handwritten on the container).

Common High Touch Surfaces

- Side rails
- Over-bed table
- Nightstand
- Call light
- Remote control devices
- Telephone
- Cubicle curtain
- Light switches
- Doorknobs, handrails, other handles
- Rails, sink, toilet, and other bathroom fixtures
- Computer keyboards and tablets
- Grips, armrests, handles for wheelchairs, walkers, and other mobility equipment

MICROFIBER TECHNOLOGY

Cleaning products are now available using microfiber—extremely fine polyester and nylon materials. Microfiber can be woven into textiles with the texture and drape of natural-fiber cloth but with enhanced washability, breathability, and water repellency.[9] In LTCFs, microfiber technology is often used in disposable wipes and mop heads. Although it is more expensive to purchase than cotton fiber alternatives, studies have confirmed multiple advantages of the microfiber technology. An EPA-funded study comparing microfiber to conventional string mop found that microfiber produced a 60 percent lifetime cost savings, 95 percent reduction in chemical costs, and 20 percent reduction in labor costs per day.[10] In addition, a study conducted at the University of North Carolina demonstrated that microfiber systems showed better microbial removal (95 percent) when compared to traditional cotton mops (68 percent) and using a detergent cleaner.[11]

TERMINAL ROOM CLEANING[8,12]

- Terminal cleaning occurs after a resident is discharged or transferred. All surfaces that came in contact with the resident or might have been contaminated during resident care must be cleaned and disinfected. This includes not only high touch surfaces but also mattresses, headboards, furniture, and privacy curtains, if used in the room.
- Unused items such as toilet paper, towels, etc. are considered contaminated and should be discarded if disposable or cleaned if reusable.
- All linen that is found in a resident's room, used or unused, is considered contaminated and must be sent to the laundry.
- Inspect pillows and mattress. If holes are found, they must be replaced.
- Use a hospital-grade EPA-approved disinfectant or combination cleaner/disinfectant during all steps of the terminal cleaning process.
- EVS staff must use PPE, including a gown, when performing terminal cleaning. All PPE must be removed and discarded and hand hygiene performed upon exiting the cleaned room.

For discharged or transferred residents with known colonization or recovering from a multidrug-resistant infection, LTCF infection prevention procedures may direct that the room undergo more rigorous terminal cleaning. The methods, thoroughness, and frequency of cleaning and the products used are determined by facility policy.[13]

Terminal Cleaning and *Clostridium difficile*

C. difficile spores are challenging to eradicate. Studies have shown that asymptomatic carriers remain an important reservoir and that person-to-person transmission presents the greatest threat to LTC residents. They can be resistant to commonly used cleaner/disinfectants and can persist in the environment for long periods of time. For that reason, EVS staff must use an EPA-registered sporicidal agent. The most common disinfectant used for *C. difficile* is a hypochlorite dilution of 1:10. Some newer disinfectants use hydrogen peroxide for elimination of *C. difficile*. However, precleaning to remove organic matter is required before using any approved disinfectant. Meticulous environmental cleaning and disinfecting practices are essential to prevent cross contamination within the LTCF.[3]

Emerging Technologies for Enhanced and Terminal Cleaning

In recent years, a number of promising new technologies have been developed for enhanced and/or terminal cleaning in healthcare settings. These technologies seek to provide a more thorough level of room disinfection than typically achieved through manual methods and emphasize the elimination of potentially transmissible pathogens. There are currently four categories of emerging technology:

- **Ultraviolet (UV) light:** UV-C destroys microorganisms by creating thymine dimers and inhibiting replication. This process has been used for years to reduce microbial contamination.[14] Newer adaptations provide a mobile unit that can effectively decontaminate a cleaned, unoccupied room.
- **Hydrogen peroxide vaporization:** This method generates vapor of hydrogen peroxide that is completely dispersed throughout the room. At the end of the process, the hydrogen peroxide is broken down catalytically to water vapor and oxygen. EPA considers this process a fumigant.[15] A portable unit is placed in a closed unoccupied room after cleaning.
- **Hydrogen peroxide aerosolization:** This method generates a fine mist by aerosolizing a solution containing 5 percent hydrogen peroxide. The EPA considers this to be a "fogging" process. After exposure, the aerosol is left to decompose spontaneously.[15]
- **Antimicrobial-coated surfaces:** Coating or impregnating copper or silver into hard surfaces seeks to provide a self-disinfecting process independent of the user. Studies are limited and application of the implications of this new technology in LTCFs are not yet fully understood or documented.

In 2013, the Centers for Disease Control and Prevention (CDC) issued the clarification regarding fogging.

These recommendations refer to the spraying or fogging of chemicals (e.g., formaldehyde, phenol-based agents, or quaternary ammonium compounds) as a way to decontaminate environmental surfaces or disinfect the air in patient rooms. The recommendation against fogging was based on studies in the 1970s that reported a lack of microbicidal efficacy (e.g., use of quaternary ammonium compounds in mist applications) but also adverse effects on healthcare workers and others in facilities where these methods were utilized. Furthermore, some of these chemicals are not EPA-registered for use in fogging-type applications.

CDC and HICPAC have recommendations in both 2003 *Guidelines for Environmental Infection Control in Health-Care Facilities* and the 2008 *Guideline for Disinfection and Sterilization in Healthcare Facilities* that state that the CDC does not support disinfectant fogging. Specifically, the 2003 and 2008 guidelines state:

- **2003:** "Do not perform disinfectant fogging for routine purposes in patient-care areas. Category IB"
- **2008:** "Do not perform disinfectant fogging in patient-care areas. Category II"

These recommendations do not apply to newer technologies involving fogging for room decontamination (e.g., ozone mists, vaporized hydrogen peroxide) that have become available since the 2003 and 2008 recommendations were made. These newer technologies were assessed by CDC and HICPAC in the 2011 *Guideline for the Prevention and Control of Norovirus Gastroenteritis Outbreaks in Healthcare Settings,* which makes the recommendation:

> "More research is required to clarify the effectiveness and reliability of fogging, UV irradiation, and ozone mists to reduce norovirus environmental contamination. (No recommendation/unresolved issue)"[16]

The 2003 and 2008 recommendations still apply; however, CDC does not yet make a recommendation regarding these newer technologies.[3,8]

TABLE 10.2: A COMPARISON OF THE ADVANTAGES AND DISADVANTAGES OF EMERGING TECHNOLOGIES FOR CLEANING AND DISINFECTION

Use	Advantages	Disadvantages
UV LIGHT		
Terminal disinfection method	• Active against a wide range of organisms relatively easy to use. • Published evidence of use in clinical settings • To reduce environmental contamination and infection rates • No need to seal off air ducts	• Expense • Must use in unoccupied room • Correct placement in room • Must move furniture • Needs to be correctly placed in the room
HYDROGEN PEROXIDE		
Terminal disinfection method	• Active against many pathogens • More effective than manual cleaning/disinfection (even distribution) • Great for disinfecting complex equipment • No toxic by-products; breaks down to water and oxygen • Published evidence of use in clinical settings to reduce environmental contamination and infection rates	• Does not remove dust and visible dirt/debris • Room must be empty and sealed • Logistical complexity (travel, FTEs, sealing air supply) • Time
COPPER		
Self-disinfecting surface	• Not use dependent • Continuous action	• Modest studies • Corrosion
SILVER		
Self-disinfecting surface	• Not use dependent • Continuous action	• Lack of studies in healthcare environment

Courtesy of Linda R. Greene, RN, MPS, CIC

Technology continues to focus on the environment, and new products, especially the "no touch" approaches, are in development. The IP must recognize that EVS is a dynamic field and new options are continuously proposed. The ability to critically evaluate emerging technologies will be increasingly important to weigh the advantages and disadvantages in coming years. A current comparison of the advantages and disadvantages is represented in Table 10.2.[5]

MONITORING CLEANING AND DISINFECTING PRACTICES

The EVS department is responsible for ensuring the quality of cleaning. However, ensuring that cleaning practices are complete and effective present special challenges for the LTCF IP. Multiple studies have shown that EVS personnel wipe only about 50 percent of surfaces targeted for cleaning.[17-19] Environmental rounds and regular visual inspection can detect obvious problems but are insufficient to ensure the removal of potential pathogens. For that reason, the use of environmental monitoring systems is being incorporated into quality improvement programs.

The first step in quality monitoring usually includes the use of checklists or other audit tools. Including staff in the use of these tools encourages a sense of shared responsibility. In addition, providing feedback to EVS staff has been shown to increase motivation and engagement with resulting improvements. An example of an environmental monitoring checklist for routine cleaning is in Table 10.6 as well as on the CD-ROM.[17]

There are several methods to determine if effective cleaning has taken place, each with its own advantages and disadvantages. Table 10.3 outlines these methods and the advantages and disadvantages of each. These methods fall under the following three categories:

- **Direct and indirect observation** (e.g., visual assessment, observation of performance, resident satisfaction surveys)
- **Detection of residual bioburden** (e.g., environmental culture, adenosine triphosphate-ATP bioluminescence)
- **Environmental marking** (e.g., fluorescent marking of hard surfaces)

TRASH

Routine infection prevention rounds should include ongoing inspection of timely trash removal not only from resident rooms, but also from all other areas of the LTCF. Facility trash must be removed per an established schedule and placed in a dumpster or other designated trash receptacle.

The IP should monitor that the steps below are being followed:

- Facility trash containers should be lined and EVS staff instructed to lift the liner rather than reaching into containers.
- Trash bags should be removed when ¾ full and tied (or otherwise secured).
- Trash bags should not be left on the floor; they must be removed in an approved holding bin or dumpster.
- Medical waste, especially biohazard containers, cannot be mixed with regular trash.
- A procedure for responding to any exposed sharp object discovered in regular trash must be in place and communicated to all staff.

MEDICAL WASTE

There is no uniform national standard for defining the wastes that comprise the category of regulated medical waste. However, in the United States, there are five federal agencies that have established regulated waste definitions. These agencies are as follows:

- **U.S. Environmental Protection Agency** (EPA; 40 CFR Part 60.51c)
- **U.S. Department of Transportation** (DOT; 49 CFR Part 173.134)
- **Occupational Health and Safety Administration** (OSHA; 29 CFR Part 1910.1030(b)
- **United States Postal Service** (USPS; 39 CFR Part 111.1)
- **U.S. Public Health Service** (PHS; 42 CFR Part 72.3).[13]

OSHA published a definition for what it has termed "regulated waste." This definition specifically includes wastes that meet the following criteria[20]:

- Liquid or semi-liquid blood or other potentially infectious materials ("other potentially infectious materials" means the following: human body fluids; semen, vaginal secretions, cerebrospinal fluid, synovial fluid, pleural fluid, pericardial fluid, peritoneal fluid, amniotic fluid, saliva in dental procedures, and all body fluids where it is difficult or impossible to differentiate between body fluids).
- Contaminated items that would release blood or other potentially infectious materials in a liquid or semi-liquid state if compressed.
- Items that are caked with dried blood or other potentially infectious materials and are capable of releasing these materials during handling.
- Contaminated sharps.
- Pathological and microbiological wastes containing blood or other potentially infectious materials.

Medical waste requires careful disposal and containment before collection. OSHA mandates that a single leak-resistant biohazard-labeled bag is usually adequate for containment of regulated waste provided the bag is sturdy and the waste can be discarded without contaminating the exterior of the bag. All bags should be securely closed for disposal. Puncture-resistant containers located at the point of use (i.e., sharps containers) are used as containment for discarded items with small amounts of blood (e.g., scalpel blades, needles, syringes, lancets). To prevent needlestick injuries, needles and other contaminated sharps should not be recapped, purposefully bent, or broken by hand. CDC has published general guidelines for handling sharps.[8,20]

TABLE 10.3: ADVANTAGES AND DISADVANTAGES OF CLEANLINESS ASSESSMENT METHODOLOGIES[10,17,19]

Advantages	Disadvantages
OBSERVATION AND INSPECTION	
• Ease of use • Cost-effective • Encourages staff participation	• Difficulty in standardizing methodology • May be viewed as punitive or "policing" activity • Results might be impacted by Hawthorne effect* • Subjective
RESIDENT SATISFACTION SURVEY	
• Encourages resident participation • Can include feedback from facility and visitors • Minimal cost	• Subjective data may not be reliable • Feedback tends to emphasize cleanliness; disinfection practices may be less obvious to residents • No benchmarks for comparison
ENVIRONMENTAL CULTURE	
• May be helpful as part of an epidemiological or outbreak investigation • Provides quantitative measure	• Not recommended by CDC as routine measure • High cost to LTCF • Presence of organism(s) may not correspond to resident infections or outbreak • Results not available for 48-72 hrs
ATP LUMINESCENCE	
• Easy to use system • Provides immediate feedback • Can be helpful when evaluating new/novel cleaning methods	• Detection of organic matter (bioburden) is not a reliable predictor of infection risk • Cost of testing equipment and supplies
FLUORESCENT MARKING TOOLS	
• Inexpensive • Easy to perform with minimal equipment • Results readily available	• Does not identify potential pathogens • Only detects whether a surface has been cleaned (yes/no methodology) • No quantitative assessment of cleanliness • Requires a team approach to avoid staff perception of "policing"

*Hawthorne effect: refers to a phenomenon that is thought to occur when people observed during an inspection, audit, or research study temporarily change their behavior or performance to reflect the desired outcome.

See Chapter 9 for additional information on sharps safety.

Healthcare facilities are instructed to dispose of medical waste regularly to avoid contamination. Medical waste requiring storage should be kept in labeled, leak-proof, puncture-resistant containers under conditions that minimize or prevent foul odors. The storage area should be well ventilated and be inaccessible to pests. Any facility that generates regulated medical wastes should have a regulated waste management plan to ensure health and environmental safety as per federal, state, and local regulations.[8]

In addition to federal definitions, the regulated community must also consider the definitions developed by the individual state legislatures and governments. Before developing a medical waste management plan, each facility should obtain and review all pertinent local and state regulations.

HAND HYGIENE SUPPLIES

In most LTCFs the EVS staff is responsible for replenishing hand hygiene supplies. This includes the soap, paper towels, and alcohol-based hand products used throughout the facility. During routine rounds, the IP should check that:

- Dispensers are in working order and there is no leakage onto the counter or the floor.
- All dispensers have sufficient product for at least another 24 hours of use.
- Paper towel dispensers, if used, are refilled.
- Waste receptacles for paper towels are emptied per schedule and are not overflowing.

PREVENTION OF LATEX ALLERGIES[21]

EVS staff, like other employees who routinely use disposable gloves, are at risk for an allergic reaction to latex. Reports of latex allergies have increased in recent years, prompting the National Institute for Occupational Safety and Health to issue guidance on how to recognize and prevent these adverse events.

Latex allergy is a reaction to certain proteins in latex rubber. The amount of latex exposure needed to produce sensitization or an allergic reaction is unknown. Mild reactions to latex involve skin redness, rash, hives, or itching. Contact dermatitis is the most common reaction; it may resemble a poison ivy skin reaction. More severe reactions may involve respiratory symptoms such as runny nose, sneezing, itchy eyes, scratchy throat, and asthma (difficult breathing, coughing spells, and wheezing). Shock rarely occurs; however, a life-threatening reaction is seldom the first sign of latex allergy. Skin contact is not the only means of exposure. When HCP change gloves, the protein/powder particles become airborne and can be inhaled. Inhalation can also trigger allergic symptoms.

For employees who develop a latex sensitivity, avoidance of latex products, while difficult, is the best approach. Additional prevention measures should include:

- If latex gloves must be used, use powder-free gloves with reduced protein content. Such gloves reduce exposures to latex protein and thus reduce the risk of latex allergy.
- Understand that "hypoallergenic" latex gloves do not reduce the risk of latex allergy. However, they may reduce reactions to chemical additives in the latex (allergic contact dermatitis).
- If latex gloves must be worn, do not use oil-based hand creams or lotions (which can cause glove deterioration).
- After removing latex gloves, wash hands with a mild soap and dry thoroughly.
- Frequently clean areas and equipment contaminated with latex-containing dust.

EQUIPMENT AND SUPPLIES

The proper handling, cleaning, disinfection, transportation, and storage of resident care items and equipment used for both personal needs and medical treatment are critical to promote health and prevent pathogen transmission. There have been documented instances of infection transmission from improper or insufficient cleaning and disinfection of resident care items or equipment. For example, a CDC report in 2005 linked breakdowns in cleaning and disinfection of glucometers to transmission of Hepatitis B in long-term care residents.[22]

The Centers for Medicare & Medicaid Services (CMS) requirements emphasize reducing infection risk from medical equipment, devices, and supplies through proper cleaning and disinfection and correct storage strategies. An LTCF could receive a regulatory citation for not being in compliance and for placing residents at risk. In addition to citations, facilities that do not properly manage resident care items may also face financial loss due to inadvertent contamination or breakage.[23]

The IP faces a variety of factors when implementing policies and best practices for cleaning, disinfection, and storage of supplies and equipment. Staffing challenges and increased complexity of residents care needs can result in breakdowns in policy and procedure. Space constraints in both the resident's room and the facility can make it challenging to meet requirements. To ensure the safety of staff and residents, HCP need education on best practices, policies, and procedures.

Infection prevention program policies must identify what items need to cleaned, disinfected, or sterilized and by whom. Policies should be based on regulatory requirements and guidelines as well as the manufacturer's recommendations and should include computers and

TABLE 10.4: TYPE OF RESIDENT CARE ITEMS AND CLEANING/DISINFECTING CONSIDERATIONS

Resident Care Items	Considerations
Equipment made of metal, plastic, vinyl, rubber	Check with the manufacturer as needed to ensure compatibility with the cleaning/disinfecting agent
Hard to clean items made of fabric, foam (e.g., wheelchair cushions, slings)	Resident care items such as slings or gait belts should either be washable or dedicated to the use of a single individual Furniture upholstery that cannot be easily cleaned should be covered with a sheet and/or waterproof pad prior to use Items with fabric breakdown and/or tears should be immediately repaired or replaced Uncovered foam items cannot be properly cleaned and disinfected; covering foam is highly recommended
Specialty items that may be sensitive to standard cleaning and disinfection agents (e.g., computer screens, handheld electronic devices)	Check with the manufacturer to determine the cleaning and disinfecting agent to prevent unintended damage to the item

other electronic equipment. See Table 10.4 for cleaning considerations for different types of resident care items.

THE SPAULDING CLASSIFICATION SYSTEM IN LONG-TERM CARE FACILITIES

Equipment used in healthcare settings, including the LTCF, is cleaned and disinfected according to the Spaulding classification system (Table 10.5). The system classifies a medical device as critical, semicritical, or noncritical, based on the use of the device. The system also established three levels of germicidal activity (sterilization, high-level disinfection, and low-level disinfection) for strategies with the three classes of medical devices (critical, semicritical, noncritical).[3] To apply Spaulding criteria to specific types of pathogens, see Figure 10.2. Because LTCFs perform few procedures that require critical or semicritical instruments and/or devices, the noncritical classification is most relevant.

Critical Equipment

The LTCF may store some types of disposable, critical equipment from different manufacturers such as sterile scalpels, irrigation sets, or lancets. Other types of critical equipment such as surgical instruments are beyond the LTCF scope of practice and are not covered in this chapter. Critical equipment reprocessing requires chemical sterilization or steam under pressure (autoclave).

Some items have no expiration date or event-related sterility whereas other items do have set expiration dates (and may contain medications) that define their estimated shelf life. These items should not be used beyond this date. Staff should be knowledgeable about expiration dates and a process should be in place to ensure outdated items are removed from the resident care areas.

Semicritical Equipment

Semicritical items such as endoscopes and intracavity ultrasound probes are not frequently used in the LTCF setting. Instead, residents needing procedures that require semicritical items are usually transferred to an acute care or outpatient treatment setting. Semicritical equipment reprocessing requires high-level disinfection or sterilization—processes usually unavailable in LTCFs.

Noncritical Equipment

Noncritical equipment comes in contact with intact skin only. Healthy, intact skin is an effective barrier to microorganisms. Items coming in contact with the resident's intact skin do not have to be sterile.[3]

Noncritical items can be divided into resident care items and environmental surfaces. Examples of resident

Can LTCFs Reprocess Single Use Devices?[3]

The reuse of single-use medical devices began in the late 1970s. Reuse of single-use devices increased as a cost-saving measure and involves regulatory, ethical, medical, legal, and economic issues. It has been extremely controversial for more than two decades. The U.S. public has expressed increasing concern regarding the risk of infection and injury when reusing medical devices intended and labeled for single use.

The U.S. Food and Drug Administration (FDA) regulates the reprocessing of single use devices and currently this practice is limited to hospitals and third party reprocessors who meet the standards for the types of items they seek to reprocess. Reprocessing of single use devices is not done in LTCFs. For more information, visit www.fda.gov.

noncritical items include bedpans, blood pressure cuffs, and pulse oximetry probes. These items can be discarded after use or decontaminated at the point of care and do not require transportation to a centralized processing area. Noncritical environmental surfaces include side rails, room furniture, and floors.

Personal care items such as toothbrushes and electric/blade razors are for single resident use only and should never be shared among other residents. This is due to the risk of bloodborne and other pathogen transmission. When possible, resident care items should have an identifier, such as the resident's name, to prevent accidental use by another resident.

MAINTAINING EQUIPMENT

All equipment approved for use in the LTCF must be cleaned and disinfected according to manufacturer instructions and included in the facility's policies and procedures. Using unapproved chemical and/or processes will invalidate the equipment warranty and potentially cause damage. All equipment polices should contain the following essential infection prevention elements:

- Immediately clean/disinfect all equipment with the facility-approved EPA hospital grade disinfectant when visibly soiled or after use with residents.
- Verify that the disinfectant's SDS is on file at the facility and is readily accessible to the staff.
- Clearly identify reusable equipment that has been cleaned/disinfected with a removable tag or label and cover with a dust cover or plastic bag.
- Always follow manufacturer's cleaning and disinfection recommendations.
- Monitor that wet contact time of the disinfectant follows EPA recommendations.
- Discourage applying tape to equipment; equipment with tape residue is not considered clean.
- Ensure staff uses PPE that is appropriate for the cleaning/disinfecting task.
- Ensure eyewash stations are located close to where chemicals are being used.

EQUIPMENT CLEANING AND SAFETY PLAN

A facility's infection prevention plan should include a process for cleaning and disinfecting noncritical equipment. This should include:

- A service/maintenance/replacement schedule should be instituted and maintained.
- Damaged or malfunctioning equipment is promptly removed from service and reported to the appropriate department for repair or disposal.
- Noncritical equipment or personally owned care items should not be shared among residents.
- Confirm that disposable equipment is discarded per policy.
- Include resident care equipment in periodic environmental monitoring activities.

Assigning responsibilities will clarify which department has ownership of cleaning and disinfecting equipment. Consider working with the interdisciplinary team to develop a cleaning grid to track all items. The grid can indicate products or chemical agents to be used, timing and frequency of cleaning and disinfection, and the department that is responsible for completing each task.

TABLE 10.5: SPAULDING CLASSIFICATION CATEGORIES

Device Classification	How Used in Resident Care	Examples	Type of Disinfection	Application in LTCFs
Critical	Enters sterile body tissue or bloodstream	• Surgical instruments • Intravascular devices • Biopsy forceps	Sterilization	Uncommon
Semicritical	Mucous membrane contact	• Dental instruments • Vaginal specula • Endoscopes • Ultrasound probes (intracavity)	High-level disinfection	Depends on level of services provided
Noncritical	Intact skin contact	• Blood pressure cuffs • Stethoscopes • Bedpans • Walkers, other mobility aids	Intermediate or low-level disinfection	Commonly used

FIGURE 10.2. DECREASING ORDER OF RESISTANCE OF MIRCOORGANISMS TO DISINFECTION AND STERILIZATION AND THE LEVEL OF DISINFECTION AND STERILIZATION[3]

Resistant	Level
Prions (Creutzfeldt-Jakob Disease)	Prion reprocessing
Bacterial spores (*Bacillus atrophaeus*)	Sterilization
Coccidia (*Cryptosporidium*)	
Mycobacteria (*M. tuberculosis, M. terrae*)	High
Nonlipid or small viruses (polio, coxsackie)	Intermediate
Fungi (*Aspergillus, Candida*)	
Vegetative bacteria (*S. aureus, P. aeruginosa*)	Low
Lipid or medium-sized viruses (HIV, herpes, hepatitis B)	
Susceptible	

STORING CLEAN EQUIPMENT AND CLEAN/STERILE SUPPLIES

The goal of supply storage is to prevent product damage, contamination, and pathogen transmission. Only clean and sterile equipment should be stored in the clean utility room. This area should be designed to protect items from contamination and damage. An alcohol-based hand sanitizer/dispenser should be available in this room. There should be no trash, boxes, or fluids on the floor.

If there are physical space constraints with clinical storage area, alternative storage areas may need to be identified for excess equipment and materials. Discard all unused, outdated, or unsafe equipment.

Clean and sterile disposable products may arrive at the LTCF in a shipping container. To ensure maximum cleanliness during storage, remove the shipping container prior to placing the supplies in the clean storage room. The boxes or soft packaging of the products inside are considered clean; the outer shipping container is not.

CDC guidelines for disinfection and sterilization outline the following criteria for storing sterile disposable items:

- Store 8 to 10 inches from the floor and 2 inches away from outside walls.
- Protect items from direct sun exposure, temperature extremes, and excess moisture.
- Keep away from the ceiling and sprinkler system (5 inches unless near a sprinkler head, then 18 inches from sprinkler head) to allow for adequate cleaning, air circulation, and compliance with the fire code.[3]
- Never prop open the entrance door to the sterile/clean supply storage room.

Additional considerations for the safe storage of equipment and supplies include the following:

- A stock rotation procedure must be in place to ensure that supplies with an expiration date are regularly placed so that staff will use them in a timely manner.
- Equipment must not be stored on or around the sink due to the potential for water damage/contamination from splashing. Sterile items that become wet are considered contaminated even if the interior of the packaging does not appear to be compromised.
- Clean and sterile items must not be stored under the sink due to potential plumbing leaks.
- Products should be stored in designated shelving, carts, or cabinets. Although closed or covered cabinets are ideal to prevent contamination, open shelving may be used.
- Supplies stored on the bottom of a wire, open-shelf cart need a physical barrier between the shelf and the floor for protection against cleaning chemicals.[24]

To protect the integrity and cleanliness of equipment and supplies, most LTCFs will restrict access to the clean holding areas.

Blood Glucose Monitoring and Supplies

Outbreaks of Hepatitis B virus (HBV) infection associated with blood glucose monitoring have been identified with increasing regularity, particularly in long-term care settings, such as nursing homes and assisted living facilities, where residents often require assistance with monitoring of blood glucose levels and/or insulin administration. In the last 10 years alone, there have been at least 15 outbreaks of HBV infection associated with providers failing to follow basic principles of infection prevention and control when assisting with blood glucose monitoring. Due to under-reporting and under-recognition of acute infection, the number of outbreaks due to unsafe diabetes care practices identified to date are likely an underestimate.[25]

Infection prevention practices for blood glucose monitoring and supplies must include:

- Never using lancets (fingerstick devices) for more than one person
- Cleaning and disinfecting the blood glucose meter in between uses when equipment sharing is necessary
- Never using insulin pens for more than one resident
- Always changing gloves and performing hand hygiene between fingerstick procedures

The safe use of blood glucose monitoring equipment and supplies is also a critical component of the LTCF's occupational health program. See Chapter 9 for additional information.

TABLE 10.6: ENVIRONMENTAL SERVICES CHECKLIST FOR DAILY CLEANING OF RESIDENT ROOM[26,27]

DATE: ___ / ___ /___ UNIT: ____________ ROOM: ____________ INITIAL OF EVS STAFF (OPTIONAL) ________

EVALUATE THE FOLLOWING PRIORITY SITES FOR EACH RESIDENT ROOM			
Cleaning Task	Cleaned	Not Cleaned	Not present in room
High dusting performed:			
Use high duster/mop head: wipe ledges (shoulder high and above)			
Vents			
Lights (do not high dust over the resident)			
Dust TV: rotate and dust screen and wires			
Damp dust: Cloths and spray bottle of disinfectant for damp wipe:			
Ledges (shoulder high)			
Door handles			
Room furniture (bureaus, chairs, etc.)			
Bedside table: disinfect surface			
Equipment per policy			
Glass surfaces			
Bathroom: All surfaces:			
Toilet			
Ledges in bathroom			
Door handles			
Sink (especially faucet handles)			
Shower stall			
Clean mirrors and chrome			
Waste basket:			
Liner bags: close before removing			
Clean and disinfect if can is visibly soiled			
Sharps container:			
Check level of sharps (remove if ¾ full)			
Take to soiled utility room after securely closing			
Clean and disinfect high-touch surfaces near resident:			
Siderails			
Call light			
Remote control unit			
Telephone			
IV pole and controls			
Bedside table handle			
Floor cleaning and disinfection:			
Sweep floor before wet mopping			
With wet mop, start farthest from door; half of room first then the other half			
Bathroom shower floor			
Bathroom floor			

A customizable version of this document is available on the CD-ROM.

Adapted from Bryce E, Simor A, Zoutman D, et al. Safe healthcare now! Campaign how-to-guide: Reduce MRSA. Getting started kit: Reduce MRSA infection How-to-guide, 2006. Safer Healthcare Now website. 2006. Available at: http://www.saferhealthcarenow.ca.

REFERENCES

1. Weber DJ, Rutala WA, Miller MB, Huslage K, Sickbert-Bennett E. Role of hospital surfaces in the transmission of emerging health care-associated pathogens: norovirus, *Clostridium difficile*, and *Acinetobacter* species. *Am J Infect Control* 2010 Jun; 38(5 Suppl 1): S25-33.
2. Otter J, Yezli S, French GL. The role played by contaminated surfaces in the transmission of nosocomial pathogens. *Infect Control Epidemiol* 2011 July; 32(7): 687-699.
3. Rutala WA, Weber DJ. *Guideline for disinfection and sterilization in health-care facilities.* CDC website. 2008. Available at: http://www.cdc.gov/hicpac/disinfection_sterilization/toc.html.
4. Rutala WA. Guideline for selection and use of disinfectants. *Am J Infect Control* 1996 August; 24(4): 313-342.
5. Garrett JH, Greene L, Homan L. *Practice Guidance for Healthcare Environmental Cleaning,* 2nd ed. Chicago: Association for the Healthcare Environment, 2012.
6. Sattler B, Hall K. Healthy choices: transforming our hospitals into environmentally healthy and safe places. *Online J Issues Nurs* 2007 May 31; 12(2): 3.
7. Rutala WA, Weber DJ. Disinfectants used for environmental disinfection and new room decontamination technology. *Am J Infect Control* 2013 May; 41(5 Suppl): S36-41.
8. Sehulster LM, Chinn RYW, Arduino MJ, Carpenter J, Donlan R, Ashford D, et al. *Guidelines for environmental infection control in health-care facilities.* Recommendations from CDC and the Healthcare Infection Control Practices Advisory Committee (HICPAC). Chicago: American Society for Healthcare Engineering/ American Hospital Association, 2003.
9. *The American Heritage Dictionary of the English Language,* 4th ed. Boston: Houghton Mifflin Harcourt, 2000.
10. Environmental Protection Agency (EPA). *Using microfiber mops in hospitals.* Environmental Best Practices for Healthcare Facilities. EPA website. 2002. Available at: http://www.epa.gov/region9/waste/p2/projects/hospital/mops.pdf.
11. Rutala, WA, Gergen MF, Weber DJ. Microbiological evaluation of microfiber mops for surface disinfection. *Am J Infect Control* 2007; 35(9): 569-573.
12. Virginia Department of Health. *Frequently asked questions about... environmental cleaning and disinfection.* WDH website. 2011. Available at: http://www.vdh.virginia.gov/epidemiology/surveillance/environmentalcleaning/factsheet.pdf.
13. Siegel JD, Rhinehart E, Jackson M, Chiarello L, and the Healthcare Infection Control Practices Advisory Committee. *Guideline for isolation precautions: Prevention of transmission of infectious agents in healthcare settings, June 2007.* CDC website. Available at: http://www.cdc.gov/hicpac/pdf/isolation/Isolation2007.pdf.
14. Boyce J. *When the patient is discharged: Terminal disinfection of hospital rooms.* Medscape. June 11, 2010. Available at: http://www.medscape.com/viewarticle/72321.
15. Otter JA, Havill NL, Boyce JM. Hydrogen peroxide vapor is not the same as aerosolized hydrogen peroxide. *Infect Control and Hosp Epidemiol* 2010 November; 31(11): 1201-1202.
16. MacCennell T, Umscheid CA, Agarwal RK, Lee I, Kuntz G, Stevenson KB, et al. *Guideline for the Prevention and Control of Norovirus Gastroenteritis Outbreaks in Healthcare Settings, 2011.* CDC website. Available: at http://www.cdc.gov/hicpac/pdf/norovirus/Norovirus-Guideline-2011.pdf.
17. Vearncombe M, Armstrong I, Baker D, Card ML, Cividino M, Katz K, et al. Provincial Infectious Diseases Advisory Committee (PIDAC). *Best practices for environmental cleaning for prevention and control of infections in all healthcare settings.* CAEM website. 2009. Available at: http://www.caenvironmentalmanagement.com/PIDAC%20best%20practice.pdf.
18. Carling PC, Briggs JL, Perkins J, Highlander D. Improved cleaning of patient rooms using a new targeting method. *Clin Infect Dis* 2006; 42: 385-388.
19. Boyce JM, Havill NL, Havill HL, Mangione E, Dumigan DG, Moore BA. Comparison of fluorescent marker systems with 2 quantitative methods of assessing terminal cleaning practices. *Infect Control Epidemiol* 2011 July; 32(12): 1187-1193.
20. Salkin IF, Krisiunas E, Turnberg WL. Medical and infectious waste management. *J Am Biol Safety Assoc* 2000; 5(2): 54-69.
21. National Institute for Occupational Safety and Health. *Latex allergy: a prevention guide.* CDC website. 1998. Available at: http://www.cdc.gov/niosh/docs/98-113/.
22. Centers for Disease Control and Prevention (CDC). Transmission of Hepatitis B Virus among persons undergoing blood glucose monitoring in Long Term Care Facilities-Mississippi, North Carolina, and Los Angeles County, California, 2003-2004. *MMWR Recomm Rep* 2005; 54: 220-223.
23. Centers for Medicare & Medicaid Services (CMS). *CMS Manual. Interpretive guidelines for long-term care facilities.* CMS website. 2009. Available at: http://www.cms.gov/Regulations-and-Guidance/Guidance/Transmittals/downloads/R51SOMA.pdf.
24. American National Standard. *Comprehensive guide to steam sterilization and sterility assurance in health care facilities.* Arlington, VA: Association for the Advancement of Medical Instrumentation, 2010: 87.
25. Centers for Disease Control and Prevention (CDC). *Infection prevention during blood glucose monitoring and insulin administration.* CDC website. 2012. Available at: http://www.cdc.gov/injectionsafety/blood-glucose-monitoring.html.
26. Guh A, Carling P. *Options for evaluating environmental cleaning.* CDC website. 2010. Available at: http://www.cdc.gov/hai/toolkits/evaluating-environmental-cleaning.html.
27. Bryce E, Simor A, Zoutman D, Hutchinson J, Johnston L, Mulvey M, et al. Safe healthcare now! Campaign how-to-guide: Reduce MRSA. *Getting started kit: Reduce MRSA infection How-to-guide, 2006.* Safer Healthcare Now website. 2006. Available at: http://www.saferhealthcarenow.ca.

REFERENCES

ADDITIONAL RESOURCES

1. Carrico RM, Bryant K, Lessa F, Limbago B, Fauerbach LL, Marx JF. *Guide to Preventing Clostridium difficile Infections.* Washington, DC: Association for Professionals in Infection Control and Epidemiology, 2013.

2. Provincial Infectious Diseases Advisory Committee. *Best Practice for Environmental Cleaning for Prevention and Control of Infections in all Health Care Settings,* 2nd edition. Public Health Ontario website. 2009. Available at: http://www.publichealthontario.ca/en/eRepository/Best_Practices_Environmental_Cleaning_2012.pdf.

CHAPTER 11

Infection Prevention for Interdisciplinary Services

Patricia Rosenbaum, RN, CIC
Marilyn Hanchett, RN, MA, CPHQ, CIC

KEY CONCEPTS

- Infection prevention measures should be an integral part of departmental policies and procedures for interdisciplinary services such as dietary, laundry, and rehabilitation to prevent transmission of disease.
- Residents requiring rehabilitation services present special risks for infection prevention. Although some potential risk factors have been studied, much remains unknown.
- Although most long-term care facilities use offsite lab services, the infection preventionist should be knowledgeable of those services and establish communication processes with the laboratory staff.
- The infection preventionist should work with the pharmacy provider and nursing staff to ensure safe delivery and handling of medications.
- If a facility has an antimicrobial stewardship program, it should include representatives from the interdisciplinary team—including laboratory and pharmacy—whether those services are contracted or provided in-house.

This chapter focuses on the primary interdisciplinary services most often encountered in long-term care (LTC) settings. If additional types of services are used, the infection preventionist (IP) should follow the basic principles described in the following text. Coordination with the manager of all interdisciplinary services is essential. For information regarding social and life enrichment services, see Chapter 12.

DIETARY DEPARTMENT

Preventing foodborne illness and food contamination are essential for the health and safety of long-term care facility (LTCF) residents, staff, and visitors. The LTCF IP must work with the dietary services department director to ensure that policies and procedures incorporate infection prevention best practices and to monitor practices accordingly. Areas to address include food handling, preparation, and storage; employee health for food service workers; and proper cleaning, disinfection, and maintenance of food prep areas, utensils, and equipment.[1]

The Centers for Disease Control and Prevention (CDC) estimates that each year roughly one in six Americans (or 48 million people) become ill, 128,000 are hospitalized, and 3,000 die of foodborne diseases. The most common foodborne illnesses are summarized in Figure 11.1. LTCF residents are particularly at risk for viral and bacterial gastroenteritis due to age-related decrease in gastric acid. In addition, risk of rapid transmission within the LTCF is increased due to shared living spaces such as bathrooms, dining rooms, and rehabilitation facilities.[1] The IP in LTC should be especially aware of the following types of foodborne illnesses: norovirus, *Salmonella, Clostridium perfringens, Campylobacter,* and *listeriosis.*

Norovirus[2]

Norovirus is the most common cause of gastroenteritis in the United States. CDC estimates that each year more than 20 million cases of acute gastroenteritis are caused by noroviruses. That means about 1 in every 15 Americans will get norovirus illness each year. Norovirus is also estimated to cause more than 70,000 hospitalizations and 800 deaths each year in the United States.

Norovirus is a leading cause of disease from contaminated foods in the United States. Foods that are most commonly involved in foodborne norovirus outbreaks include leafy greens (e.g., lettuce), fresh fruits, and shellfish (e.g., oysters). Norovirus can be spread either by direct person-to-person contact or by fecal contamination of food or water. Residents can be infected by touching facility surfaces or objects contaminated with norovirus and by having contact with residents who are infected.

Although most individuals recover within 1 to 2 days, norovirus can pose a much more serious threat to the elderly due to the risk of dehydration. Without rapid intervention, elderly residents may require hospitalization. In addition, norovirus spreads quickly within institutions, including LTCFs. There is neither immunization to prevent nor medication to treat an infected resident with norovirus. Prevention based on Standard Precautions, safe food handling, preparation, and storage criteria described in this chapter offer the best measures for resident safety.

Salmonella[3]

Salmonella gastrointestinal infections are characterized by diarrhea, fever, and abdominal cramping and are acquired from eating contaminated foods. These infections usually resolve in 5 to 7 days and most do not require treatment other than oral fluids. Residents with severe diarrhea may require rehydration with intravenous fluids.

Antibiotic therapy can prolong the duration of excretion of non-typhoidal *Salmonella* and is recommended only for individuals with severe illness (e.g., those with severe diarrhea, high fever, bloodstream infection, or who need hospitalization) or those at risk of severe disease or complications, including older adults (over 65 years old) and immunocompromised persons. Antibiotic resistance is increasing among some *Salmonella* bacteria; therefore, susceptibility testing can help guide appropriate therapy. Choices for antibiotic therapy for severe infections include fluoroquinolones, third-generation cephalosporins, and ampicillin (for susceptible infections).

FIGURE 11.1: TOP PATHOGENS CONTRIBUTING TO DOMESTICALLY ACQUIRED FOODBORNE ILLNESSES AND DEATHS, 2000–2008

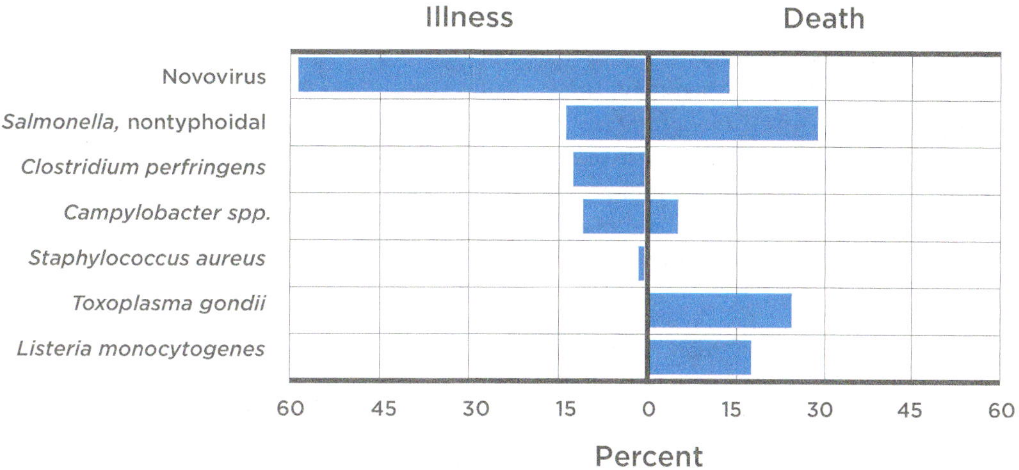

From Centers for Disease Control and Prevention. *Estimates of foodborne illness in the United States.* CDC website. 2013. Available at: http://www.cdc.gov/foodborneburden/index.html.

Salmonella may also be found in the feces of some animals, especially those with diarrhea. Hand hygiene reduces transmission after contact with animals. Reptiles and young birds are particularly likely to harbor *Salmonella* even if they appear healthy. LTCF residents who participate in pet therapy and or other animal visitation programs must perform thorough hand hygiene at the end of the activity.

Clostridium perfringens[4]

Clostridium perfringens is a spore-forming gram-positive bacterium that may produce toxins in the intestine causing disease. It is found in many environmental sources as well as in digestive tracts of humans and animals. It is one of the most common causes of foodborne illness in the United States accounting for nearly a million cases of foodborne illness each year.

Persons infected with *C. perfringens* develop diarrhea and abdominal cramps within 6 to 24 hours (typically 8 to 12). The illness usually begins suddenly and lasts for less than 24 hours. This illness is not transmitted from one person to another. People infected with *C. perfringens* usually do not have fever or vomiting. The elderly are most at risk of more severe symptoms resulting from *C. perfringens* infections. Complications, including dehydration, may occur and symptoms may last for 1 to 2 weeks in severe cases.

Beef, poultry, gravies, and dried or precooked foods are common sources of *C. perfringens* infections. *C. perfringens* infection often occurs when foods are prepared in large quantities and kept warm for a long time before serving. Outbreaks often happen in institutions such as hospitals and nursing homes, or at events with catered food.

Foods such as beef, poultry, and gravies should be cooked to recommended temperatures. Foods should then kept warmer than 140°F (60°C) or cooler than 4°F (5°C) to prevent the growth of *C. perfringens* spores that might have survived the initial cooking process. Meat dishes should be served hot right after cooking. Leftover foods should be refrigerated at 40°F (4°C) or below as soon as possible and within 2 hours of preparation. IPs inspecting food preparation area must be vigilant regarding consistent use of cooking, reheating, and cooling temperatures for all foods.

Campylobacter[5]

Campylobacteriosis is an infectious disease caused by bacteria of the genus *Campylobacter*. Most people who become ill with campylobacteriosis get diarrhea, cramping, abdominal pain, and fever within 2 to 5 days after exposure to the organism. The diarrhea may be bloody and can be accompanied by nausea and vomiting. The illness typically lasts about 1 week. Some infected persons do not have any symptoms. In persons with compromised immune systems, *Campylobacter* occasionally spreads to the bloodstream and causes a serious life-threatening illness. *Campylobacter* is one of the most common causes of diarrheal illness in the United States. Most cases occur as isolated, sporadic events, not as part of recognized outbreaks. Although anyone may be susceptible to this infection, it is more common in younger people than in the elderly.

Almost all residents infected with *Campylobacter* recover in less than 1 week without any specific treatment. Individuals should drink extra fluids as long as the diarrhea lasts. Antimicrobial therapy is warranted only in cases of severe disease or those at high risk for severe disease, such as those with immune systems severely weakened from medications or other illnesses. Azithromycin and fluoroquinolones (e.g., ciprofloxacin) are commonly used for treatment of these infections, but resistance to fluoroquinolones is common. Antimicrobial susceptibility testing can help guide appropriate therapy.

Listeriosis[6]

Listeriosis is a serious infection usually caused by eating food contaminated with the bacterium *Listeria monocytogenes* and is an important public health problem in the United States. The disease primarily affects older adults, pregnant women, newborns, and adults with weakened immune systems. However, rarely, persons without these risk factors can also be affected.

A resident with listeriosis usually has fever and muscle aches, sometimes preceded by diarrhea or other gastrointestinal symptoms. Almost everyone who is diagnosed with listeriosis has "invasive" infection, in which the bacteria spread beyond the gastrointestinal tract. The symptoms vary with the infected person. In older adults and persons with immunocompromising conditions, septicemia, and meningitis are the most common clinical presentations.

In addition to the general safe food handling recommendations described in this chapter, the CDC has issued specific recommendations for persons at higher risk, including persons with weakened immune systems and older adults. These recommendations include:

Meats

- Do not eat hot dogs, luncheon meats, cold cuts, other deli meats (e.g., bologna), or fermented or dry sausages unless they are heated to an internal temperature of 165°F (74°C) or until steaming hot just before serving.
- Avoid getting fluid from hot dog and lunch meat packages on other foods, utensils, and food preparation surfaces, and wash hands after handling hot dogs, luncheon meats, and deli meats.
- Pay attention to labels. Do not eat refrigerated pâté or meat spreads from a deli or meat counter or from the refrigerated section of a store. Foods that do not need refrigeration, like canned or shelf-stable pâté and meat spreads, are safe to eat. Refrigerate after opening.

Cheeses

- Do not eat soft cheese such as feta, queso blanco, queso fresco, brie, Camembert, blue-veined, or panela (queso panela) unless it is labeled as made with pasteurized milk. Make sure the label says, "made with pasteurized milk."

Seafood

- Do not eat refrigerated smoked seafood, unless it is contained in a cooked dish, such as a casserole, or unless it is a canned or shelf-stable product.
- Refrigerated smoked seafood, such as salmon, trout, whitefish, cod, tuna, and mackerel, is most often labeled as "nova-style," "lox," "kippered," "smoked," or "jerky."
  - These fish are typically found in the refrigerator section or sold at seafood and deli counters of grocery stores and delicatessens.
- Canned and shelf stable tuna, salmon, and other fish products are safe to eat.

General U.S. Food and Drug Administration Advice for Melon Safety

- Consumers and food preparers should wash their hands with warm water and soap for at least 20 seconds *before* and *after* handling any whole melon, such as cantaloupe, watermelon, or honeydew.
- Scrub the surface of melons, such as cantaloupes, with a clean produce brush under running water and dry them with a clean cloth or paper towel before cutting. Be sure that the scrub brush is sanitized after each use to avoid transferring bacteria between melons.

- Promptly consume cut melon or refrigerate promptly. Keep cut melon refrigerated at 40°F (4°C) (32° to 34°F/0° to 1°C is best) or less for no more than 7 days.
- Discard cut melons left at room temperature for more than 4 hours.

FOOD SERVICE EMPLOYEES

Employees who handle food cannot have communicable diseases or infected skin conditions. Persons who are carriers of enteric infection are not allowed to work with food. Any food service employee with signs of illness such as colds, boils, fever, rashes, or active gastrointestinal symptoms must be sent home and cleared by employee/occupational health or a physician before returning to work. Food service personnel need to be educated about personal hygiene: hand washing, glove use, foodborne illness prevention, transmission, as well as regulations and standards that apply to food preparation, sanitation, and storage. Bare hand contact with food is not recommended for food handlers. Hand washing with soap and water is required; alcohol-based hand rubs (ABHR) cannot be used in place of hand washing with soap and water in food preparatory areas.[7,8]

Hygiene for food handlers:

- Hair restraints such as hairnets must be worn by kitchen employees according to facility policy.
- Fingernails must be clean and well-trimmed.
- Do not wear dangling jewelry such as earrings and necklaces.
- Wear clean uniforms.
- Beards must be covered.
- Hands must be washed:
    a. After performing bodily functions (using the bathroom, blowing or wiping the nose, etc.)
    b. On reentering the kitchen
    c. Before handling food or clean utensils
    d. After handling raw meats or soiled equipment or utensils
    e. Before and after glove use
- Eating, drinking, or smoking is not allowed in the kitchen area.
- Gloves must be changed between food preparatory tasks to prevent cross contamination of food and kitchen items.[7]

The LTCF food service director or manager is responsible for the safety of food and food service workers. The IP should work with the director/manager to develop policies and procedures and employee education to promote food safety for everyone in the facility. The food service director must ensure the following[8]:

- Maintain daily records of temperatures for refrigeration and ensure proper functioning of refrigeration equipment.
- Obtain food only from approved sources.
- Provide for the proper receipt and storage of all food supplies.
- Maintain cold foods at 41°F (5°C) or below.
- Store frozen food at or below 0°F.
- Provide for proper waste disposal from the kitchen area.
- Place leftover hot foods in containers that allow them to cool quickly.
- Keep raw animal products separated from each other and stored on shelves below other foods to prevent meat juices from dripping on them.
- Label, date, and monitor all refrigerated food to ensure use in proper time frames.
- Do not store food on the floor of walk-in refrigeration areas.

Food Handling and Monitoring[8]

- Thermometers and logs must be kept and placed in areas that must be monitored.
- All raw foods must be washed before use.
- Foods cannot be thawed and refrozen.
- Ice should not be handled by staff with bare hands.
- Hot foods should be held at temperatures of at least 140°F (60°C).
- Food should be transported in temperature-controlled carts.
- Dry food storage should be off the floor and protected from any pests or moisture, clear of sprinkler systems, disposal pipes, and air vents.
- Dry foods should be handled to maintain packaging integrity and supplies properly dated and rotated.

- Eggs should be purchased from a U.S. Department of Agriculture (USDA)-approved source.
- Adequate dishwashing facilities should be available and all machines maintained according to manufacturer's recommendations.
- All food preparation equipment should be cleaned between uses.
- Separate cutting boards should be used for meats and vegetables.
- Garbage should not be allowed to reach overflow conditions; it should be in leak-proof containers with lids.
- Uncooked food should not be stored above cooked food.
- Food must be monitored for expiration dates.
- Chemicals and cleaning supplies should not be stored near food.[8]

Food Service Equipment

Refrigerators

Refrigerators must be cleaned and maintained according to manufacturer's instructions. Temperatures at or below 41°F (5°C) are checked and recorded on a log daily. Refrigerators on the resident units must be kept clean and used only to store food. All food should be labeled with date and resident's name.

Refrigerators or cool boxes for laboratory specimens should be kept clean. Refrigerators temperatures should be between 36° and 41°F (2° and 5°C). Temperatures must be monitored and logged daily. A biohazard label should be placed on the outside of the refrigerator or cool box. The maintenance and inspection of refrigerators dedicated to laboratory items is not usually the responsibility of dietary personnel.

Refrigerators for medications, usually located in medication rooms also should be cleaned and temperature monitored and logged daily. Temperature should be between 36°F (2°C) and 41° F (5°C). Inform the pharmacy if the safe temperature range is not maintained. Medications may have to be discarded and replaced. Responsibility for cleaning, maintaining, and inspecting medication refrigerators should be described in a facility policy.[8]

Dishwashing Machines

LTCFs use commercial dishwashing machines for most food service dishes and utensils. Commercial equipment is generally faster than residential units and provides a higher level of sanitization than is usually needed for home use. Commercial dishwashers are designated as either high or low temperature.

- High-temperature dishwashers use heat sanitization. The washing temperature is 150° to 165°F (66° to 74°C) and the final rinse is 180°F (82°C). They use shorter cycle times than low temperature machines and do not need chemicals beyond detergent. These dishwashers are initially more expensive than low temperature models but are highly efficient, even though the required booster heater increases the amount of energy needed to heat the wash water.
- Low-temperature dishwashers that provide chemical sanitization and cycles must include the chemical indicated by the manufacturer. These machines process items at lower temperatures than the high temperature counterparts, but items may require multiple cycles to remove staining or highly adherent particles. They do not require a booster heater and usually produce less steam.[8]

Ice Machines[9]

Ice, ice storage chests, and ice making machines may have microorganisms present. There are two primary sources of microorganisms in ice: the potable water from which it is made and transfer of microorganisms from hands. Ice that has become contaminated has been associated with colonization and infections. Contaminated ice can also contaminate specimens and medical solutions when used for cooling. Some organisms identified in ice have been *Enterobacter, Pseudomonas, Cryptosporidium,* and *Legionella.*[9]

General infection prevention practice for maintaining ice machines include:

- Clean, disinfect, and maintain ice machines and ice storage chests on a routine basis. This is usually quarterly for ice machines and daily for ice chests.
- Keep ice scoops on a chain short enough that the scoop would not touch the floor if dropped; store the scoop on a hard clean surface when not in use. Do not store the scoop in the ice bin. Ice scoops should be cleaned daily.

- Ice container doors or lids must be kept closed except when removing ice. Ice should never be handled with bare hands.
- Always follow manufacturer's instructions for cleaning ice machines. Document that the cleaning and disinfecting of these machines is done according to manufacturer recommendations and LTCF policy.
- Ice machines and dispensers must be cleaned and disinfected if they have been disconnected before water disruptions, temporarily taken out of service, or shut down for relocation within the facility.
- When cleaning make sure to clean all door hinges and any groves and uneven surfaces.
- Microbiologic sampling of ice, ice chests, and ice-making machines and dispensers is only done when indicated during an epidemiologic investigation.

Transported Food

Foods transported to resident care area and dining rooms is best accomplished using temperature-controlled carts. Temperatures should be monitored randomly to ensure food safety. All carts whether or not they control temperatures must be cleaned per an established schedule and according to manufacturer's recommendations. Any food service cart that is visibly soiled must be cleaned immediately. The responsibility for cleaning food service carts should be described per facility policy.[8]

Foodborne Outbreak Investigation

Foodborne illness outbreaks can be a common occurrence in LTCFs.[1] More than half of all reported norovirus outbreaks in the United States have occurred in this setting.[10] Issues related to outbreaks are incorrect holding of food and improper food temperatures. Many types of foods can become contaminated. Some of the foods that have been linked to outbreaks are eggs, fish and shellfish, meat, nuts, poultry, raw (unpasteurized) milk, and raw fruits and vegetables. Foodborne illnesses may be spread by infected facility staff, even if their symptoms appear mild.

Because the symptoms of foodborne illness can be non-specific, the early recognition of a possible outbreak can be very challenging. According to the CDC, available outbreak statistics may underreport the actual incidence of infections. For that reason, the IP in LTCF must carefully investigate any cases suggesting a foodborne infection. The IP should follow the steps outlined in Figure 11.2. Due to complexity of these types of outbreaks, many of the steps may occur simultaneously. As in any outbreak investigation, mobilization of the LTCF interdisciplinary team and notification of the local health department are essential in identifying the cause and managing situation to prevent further transmission. Table 11.1 follows the steps of the investigation process and includes sample questions that can help the IP identify the source and determine the necessary course of action.[11]

Food Recalls

The dietary department and the IP must be aware of food alerts and recalls and coordinate the facility response plan, as needed. The website http://www.recalls.gov/food.html is maintained by the U.S. Department of Health and Human Services, CDC, the U.S. Food and Drug Administration (FDA), and the Food Safety and Inspection Services and is a useful resource when monitoring food related alerts and recalls.

The IP can also reference the Hazard Analysis Critical Control Points (HACCP) website (http://sop.nfsmi.org/HACCPBasedSOPs.php) for food safety management. The National Food Service Management Institute (NFSMI) has developed HACCP-based standard operating procedures (SOPs) in conjunction with USDA and FDA to contribute to providing safe food. The site offers information on food and provides multiple samples of checklists logs that can be used as an adjunct to infection prevention monitoring.

LAUNDRY SERVICES

The LTCF is required to provide clean linen and must clean residents' clothing. This requirement is described in the Centers for Medicare & Medicaid Services (CMS) F tag 441 regulation §483.65 (C) Linens – Personnel must handle, store, process, and transport linen so as to prevent the spread of infection.[12] The facility may choose to operate an onsite laundry service or utilize a contractor. There are infection prevention advantages and disadvantages to both options (see Table 11.2).

FIGURE 11.2: STEPS IN A FOODBORNE OUTBREAK INVESTIGATION

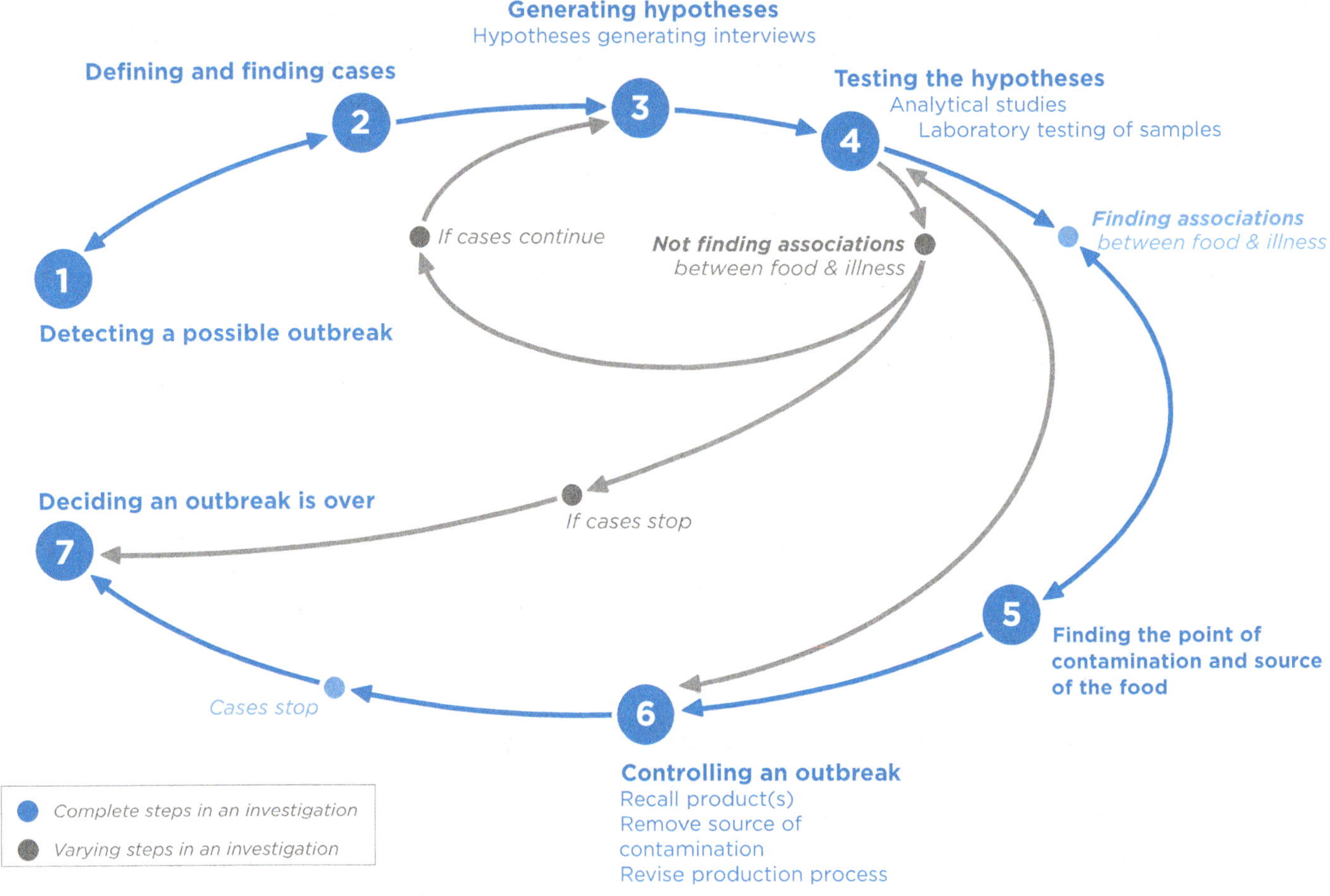

From Centers for Disease Control and Prevention. *Foodborne outbreak investigations.* CDC website. 2013. Available at: http://www.cdc.gov/outbreaknet/investigations/figure_outbreak_process.html.

Resident Clothing and Washable Personal Items

Personal clothing should be labeled with the resident's name to ensure prompt return to the correct individual. Additional considerations include[13]:

- The resident and the family should be encouraged to purchase washable items.
- Clothing should be sufficiently durable to withstand repeated commercial laundering.
- Personal items such as blankets, throws, pillows, etc. should be suitable for regularly processing in a commercial laundry.
- Resident items that cannot be processed in a commercial laundry may be washed by family members/caregivers, but should be bagged prior to removal from the resident's room. The same bag should not be used when the item is returned to the resident.
- Staff should be alert to resident belongings that may be in the linen, such as hearing aids, glasses, and dentures.

Monitoring Laundry Services

No matter how laundry is processed by the LTCF, the IP should include periodic inspection and monitoring

TABLE 11.1: OUTBREAK INVESTIGATION PROCESS

Process	Sample Questions
1. Detecting a possible outbreak	
2. Defining and finding cases	• What is the nature of the infection? • What is the onset and common symptoms? • How many individuals has been infected and within what time frame?
3. Generating the hypotheses about likely sources	• Was the infection due to a specific type of food product? • Was the food contaminated during cooking? • Was it contaminated during storage?
4. Testing the hypothesis	• Do any suspected food items show evidence of pathogens? Have these been identified through laboratory testing? • Do any food service employees have signs of infection? Have any been tested and if so, for what illnesses? What are the results?
5. Finding the point of contamination and source of the food	• Did the identified contaminated food item arrive at the LTCF contaminated? • Was the food item compromised during delivery?
6. Controlling the outbreak	• Has all contaminated food been removed from the LTCF? • Have all cases of infection among residents (or family, visitors) been discovered and reported? • Has treatment for all affected individuals been initiated?
7. Determining that the outbreak has been resolved	• How much time has passed since the last case of infection was identified? • Are previously infected residents showing signs of improvement? • Has any individual required urgent or emergency treatment? • What measures have been implemented to assure that the contaminated food has been removed and future contaminated prevented?

Source : Adapted from Centers for Disease Control and Prevention. *CDC Guide to Investigating Foodborne Outbreaks*. CDC website. 2013. Available at: http://www.cdc.gov/outbreaknet/investigations/detection.html.)

of the products and processes used. General inspection criteria for fabrics should include:

- Levels, if any, of permissible stains present after processing
- Type and extent of damage (holes, tears, frayed edges) permissible after processing
- Maximum number of mends or other repairs permissible in recycled fabrics
- Description of conditions (general wear, fading) when fabrics must be removed from inventory

Routine microbiologic sampling of clean linen is not recommended, although microbiologic sampling may be necessary in an outbreak if evidence suggests linen, textiles, or clothing as a source of disease transmission.[9] Visual inspection helps ensure that routine cleaning achieves acceptable standards and that fabric damage does not increase the risk of incomplete cleaning.

General inspection criteria for laundry facilities should include[9]:

- A physical barrier between the clean and soiled linen area.
- To avoid recontamination of clean linen, areas for receiving soiled linen should have negative pressure ventilation.

TABLE 11.2: FACILITY-BASED AND CONTRACTED LAUNDRY SERVICES: ADVANTAGES AND DISADVANTAGES

FACILITY-BASED SERVICES		CONTRACTED SERVICES	
Advantages	Disadvantages	Advantages	Disadvantages
• Onsite laundry may speed processing and availability. • More control over the cleaning of specialty fabrics, clothing may be possible. • Greater control over potential loss or damage to fabrics and clothing. • IP able to inspect at any time. • IP can participate in laundry staff orientation and ongoing training.	• LTCF must provide space, plumbing, and ventilation per commercial laundry standards. • May not be able to respond to sudden increases in loads or changing intrafacility demands. • Must be secured to prevent unintended entry by at-risk or cognitively impaired residents. • Costs associated with equipment purchase, routine maintenance, and repairs. • Increases cost of utilities. • Requires staff time and training. • LTCF must have quality monitoring systems in place. • IP must be knowledgeable in inspection and monitoring requirements.	• Eliminates need for LTCF staff training and anticipated turnover. • Quality monitoring done by the contractor. • Usually able to quickly respond to increased demands. • Convenient for LTCF staff. • Responsible for transport and deliveries. • Available to consult with the LTCF IP.	• LTCF must plan for periodic delivery and pickup. • Potential for incomplete or missed deliveries, resulting in shortages. • Must maintain adequate holding area for soiled items awaiting pickup. • Commercial chemicals may damage or degrade fabrics, clothing. • IP must visit an offsite facility for inspections, consultations.

- Any carts, shelves, and folding tables should be cleaned and disinfected on a regular basis.
- The laundry must have a procedure for safely responding to any needles or other sharp items discovered in soiled linen. This includes the availability of one or more accessible sharps containers.
- Hand hygiene products and hand washing sinks must be available to laundry personnel.
- Laundry personnel must be trained in and demonstrate the correct use of personal protective equipment, including circumstances in which eye protection must be used.
- If the laundry permits the use of utility gloves, there is a procedure for their cleaning and disinfection between periods of use.
- Laundry equipment is checked and maintained per institutional policy and manufacturer recommendations. These monitoring activities are documented.
- The area should have proper ventilation to direct the air flow from the clean linen area (positive pressure) to the soiled linen area (negative pressure).[14]

If the facility has a laundry chute, all soiled linen should be placed in bags and closed and secured before being placed in the chute.[9] Laundry chutes should be properly designed and maintained to minimize dispersion of aerosols from contaminated laundry. For resident safety, all laundry chutes should be kept locked (if in open areas accessible to residents) or be behind locked doors.

Monitoring the Laundry Process[9,12,15]

- Washing machines and dryers must be used and maintained according to the manufacturer's recommendations.
- Damp linen must not be left in machines overnight.
- Detergent and water (process dilution) physically will remove many microorganisms during the wash cycle.
- Facilities may select any detergent designated for use in laundry processing. Laundry detergents are not required to state they are antimicrobial.
- Laundry processing in a low-water temperature situation does not always require a chlorine bleach rinse, and it is not required for all laundry. Some

laundry detergents are able to hygienically clean fabric without the presence of chlorine bleach.

- Chlorine bleach rinse may be used for laundry composed of materials such as cotton.
- Hot water is an effective means of destroying microorganisms. The water should be at the temperature of 160°F (71°C) or higher for a minimum of 25 minutes.
- Low-water temperature washing at 71° to 77° F (22° to 25°C) with a 125 part-per-million (ppm) chlorine bleach rinse effectively process laundry.
- Bleach can be used as a disinfectant laundry but can potentially damage many fabrics.
- All laundry chemicals must be used according to manufacturer's instructions.
- LTCFs are not required to maintain a record of water temperatures during the laundry process.
- The CDC and CMS recommend leaving washing machines open to air when not in use.
- Ozone cleaning systems (ozonated water) are an acceptable means of processing laundry. These systems must be used according to manufacturer's instructions.

Handling Soiled Linen and Resident Clothing

- Soiled linen should be handled as little as possible and with minimal agitation to prevent microbial contamination of the air and any healthcare personnel/other individuals in the adjacent area.[16]
- All soiled linen should be handled as if contaminated and should be bagged and put into carts at the location where it is collected.
- Soiled linen should not be sorted in resident rooms, hallways, or other open access areas.[13]
- Soiled linen should be placed in impervious bags, placed in designated carts, and transported to a holding area for either on site processing or scheduled pick up by the contracted laundry service.
- Facilities that provide hampers in resident rooms for soiled clothing must be emptied per schedule; clothing should be bagged prior to removal from the room.

Linen from Isolation Rooms

All used linen is considered contaminated, and there is no need to separate or label it. Linen from isolation rooms is treated the same as other soiled linen. Double bagging is only done if the original bag leaks or has become contaminated on the outside. Leak-resistant bags should be used. Unused linen removed from isolation rooms, however, must always be treated as soiled. These items can potentially transmit pathogens to other residents if not thoroughly cleaned before reuse.[9]

Linen Infested with Lice or Scabies

Facility linen can become contaminated with lice or scabies from residents, especially during an outbreak. In these situations, linen and clothing from infected residents must be washed and dried at high temperatures. It is not necessary to treat fabrics with an insecticide. Processing all fabrics in commercial wash and dryer cycles provides sufficient heat to kill these parasites.[15]

Linen Transport[9]

- Soiled linen carts should be cleaned and disinfected whenever visibly soiled and according to a scheduled described in facility policy.
- Separate carts should be used for transporting clean and soiled linen. If this is not possible, the soiled cart must be thoroughly cleaned and disinfected per facility protocol before being used to move clean items.
- Clean linen must always be kept separate from soiled linen. The use of separate rooms, closets, or other designated spaces with a closing door provides the most secure method for reducing the risk of accidental contamination.
- Clean linen must be transported in clean covered carts.
- Resident clean clothing must be transported in covered carts if folded or covered rods if hanging.

Mattresses and Pillows[9]

- Mattress and pillow covers with tears or holes must be replaced.
- Mattresses that have tears or other exterior damage and/or that are suspected to have interior microbial contamination must be replaced.
- Mattress covers that are moisture resistant should be disinfected between residents or whenever visibly soiled with an Environmental Protection Agency-approved germicidal detergent.

- Fabric mattress covers should be laundered per an established cleaning schedule. Minimally, this must occur between residents or whenever the fabric covers are visibly soiled.
- Pillows and pillow covers should be laundered per an established cleaning schedule and should be sufficiently durable for repeated commercial laundering. Pillows and pillow covers are always cleaned between use by different residents.

REHABILITATION SERVICES

Rehabilitation services are specialized programs designed to maintain and, when possible, improve independent function and support self-care. Depending on the provider, these services may include physical medicine, speech and audiology services, care for amputees and prosthetic services, sensory aids, and blind rehabilitation. In some programs, therapeutic recreational services may be included. Specialized programs may focus on a specific type of rehabilitation such as the Veterans Affair's (VA) polytrauma or traumatic brain injury services. In LTCFs, the services most often provided onsite are physical and occupational therapy.

Infection prevention in any rehabilitation program presents special challenges due to the number of risk factors associated with these residents. Longer lengths of stay, high incidence of urinary tract problems and infections, and high incidence of skin lesions, including decubitus ulcers and stump wounds, differentiate this group from the general nursing home population.[17] Some studies have reported a higher incidence of healthcare-associated infections (HAIs) in chronic and rehabilitative settings even after case mix adjustment than in acute care.[18,19] Independent variables associated with HAIs in rehabilitation settings have also been more closely linked to female gender and glycosuria rather than underlying medical conditions. Urinary catheter use and bedridden status have also been reported as statistically significant risk factors. However, further studies are needed to better understand the incidence and prevalence of HAIs among those receiving rehabilitative services in LTCFs.[20]

Infection Prevention Considerations

LTCF staff must use hand hygiene when entering the department and between caring for each resident. Hand washing facilities should be located either within or adjacent to each treatment space. ABHR products should be conveniently located to provide easy access for personnel.[21] Although all standard prevention practices are applicable in rehabilitation programs, the IP should pay extra attention to the following.

Use of Urinary Catheters and Supplies

Residents requiring rehabilitative therapies often have decreased sensation, limited mobility, and other neurological impairment related to bladder function. Indwelling catheters must be positioned and secured to prevent urine reflux and avoid the risk of drainage tubing and/or the collection bag becoming tangled in equipment or contacting the floor. The IP should be aware if the LTCF is utilizing a combined intervention approach, often called a "bladder bundle," to reduce these types of risks.[22] Antimicrobial catheters have also been proposed as a prevention approach for high-risk residents. However, research has not shown a sustainable reduction in asymptomatic bacteruria when antibiotic-impregnated catheters remained in place for longer than 1 week.[23]

Because residents receiving rehabilitation often require long-term indwelling catheters, blockage is a recurrent risk. Catheter irrigation or "washout" practices have been studied but results are inconclusive. Rigorous studies of different types of irrigants, volumes, frequency, and techniques are needed to validate routine use of this procedure.[24] According to the CDC, further research is needed on the benefit of irrigating the catheter with acidifying solutions or use of oral urease inhibitors in long-term catheterized patients who have frequent catheter obstruction.[2]

Intermittent catheterization may be used in lieu of an indwelling device. When intermittent catheterization is done using aseptic technique, infection risks are low. Infection risks are also low when catheters are re-used per aseptic technique for the same resident.[26]

The effectiveness of antibiotic prophylaxis for residents requiring long-term indwelling or intermittent catheterization is sparse. Although the number of studies is small, most reflect limited or no evidence that prophylactic antibiotics reduce the rate of asymptomatic and symptomatic bacteriuria.[27]

LCTFs may have policies to decontaminate urinary collection bags. These policies are intended to reduce the bioburden associated with the extended use of drainage systems, as well as limit the costs of frequent replacement of disposable products. In the few studies of urinary draining bag decontamination conducted between 1985 and 1994, most of the studies did not provide standardization of definitions and outcome measures. Bleach solutions in various concentrations have been most often studied and their use has demonstrated a reduction in microbial contamination.[28] However, the use of a vinegar solution for routine cleaning and infection reduction is not supported in the literature.[29]

Respiratory Infection Risks

Although respiratory infections are common across all healthcare settings, they are especially dangerous for the elderly. The microbial cause of respiratory tract infections vary depending on the nature of the infection (pneumonia compared to bacterial sinusitis), care setting (skilled nursing compared to residential care), as well as resident-specific risks associated with smoking, alcoholism, multiple comorbidities, and immunosuppression.[30]

Respiratory hygiene and other prevention practices should be applied in rehabilitation programs in the same manner in which they are used throughout the LTCF. However, due to the risk factors associated with this group of residents, outbreaks of streptococcal infections have been reported. Transmission has occurred through direct contact between residents.[31] Staff turnover and inadequate employee education have also been associated with streptococcal infection among both residents and staff. However, most studies indicate that suboptimal infection prevention practices, including inconsistent use of hand hygiene, are frequent contributing factors to outbreaks among skilled nursing and rehabilitation residents.[32,33]

Increased risks of respiratory infections and facility outbreaks have also been linked to lack of vaccination programs. Reported outbreaks have focused on the need for both seasonal influenza as well as pneumococcal immunization programs.[34,35] (For more information on immunizations, see Chapters 8 and 9.) The IP should verify that residents participating in rehabilitation programs have been appropriately vaccinated.

Older residents with respiratory tract infections are also at risk for inappropriate use of antibiotics. Antibiotics are frequently overprescribed for treatment of bronchitis.[36] Since rehabilitative services are often performed in groups or in common therapy areas, the potential risk of transmission for respiratory infections requires vigilance by both the therapists and the IP. These residents should also be included in medication monitoring and antimicrobial stewardship programs maintained by the LTCF.

Protection of Skin and Soft Tissue

As discussed in Chapter 6, age-related changes in skin and soft tissue are common. In fact, some studies suggest that as many as 90 percent of older adults have some type of skin disorder. However, impaired sensation and mobility increase the risks of skin damage among rehabilitation residents. Fortunately most pressure ulcers do not become infected. However, when they do, empiric therapy is typically used to cover *Staphylococcus aureus*, gram-negative bacilli, and anaerobes.[37]

The IP should be aware of the types of supportive devices and surfaces used at the LTCF. Optimal weight and pressure distribution are key considerations in protecting skin integrity. The IP should collaborate with the therapist to ensure that supportive devices such as braces and splints fit comfortably and do not increase the risk of skin pressure or damage. Pads and cushions should be waterproof with sealed seams to prevent inadvertent contamination of interior spaces and allow for frequent, thorough cleaning and disinfection. Pads, cushions, or other soft surfaces that become damaged must be evaluated to determine if repair is feasible or, if not, promptly replaced. Dedicating supportive equipment to individual residents provides the optimum infection prevention approach but may not be possible in all rehabilitation programs.

Cleaning and Disinfection of Rehabilitative Equipment

Hydrotherapy

Hydrotherapy tanks such as whirlpools or Hubbard tanks are closed water systems in which hydro jets circulate water. In these hydrotherapy systems, warm water temperature and aeration provide an ideal condition for bacterial proliferation if the equipment is not properly cleaned and disinfected. All equipment used should be routinely cleaned and disinfected per manufacturers' instructions after use, even if tub liners are used. The cleaning and disinfecting process should also include the drain and the agitator. Equipment should be allowed to dry prior to the next use. When evaluating hydrotherapy equipment for purchase, the IP should help evaluate the overall design and any components that would be difficult to clean or disinfect or that would remain wet. Equipment evaluation should also asses the risk of spilling and splashing, as potential pathogens from tub water can spread to walls, floors, and drains.[38]

Hydrocollators

Hydrocollators are liquid heating systems designed to warm reusable packs for therapeutic use. The hydrocollator unit keeps the packs hot and ready for use. The recommended operating temperature (usually 160°F to 166°F) and the water level should be monitored and recorded daily. Bleach or high-chorine content products are not recommended for disinfection as they may damage the unit. The IP should make sure that the manufacturer's cleaning and disinfecting instructions are readily accessible to the therapy team and fully implemented. The unit should be drained and cleaned at least every 2 weeks or per LTCF policy. Individual hot packs should be wrapped in a towel or covered in another way before placing them against the resident's skin. These covers should only be used once and not transferred from one resident to another.

Physical or Occupational Treatment Tables

Treatment tables may also be called mats or platform tables and are routinely used in physical therapy programs. These tables must be cleaned and disinfected between each resident with manufacturers' approved chemicals that will not damage the hard and/or soft surfaces. If a sheet is placed between the resident and the table surface during the therapy session, it should be changed after each use. The table surface should be monitored for cracks and tears that could potentially harbor pathogens.

Gait Belts

Gait belts are used to provide stability and security when ambulating residents. They are also used when assisting residents to move from a chair, wheelchair, or bed. Gait belts should be cleaned between use with each resident. If feasible, the facility may consider having dedicated gait belts for each resident.[39] Belts made with antimicrobial-coated materials will still require regular cleaning between use with different residents.

Walking Rails

Parallel bars, often called walking rails, are frequently used in mobility training. The rails should be wiped with a cleaner/disinfectant after use with each resident.

Paraffin Wax

Heated wax is used for hand, elbow, or foot pain relief. A machine contains a heat source that melts the paraffin wax and maintains it in a liquid state at a safe temperature. Residents with skin lesions or other skin infections should be excluded from this type of therapy until the risk of transmission has passed. The IP should monitor that the unit is cleaned and disinfected per manufacturer instructions per facility policy and schedule.

Mobility Aids

Aids such as walkers, wheelchairs, leg scooters, and motorized scooters should be cleaned between residents if the equipment is shared. Even when residents own their mobility equipment, a regular cleaning and disinfection schedule should be in place, as these items can quickly become contaminated as residents move within and without the facility. A more rigorous cleaning procedure may be required based on individual resident needs and the need for stringent containment measures during outbreaks.

In-Room Rehabilitation Services

Although LTCFs strive to maximize resident independence and social interaction, health issues may occasionally restrict the individual to his or her room or limit participation in group activities. In these instances, rehabilitative services may be provided in the resident's room. All isolation precautions should be followed. Any equipment taken into the room must be thoroughly cleaned and disinfected upon removal. If possible, equipment should remain within the room until the isolation is discontinued. Any fabric items should be contained and laundered per facility policy and disposable items discarded prior to exiting the room.

LABORATORY SERVICES

LTCFs in the United States generally do not have onsite laboratories. If the LTCF is part of a large health system, a hospital's laboratory may be used. All other LTCFs will contract with a private, often called reference, laboratory for diagnostic services. The IP must be knowledgeable about the lab services available to LTCF and maintain effective communication with designated laboratory staff. The IP's laboratory checklist should include:

- Types of tests performed by the lab and the normal ranges for each
- Expected turnaround times
- Methods of reporting results
- Specimen collection procedures
- Specimen holding and transport to the laboratory
- Types of diagnostic testing not performed by the laboratory

CLIA Waived Tests

All facilities in the United States that perform laboratory testing on human specimens for health assessment or for the diagnosis, prevention, or treatment of disease are regulated under the Clinical Laboratory Improvement Amendments of 1988 (CLIA). Waived tests are systems cleared by the FDA for home use and those tests approved for waiver under the CLIA criteria. CLIA requires that waived tests must be simple and have a low risk for erroneous results.[40]

Since CLIA was implemented, waived testing has steadily increased in the United States. Surveys conducted during 1999 to 2004 by CMS and studies funded by CDC during 1999 to 2003 evaluated testing practices in sites holding a CLIA Certificate of Waiver (CW). Although study findings indicate CW sites generally take measures to perform testing correctly, they raise quality concerns about practices that could lead to errors in testing and poor patient/resident outcomes. These issues are probably caused, in part, by high personnel turnover rates, lack of understanding about good laboratory practices, and inadequate training.[41]

Of the facilities surveyed by CMS during 2003 to 2004, 90 percent reported that they performed no more than five different waived tests. The five most commonly performed waived tests were identified as:

- Blood glucose
- Dipstick urinalysis
- Fecal occult blood
- Urine human chorionic gonadotropin (hCG) (visual color comparison)
- Group A streptococcal antigen (direct test from throat swabs)

Waived testing for influenza was also performed by some institutions, but far less frequently.

Waived testing is increasingly used in LTCF settings as well. Data from facilities with a certificate of waiver from CMS surveyed sites, 2002 to 2004 (n = 4,214), and all CW sites, 2004 (n = 109,820), indicated that nursing homes ranked second only to physicians' offices in the overall percent of waivers held.[41]

LTCFs can obtain information on how to apply for a CLIA waiver, including associated fees and program updates at www.cms.goc/clia. Because staff education in performing these tests is critical and failures have led to serious outbreaks, the CDC offers educational materials and an online training course specific to waived testing at www.cdc.gov/clia. The CDC materials are appropriate for use in long-term care.

Specimen Integrity

When testing cannot be completed at the point of care, the IP must monitor that specimen collection, handling, and transport are consistent with laboratory requirements.

A high-quality specimen is required to produce high-quality diagnostic results. Although errors can potentially occur for any test, LTCFs have two specimen collection procedures in LTCFs that are often problematic and may require focused monitoring by the IP: obtaining urine and wound cultures.

Obtaining a Urine Culture

Urine for culture must be either freshly voided or obtained directly from the urinary catheter. The specimen should not be collected from a urinary drainage bag. The specimen container must be sterile and must not be contaminated during the collection process. Residents with indwelling catheters should have the device changed prior to specimen collection because bacteria quickly ascend into the bladder and biofilm rapidly accumulates on indwelling device surfaces.[42] Urine cultures must be refrigerated after collection and kept cool during transport to the laboratory.

Obtaining a Wound Culture

Drainage and exudate must be removed before a culture is obtained. Usually this is accomplished by irrigation with a solution such as normal saline, which is indicated on the resident's wound management plan. When organic matter has been removed, the sterile swab is then applied to the wound bed. Culturing wound drainage, rather than the wound bed, increases the risk of an inaccurate result. A different swab must be used for each wound, and the specimen containers must be labeled to indicate different sites.

When troubleshooting problems associated with laboratory specimens, the IP should also evaluate:

- Incomplete or misplaced specimen labels
- Accidental contamination during collection
- Inadequate amounts in tubes, containers, or swabs sent for processing
- Missed or delayed transport times to the laboratory
- Inadvertent use of expired or otherwise compromised specimen collection supplies
- Other evidence of mishandling or improper storage that could jeopardize specimen integrity

Role of the Laboratory in LTC Antimicrobial Stewardship

Several studies have documented the overutilization of antibiotics in long-term care, as well as an increase in resistance to those antibiotics.[43] Of all the cases of antimicrobial use in nursing homes, 20 to 60 percent of cases can be attributed to UTI, even though only 30 to 60 percent of those cases are considered appropriate for antimicrobial therapy.[44] Other recent research has shown that many residents receive antibiotics for more than 7 days, and some for as long as 90 days.[45,46] Because neither physicians nor laboratory services are available onsite, the empiric use of antibiotics, such as prescribing a broad spectrum antibiotic without laboratory confirmation of the pathogen, remains a common practice. These issues support the extension of antimicrobial stewardship programs, as begun in hospitals, into long-term care.[47]

What is a PCR Test?

The **polymerase chain reaction (PCR)**, introduced in 1983, is a technique widely used in molecular testing. Unlike cultures or assays, the test is based on DNA. Because of its accuracy, PCR testing is now a widely used in many fields such as genomic research, hereditary disease, and more recently infectious diseases. Although PCR testing is more costly than other diagnostic methods, it is increasingly used to identify pathogens such as *Clostridium difficile* and methicillin-resistant *Staphylococcus aureus*. The IP in long-term care should understand the extent to which PCR testing may be needed, the laboratory's capabilities to perform such testing, and the associated turnaround times for results.[49]

The role of the laboratory should be included in any facility-based antibiotic stewardship program. In acute care settings, the laboratory usually produces antibiogram reports. These reports present summary susceptibility data to designated antibiotics by a specific strain of bacteria. The analysis of susceptibility data is useful in understanding patterns of resistance, how these patterns may or may not be changing, and if the antibiotics used in empiric therapy or initial treatment are the best choice. However, antibiograms reporting is infrequently available in LTC. Antibiograms must be based on the results of at least 30 isolates within the reporting time frame, a threshold that even skilled nursing facilities may be unable to meet.[48]

Even when antibiogram reporting is unavailable, the IP should collaborate with the laboratory staff to ensure that drug-resistant organisms are identified and that diagnostic data are used in the facility's multidrug-resistant organism (MDRO) management strategies, including the implementation of an antibiotic stewardship program. The LTCF should establish a process in which the IP reviews all culture results, and the analysis of laboratory reports should be included in the data reviewed by the LTCF's infection prevention committee.

TABLE 11.3: MOST FREQUENTLY REPORTS MEDICATIONS AMONG RESIDENTS EVALUATED FOR POLYPHARMACY: 2004 NATIONAL NURSING HOME SURVEY[51]

Medication	Frequency of Use
Gastrointestinal agents	
Laxatives	47.5%
Agents for acid/peptic disorders	43.3%
Central nervous system agents	
Antidepressants	46.3%
Antipsychotics	25.9%
Pain relievers	
Nonnarcotic analgesics	43.6%
Antipyretics	41.2%

PHARMACY SERVICES

Pharmacotherapy has become an integral and essential component of long-term care. However, the use of medications among the elderly is a complex, multifactor issue that includes more than safe, age appropriate prescribing. The following factors must be considered:

- Age appropriate drug development
- Age appropriate drug testing in clinical trials
- Reliable medication administration
- Ongoing assessment of the response to prescribed medications
- Adherence to medication programs
- Age appropriate outcomes monitoring[50]

The widespread use of multiple medications in LTCFs remains a clinical challenge. A study of more than 13,000 LTCF residents' medication use, extracted from the 2004 National Nursing Home Survey, reported a 40 percent prevalence of polypharmacy (defined as nine or more prescribed medications). This study also identified the most commonly used drugs among residents meeting the definition for polypharmacy.[51] See Table 11.3.

The 2004 National Nursing Home Survey data also revealed additional serious threats associated with high-drug utilization. For example, residents taking nine or more medications were more likely to experience a potentially preventable emergency department visit (56 percent) than other nursing home residents (50 percent).[52] Forty-four percent of residents with pain received neither standing orders for analgesia nor special services for pain management.[53]

Although there is limited research to indicate the best practices to reduce polypharmacy and the risk of drug related adverse events in the elderly, some studies have indicated that improved prescribing and enhanced medication adherence programs may be helpful. The use of some level of individual case management or an enhanced interdisciplinary team approach have also been effective, especially when multiple comorbidities have been assessed.[54] Although prevention of polypharmacy among elderly residents is by no means a precise science, the factors listed below may increase the risk of negative outcomes, including an increased risk of mortality:

- Diagnosis of dementia
- Care in a large LTCF
- High or above average turnover rates for nursing staff

- Limited physician availability to coordinate medical care
- Severe or uncontrolled resident pain[55]

LTCFs typically receive medications from an offsite, community-based provider. The IP should collaborate with the pharmacy provider to ensure that medications are dispensed and delivered to the facility in a manner that prevents possible contamination. Package integrity must be regularly checked and expiration dates, as indicated on labels, reviewed. If the LTCF has an antimicrobial stewardship program in development or in place, the contracted pharmacy must be an active participant in the interdisciplinary stewardship team. Coordination of these activities with the nursing department will also be essential.

Considerations for infection prevention may occur at any point in the drug administration process but commonly include the following:

Dose Form Modification Practices

For residents who have dysphagia or who require feeding tubes, the pharmacist should be consulted regarding the optimum form of the medication. Dose form modification—or the emptying of capsules/crushing of tablets—may need to be done: (1) if no other form of the medication exists and (2) the modification is not contraindicated by the drug manufacturer. The optimum approach is to use a form that does not require this level of manipulation, as contamination and spillage are common threats.[56,57]

Safe Handling and Storage of Liquids

The IP should inspect any medication bottles for labeling. Changes or alterations to pharmacy labels are not permissible. Containers once opened should be dated. Any reusable container or bottle can be easily contaminated during handling. Therefore, the IP should monitor hygienic practices used in pour techniques. Prepouring of liquid medications is not recommended as a routine administration practice.

Administration of Anti-infective Agents

The IP should be aware of the anti-infective agents available at the LTCF. Common categories of these drugs are antimicrobials, antimycotics, antivirals, and antiparasitics. The monitoring of hygienic or sterile administration practices will be based on the form of the drug. Anti-infective requiring intravenous infusion will require more focused surveillance (see Chapter 6). Periodic observation of medication administration practices, often known as the "med pass," will provide real time, useful data regarding the safe handling and administration of these commonly prescribed drugs. Observed errors or infection prevention discrepancies must be promptly reported to the nurse supervisor.

Safe Handling of Medication Vials

The misuse of medication vials poses serious risks across all healthcare settings. Healthcare personnel (doctors, nurses, and anyone providing injections) should **never reuse a needle** to withdraw medicine from a vial. Both needle and syringe must be discarded once they have been used. It is not safe to change the needle and reuse the syringe as this practice can contaminate the vial and transmit acute infections as well as chronic disease.

IPs in LTCFs should include monitoring and use of all medication vials on a routine basis, due to the high risk of disease infection from improper handling.

- A single-use vial contains only one dose of medication and should only be used once for one patient, using a clean needle and clean syringe. The label on the vial will clearly state that it is "for single patient use."
- A multidose vial contains more than one dose of medication and is often used by diabetic patients or for vaccinations. The label will state that the container is approved for multiple uses. A new, clean needle and clean syringe should always be used to access the medication in a multidose vial. Reuse of needles or syringes to access a multidose vial can result in contamination of the medication and is not acceptable as this practice has led to major outbreaks.

Whenever possible, CDC recommends that single-use vials be used and that multidose vials of medication be assigned to a single resident to reduce the risk of disease transmission.[58]

Safe Use of Insulin Pens

Insulin pens offer an alternative method for insulin administration. The pen-shaped injector devices contain a disposable needle and either an insulin reservoir or an insulin cartridge. The devices typically contain enough insulin for a resident to self-administer several doses of insulin before the reservoir or cartridge is empty. All insulin pens are approved only for "single-patient use" (one device for only one patient).

As with other devices contacting blood or body fluids, the IP must carefully monitor the usage of these high-risk items and include an analysis of facility risks associated with blood glucose monitoring and insulin administration. This analysis should be reviewed by the interdisciplinary team and with the pharmacy provider at least annually or whenever new/changing infection risks have been identified.

Environmentally Acceptable Means of Drug Disposal

Unused drugs in any form must be discarded by the LTCF. The method of disposal must conform to local or state environmental standards. Unused drugs should not be flushed down toilets or poured into drains, as this increases the contamination risks to waste disposal and water treatment systems. The IP should verify that safe medication disposal is incorporated into the LTCF's safety program.

> Although the FDA issued a national alert in 2009, warning that using ***one insulin pen for multiple patients has been linked to exposure of thousands of individuals and outbreaks of bloodborne disease***, these devices continue to present the potential for incorrect use.[59]

REFERENCES

1. Smith PW, Bennett G, Bradley S Drinka P, Lautenbach E, Marx J, et al. SHEA/APIC Guideline: Infection prevention and control in the long-term care facility. *Am J Infect Control.* 2008 Sep; 36(7): 504-535.
2. Centers for Disease Control and Prevention (CDC). *Norovirus.* CDC website. 2013. Available at: http://www.cdc.gov/norovirus/index.html.
3. Centers for Disease Control and Prevention (CDC). *Salmonella.* CDC website. 2013. Available at: http://www.cdc.gov/salmonella/.
4. Centers for Disease Control and Prevention (CDC). *Food Safety—Clostridium perfringens.* CDC website. 2013. Available at: http://www.cdc.gov/foodsafety/clostridium-perfingens.html.
5. Centers for Disease Control and Prevention (CDC). *National Center for Emerging and Zoonotic Infectious Diseases—Campylobacter.* CDC website. 2013. Available at: http://www.cdc.gov/nczved/divisions/dfbmd/diseases/campylobacter/#what.
6. Centers for Disease Control and Prevention (CDC). *Listeria (Listeriosis).* CDC website. 2013. Available at: http://www.cdc.gov/listeria/index.html.
7. U.S. Public Health Service—Food and Drug Administration. *Food Code 2009.* FDA website. 2009. Available at: http://www.fda.gov/downloads/Food/GuidanceRegulation/UCM189448.pdf.
8. Fauerbach L. Nutrition services. In: Carrico R, ed. *APIC Text of Infection Control and Epidemiology,* 3rd ed. Washington, DC: Association for Professionals in Infection Control and Epidemiology, Inc., 2009: 58-1–58-9.
9. Schulster LM, Chinn RYW, Arduino MJ, Carpenter J, Donlan R, Ashford D, et al. Guidelines for environmental infection control in health-care facilities: Recommendations from CDC and the Healthcare Infection Control Practices Advisory Committee (HICPAC). Chicago, IL: American Society for Healthcare Engineering/American Hospital Association, 2004: 65-67.
10. Centers for Disease Control and Prevention (CDC). *Norovirus—Trends and Outbreaks.* CDC website. 2013. Available at: http://www.cdc.gov/norovirus/trends-outbreaks.html.
11. Centers for Disease Control and Prevention (CDC). *Multistate and Nationwide Foodborne Outbreak Investigations: A Step-by-step Guide.* CDC website. 2012. Available at: http://www.cdc.gov/outbreaknet/investigations/investigating.html.
12. Centers for Medicare & Medicaid Services (CMS). *CMS Manual System Pub. 100-07 State Operations Provider Certification, Transmittal 55.* CMS website. December 2, 2009. Available at: http://www.cms.gov/Regulations-and Guidance/Guidance/Transmittals/downloads/R51SOMA.pdf.
13. Rosenbaum P, Zeller J, Franck J. Long-term care. In: Carrico R, ed. *APIC Text of Infection Control and Epidemiology,* 3rd ed. Washington, DC: Association of Professionals in Infection Control and Epidemiology, Inc., 2009: 52-1–52-18.
14. Belkin N. Laundry, patient linens, textiles, and uniforms. In: Carrico R, ed. *APIC Text of Infection Control and Epidemiology,* 3rd ed. Washington, DC: Association of Professionals in Infection Control and Epidemiology, Inc., 2009: 101-1–101-8.
15. Pien FD, Pien BC. Parasites. In: Carrico R, ed. *APIC Text of Infection Control and Epidemiology,* 3rd ed. Washington, DC: Association for Professionals in Infection Control and Epidemiology, Inc., 2009: 92-1–92-9.
16. U.S. Department of Labor, Occupational Safety and Health Administration. Occupational exposure to bloodborne pathogens – final rule. *Fed Reg* 1991; 56: 64004-64182.
17. Flaherty PJ, Liljestrand JS, O'Brien TF. Infection control surveillance in a rehabilitation hospital. *Arch Phys Med Rehabil,* 1984 Jun; 65(6): 313-315.
18. Smith MA, Duke WM. A retrospective review of nosocomial infections in an acute rehabilitative and chronic population at a large skilled nursing facility. *J Am Geriatr Soc* 1994 Jan; 42(1): 45-49.
19. Sax H, Hugonnet S, Harbarth S, Herrault P, Pittet D. Variation in nosocomial infection prevalence according to patient care setting:a hospital-wide survey. *J Hosp Infect* 2001 May; 48(1): 27-32.
20. Baldo V, Massaro C, Iaia V, Bajo M, Cristofoletti M, Belloni P, et al. Prevalence of nosocomial infections in a rehabilitation hospital. *J Prev Med Hyg,* 2002; 43: 30-33.
21. The Facility Guidelines Institute. *Guidelines for Design and Construction of Health Care Facilities,* 2010 ed. Chicago: The Facilities Guidelines Institute, 2010: 153.
22. Clarke K, Tong D, Pan Y, Easley KA, Norrick B, Ko C, et al. Reduction in catheter-associated urinary tract infections by bundling interventions. *Int J Qual Health Care* 2013 Feb; 25(1): 43-49.
23. Schumm K, Lam TB. Types of urethral catheters for management of short-term voiding problems in hospitalized adults: a short version Cochrane review. *Neurourol Urodyn* 2008; 27(8): 738-746.
24. Sinclair L, Hagen S, Cross S. Washout policies in long-term indwelling urinary catheterization in adults: a short version Cochrane review. *Neurourol Urodyn* 2011 Sep; 30(7): 1208-1212.
25. Sehulster LM, Chinn RYW, Arduino MJ, Carpenter J, Donlan R, Ashford D, et al. Guidelines for environmental infection control in health-care facilities: Recommendations from CDC and the Healthcare Infection Control Practices Advisory Committee (HICPAC). Chicago, IL: American Society for Healthcare Engineering/American Hospital Association, 2004.
26. Kannankeril AJ, Lam HT, Reyes EB, McCartney J. Urinary tract infection rates associated with re-use of catheters in clean intermittent catheterization of male veterans. *Urol Nurs* 2011 Jan-Feb; 31(1): 41-48.
27. Niël-Weise BS, van den Broek PJ, da Silva EM, Silva LA. Urinary catheter policies for long-term bladder drainage. *Cochrane Database Syst Rev* 2012 Aug 15; 8: CD004201.
28. Wilde MH, Fader M, Ostaszkiewicz J, Prieto J, Moore K. Urinary bag decontamination for long-term use: a systematic review. *J Wound Ostomy Continence Nurs* 2013 May-Jun; 40(3): 299-308.
29. Hus J, Witts K, Jacobson T. Cleaning urinary drainage bags with vinegar following radical prostatectomy surgery: is it necessary? *Urol Nurs* 2012 Nov-Dec; 32(6): 297-304.

REFERENCES

30. File TM. The epidemiology of respiratory tract infections. *Semin Respir Infect* 2000 Sep; 15(3): 184-194.

31. Harkness GA, Bentley DW, Mottley M, Lee J. Streptococcus pyogenes outbreak in a long-term care facility. *Am J Infect Control* 1992 Jun; 20(3): 142-148.

32. Dooling KL, Crist MB, Nguyen D, Bass J, Lorentzson L, Toews KA, et al. Investigation of a prolonged group A streptococcal outbreak among residents of a skilled nursing facility, Georgia, 2009-2012. *Clin Infect Dis* 2013 Sep 9 [epub ahead of print].

33. Thigpen MC, Thomas DM, Gloss D, Park SY, Khan AJ, Fogelman VL, et al. Nursing home outbreak of invasive group a streptococcal infections caused by 2 distinct strains. *Infect Control Hosp Epidemiol* 2007 Jan; 28(1): 68-74.

34. Tan CG, Ostrawski S, Bresnitz EA. A preventable outbreak of pneumococcal pneumonia among unvaccinated nursing home residents in New Jersey during 2001. *Infect Control Hosp Epidemiol* 2003 Nov; 24(11): 848-852.

35. Gleich S, Morad Y, Echague R, Miller JR, Kornblum J, Sampson JS, Butler JC. Streptococcus pneumoniae serotype 4 outbreak in a home for the aged: report and review of recent outbreaks. *Infect Control Hosp Epidemiol* 2000 Nov; 21(11): 711-717.

36. Vergidis P, Hamer DH, Meydani SN, Dallal GE, Barlam TF. Patterns of antimicrobial use for respiratory tract infections in older residents of long-term care facilities. *J Am Geriatr Soc* 2011 Jun; 59(6): 1093-1098.

37. O'Donnell JA, Hofmann MT. Skin and soft tissues. Management of four common infections in the nursing home patient. *Geriatrics* 2001 Oct; 56(10): 33-38, 41.

38. Gould CV, Umscheid CA, Agarwal RK, Kuntz G, Pegues DA, and the Healthcare Infection Control Practices Advisory Committee (HICPAC). Guideline for Prevention of Catheter-associated Urinary Tract Infections, 2009. Atlanta: Centers for Disease Control and Prevention, 2009.

39. Felix K. Rehabilitation services. In Carrico R, ed. *APIC Text of Infection Control and Epidemiology,* 3rd ed. Washington, DC: Association for Professionals in Infection Control and Epidemiology, Inc., 2009: 66-1–66-10.

40. Centers for Disease Control and Prevention (CDC). *Waived tests.* CDC website. 2013. Available at: http://wwwn.cdc.gov/clia/Resources/WaivedTests/default.aspx.

41. Howerton D, Anderson N, Bosse D, Granade S, Westbrook G. Good laboratory practices for waived testing sites: survey findings from testing sites holding a Certificate of Waiver under the Clinical Laboratory Improvement Amendments of 1988 and recommendations for promoting quality testing. *MMWR* 2005 Nov 11; 54(RR13): 1-25.

42. Siddiq DM, Darouiche RO. New strategies to prevent catheter-associated urinary tract infections. *Nat Rev Urol* 2012 Apr 17; 9(6): 305-314.

43. Montoya A, Mody L. Common infections in nursing homes: a review of current issues and challenges. *Aging health* 2011 Dec; 7(6): 889-899.

44. Nicolle LE. Resistant pathogens in urinary tract infections. *J Am Geriatr Soc* 2002; 50(7 Suppl): S230-S235.

45. Daneman N, Gruneir A, Newman A, Fischer HD, Bronskill SE, Rochon PA, et al. Antibiotic use in LTC facilities. *J Antimicrob Chemother* 2011 Dec; 66(12): 2856-2863.

46. Daneman N, Gruneir A, Bronskill SE, Newman A, Fischer HD, Rochon PA, et al. Prolonged antibiotic treatment in long-term care: role of the prescriber. *JAMA Intern Med* 2013 Apr 22; 173(8): 673-682.

47. Bonomo RA. Multiple antibiotic-resistant bacteria in long-term-care facilities: an emerging problem in the practice of infectious diseases. *Clin Infect Dis* 2000; 31: 1414-1422.

48. Clinical and Laboratory Standards Institute (CLSI). *Analysis and Presentation of Cumulative Susceptibility Test Data, Approved Guideline,* 3rd ed. CLSI document M39-A3. Wayne, PA: CLSI, 2009; 29(6): 1-68.

49. Bartlett JM, Stirling D. A short history of the polymerase chain reaction. *Methods Mol Biol* 2003; 226: 3-6.

50. Topinková E, Baeyens JP, Michel JP, Lang PO. Evidence-based strategies for the optimization of pharmacotherapy in older people. *Drugs Aging* 2012 Jun 1; 29(6): 477-494.

51. Dwyer LL, Han B, Woodwell DA, Rechtsteiner EA. Polypharmacy in nursing home residents in the United States: results of the 2004 National Nursing Home Survey. *Am J Geriatr Pharmacother* 2010 Feb; 8(1): 63-72.

52. Caffrey C. Potentially preventable emergency department visits by nursing home residents: United States, 2004. *NCHS Data Brief* Apr 2010; 33: 1-6.

53. Sengupta M, Bercovitz A, Harris-Kojetin LD. Prevalence and Management of Pain, by Races and Dementia Among Nursing Home Residents: United States, 2004. *NCHS Data Brief* Mar 2010; 30: 1-7.

54. Smith SM, Soubhi H, Fortin M, Hudon C, O'Dowd T. Interventions for improving outcomes in patients with multimorbidity in primary care and community settings. *Cochrane Database Syst Rev* 2012 Apr 18; 4: CD006560.

55. Lukas A, Mayer B, Fialová D, Topinkova E, Gindin J, Onder G, et al. Treatment of pain in European nursing homes: results from the Services and Health for Elderly in Long Term Care (SHELTER) Study. *J Am Med Dir Assoc* 2013 Jun 5 pii: S1525-8610(13)00250-8.

56. Stubbs J, Haw C, Dickens G. Dose form medication – a common but potentially hazardous practice. A literature review and study of medication administration to older psychiatric inpatients. *Int Psychogeriatr* 2008 Jun; 20(3): 616-627.

57. Morris H. Administering drugs to patients with swallowing difficulties. *Nurs Times* 2005 Sept; 101(39): 28-30.

REFERENCES

58. Centers for Disease Control and Prevention (CDC). *Injection safety – a patient safety threat – syringe reuse.* CDC website. 2011. Available at: http://www.cdc.gov/injectionsafety/patients/syringeReuse_faqs.html.

59. U.S. Food and Drug Administration (FDA). *Insulin pens and insulin cartridges must not be shared.* FDA website. 2009. Available at: http://www.fda.gov/NewsEvents/Newsroom/PressAnnouncements/ucm149546.htm.

ADDITIONAL RESOURCES

1. Centers for Disease Control and Prevention (CDC). *Foodborne outbreak online database (FOOD).* CDC website. 2013. Available at: http://wwwn.cdc.gov/foodborneoutbreaks/Default.aspx.

2. Centers for Disease Control and Prevention (CDC). Management of foodborne illnesses: a primer for physicians and other health care professionals. *MMWR* 2004; 53(No. RR-4): 1-7.

CHAPTER 12

Life Enrichment and Support Services

Deborah Patterson Burdsall, MSN, RN-BC, CIC

KEY CONCEPTS

- The infection preventionist should be aware of all life enrichment programs and activities that may introduce unexpected and novel challenges in the long-term care community.
- The infection preventionist should develop strategies and provide tools and resources to promote infection prevention and control practices during these programs and activities.

CHANGES IN LONG-TERM CARE

As recently as 20 years ago, long-term care facilities (LTCFs) had stable resident populations. There were fewer admissions and discharges to hospitals and to the community. This stability allowed for consistent and well-rehearsed activities with many of the same participants. Support services provided to traditional long-term residents were limited to barber and beauty salon services; volunteer services; transportation; pastoral care; and group activities such as religious services, games, and few planned outings.

As the traditional resident population in LTCFs has changed in the last 20 years, the services and support provided in LTCFs have become more diverse and more skilled. The familiar cohorts of residents in skilled care are being replaced with more dynamic groups that include younger and sicker rehabilitation patients with postsurgical joint replacement surgery or postacute recovery covered under Medicare or private insurance. At the same time, independent living, assisted living, and supportive living are being challenged with care needs of increasingly frail older adults. It takes a wide variety of support and services to meet the medical, biopsychosocial, and spiritual needs of the residents now residing and rehabilitating in long-term care. This is seen in the widespread adoption of a person-centered model of care in a home-like environment. This model often includes more extensive salon or spa services, fitness centers, computer labs, music therapy, intergenerational interaction, and visits by pets, companion animals, and therapy animals.

The changes in residents' needs have also introduced more interaction with hospitals, doctors' offices, dialysis centers, and infusion centers. A patient or resident may now come straight from a dialysis session to a group activity. These changes may increase the introduction of epidemiologically important organisms such as multidrug-resistant organisms (MDROs) and infectious diseases such as influenza, respiratory syncytial virus (RSV), and norovirus into the long-term care community. (See Chapter 14 for additional information about transitions in care.)

With these new activities and services, the infection preventionist (IP) will need to address potential increased risk of pathogen transmission. A comprehensive infection prevention plan must now include measures to prevent environmental contamination of items such as in-room computers, public computer keyboards, touch screens, musical instruments, and exercise and therapy equipment. In addition, the plan must anticipate increased traffic in and out of the LTCF by visitors and service providers who support these activities.

LIFE ENRICHMENT ACTIVITY PROFESSIONALS

Activity professionals are an important part of the LTCF interdisciplinary team and a vital link to residents, families, and the community. Starting in the 1960s, volunteers, nurses' aides, and other long-term care staff developed structured activities as well as psychosocial programs for older adults living in LTCFs. As activity services have gained recognition as important way for the LTCF to improve resident quality of life, the activity service profession has become more formalized and defined. In 1981, the National Association of Activity Professionals (NAAP) was formed to "provide excellence in support services to Activity Professionals through education, advocacy, technical assistance, promotion of standards, and peer and industry relations."[1]

THE ROLE OF THE INFECTION PREVENTIONIST IN LIFE ENRICHMENT ACTIVITIES

The IP needs to be aware of the types of activities that are being offered to residents at any given time. It is important that there is clear communication among life enrichment activity professionals, the IP, and nursing staff from the beginning of the activity planning process. Clear communication will decrease the accidental inclusion of an infectious individual in a group activity.

To reduce the risk of infection during life enrichment and other support service activities, the IP must develop infection prevention and control policies and procedures that are both accurate in content and consistently implemented. These policies and procedures must have an evidence and regulation basis and must be shared with the interdisciplinary team. The policies and procedures must provide clear direction and identify lines of communication between program coordinators, residents, families, and staff.

Policies and procedures for support and life enrichment activities should address the following:

- **The health of individuals participating in group activities:** Have processes in place to identify and exclude individuals with contagious illness from group activities.
- **The cleanliness and sanitation of the environment:** Have procedures in place to ensure that the environment in which an activity is to take place is properly cleaned and disinfected before and after the event. Be sure to include cleaning and disinfecting any equipment used such as computer keyboards, touchscreens, musical instruments, and exercise or therapy equipment.
- **Hand hygiene:** Encourage hand hygiene before, during, and after activities and provide easy access to soap, water, paper towels, alcohol-based hand rub, or alcohol-based hand wipes.[2]
- **Respiratory hygiene and cough etiquette:** Encourage individuals to cough into tissues or their sleeve or elbow rather than their hands. Tissues should be readily available and procedure masks provide as needed.[3]
- **Vaccination of residents and healthcare personnel (HCP), including volunteers:** All HCP need to be offered or encouraged to receive appropriate vaccinations as directed by the Centers for Disease Control and Prevention (CDC)[4] and applicable regulations, such as Centers for Medicare & Medicaid Services (CMS) interpretive guidance F tag 441 (see Chapter 9 on Occupational Health for additional information).[5]
- **Outbreak Control:** Have processes and procedures in place to limit access to the LTCF by groups or visitors during outbreaks or epidemics. Include methods of communication such as signs posted at entrances or on unit doors alerting visitors to the outbreak and any associated restrictions.
- **Visitor access and movement:** Have procedures in place to limit visitor access to certain areas within the facility; for example, control visitor access into food preparation areas, treatment areas, medication rooms, and chemical or potentially hazardous waste storage areas.
- **Record keeping:** LTCF should keep attendance records for all life enrichment programs. Activity attendance records facilitate easy identification of individuals exposed during outbreak situations.

The IP should have input into access and visitation policies, especially during increased infectious disease incidence in the LTCF or community because family members and visitors like to participate in the facility's social events and group activities. Programs should be instituted to screen visitors and family members to temporarily defer visitation when necessary.

Infection Prevention Measures during Life Enrichment Activities

Any life enrichment activity must include hand hygiene practice by staff, volunteers, and residents to prevent transmission of infection. Hand hygiene should be performed:

- When entering the LTCF or community
- When hands are visibly soiled (soap and water for 15 to 30 seconds)
- Before and after activities
- Before or after eating
- Before and after handling food or assisting with meals (soap and water for 15 to 30 seconds)
- After personal use of the toilet (soap and water for 15 to 30 seconds)
- After handling soiled equipment
- Before and after using gloves
- When leaving the LTCF or community[1,6,7]

Basic Standard Precautions must also be a part of any activity. These include:

- Ensuring there is easy access to sinks, alcohol-based hand rubs, or alcohol-based sanitizing hand wipes for every activity
- Ensuring appropriate surface cleaner/disinfectants are available and are used before and after activities
- Emphasizing hand hygiene for all participants at the start and the conclusion of activities
- Encouraging respiratory etiquette; for example, coughing into the sleeve or elbow or using tissues
- Providing activities for residents who have potentially infectious conditions and are temporarily excluded from group activities
- Ensuring easy access to and proper use of gloves and other personal protective equipment as needed; gloves should be removed promptly after use and hands should be washed or sanitized to avoid transfer of microorganisms to other individuals or the environment[1,2,6,7]

Activities that use any type of shared equipment will require routine cleaning between each resident. This includes musical instruments, video game controllers, keyboards, touch screens, and other equipment.[8] Equipment used in activity programs should be cleaned and disinfected according to the manufacturer recommendations. Cleaners and disinfectants for life enrichment activity equipment should have the following characteristics:

- A low level of toxicity (Health Hazard of 0 or 1)
- A single step clean and disinfect
- Highly effective against a variety of organisms, killing both vegetative and spore forms of bacteria and encapsulated and nonencapsulated viruses
- A short contact time
- Do not damage surfaces
- Leave a minimal film or have a film that can be easily removed after the appropriate contact time[9]

Food preparation activities can be very therapeutic to LTCF residents. It is important that all activity coordinators understand the regulatory requirements and work with the dietary department to ensure that food is prepared by residents in a safe manner (see Chapter 11 for more information about foodborne illness and food safety). It is important that:

- Hand hygiene is performed before food preparation.
- Gloves are used correctly.
- Cleanliness and correct food temperatures are maintained.
- The food is prepared and stored safely.
- Foods prepared with raw ingredients such as eggs or raw meats are not to be consumed prior to cooking. All foods should be baked or cooked according to the recommended internal food temperatures.
- Dietary services should be involved to ensure safe and proper use, cleaning, and disinfection of dishware, utensils, and equipment.
- Dishes, utensils, and objects used to prepare food must be washed and disinfected in accordance with food safety rules and regulations. To ensure proper levels of disinfection return items to the dietary department.[10]

SALON AND BARBER SHOP SERVICES

Each state has a board of regulations that governs the establishment of personal or independent contractor licensure and educational requirements for beauty salons and spas, barber shops, cosmetologists, estheticians, and manicurists. Local village or city ordinances may also have licensure requirements. Safety and sanitation guidelines and regulations are set by the state and/or local government boards and accrediting and professional organizations such as National Accrediting Commission of Cosmetology Arts and Sciences (NACCAS), the National Cosmetology Association, the Nail Manufacturers Council, and the Professional Beauty Association. These guidelines and regulations include criteria for disposable products, foot spa cleaning guidelines, chemical use and storage, and other general salon safety rules.[11,12] Appropriate cleaning and disinfecting must be done utilizing Environmental Protection Agency-approved disinfectants with the appropriate contact time.

It is important that policies and procedures for LTCF salons and barber shops take into consideration both LTCF and state cosmetology regulations. It is also important to ensure that personnel do not perform services that are outside the scope of their assigned duties, training, or licensure. Lapses in infection prevention practice in salons or barber shops can be avoided by adequate training, supervision, and regular monitoring.

Nail care and nail hygiene are activities that can improve resident hygiene and self-image as well as provide time for social interaction. CMS defines nail hygiene services as "routine trimming, cleaning, filing, but not polishing of undamaged (finger) nails."[5] The IP needs to ensure that individuals performing nail care and nail hygiene are following proper infection prevention and control procedures. Nail-care tools must be appropriately cleaned and disinfected or discarded and replaced between residents. Designating nail-care tools for each resident is ideal. Proper personal protective equipment (PPE) such as gloves, gowns, masks, and eye equipment must be utilized by any individuals providing nail care and nail hygiene services. Volunteers may be allowed to assist with nail care, depending on regulations and facility policy. Facility documentation for individuals performing nail care services should include demonstration or return demonstration of proper procedures and correct handling and storage of chemicals.

There is a significant difference in risks associated with fingernail and toenail care in older adults. ***Only authorized individuals should perform foot care or toenail care.*** Foot care is outside the scope of the life enrichment program.

INTERGENERATIONAL AND GROUP ACTIVITIES

LTCFs and communities are part of the larger social community. Intergenerational interaction is an important part of the biopsychosocial development of children and the continued connection of older adults to their community. Intergenerational activities can include onsite day care, school activities, arts and crafts, or religious groups. When planning intergenerational activities, it is important to consider the following:

- Communication with event planners
- Prescreening of participants
- Types of events
- Time of the year
- Communicable disease trends and/or outbreaks occurring in the community, schools, and LTCFs

Event planners and the participants themselves must communicate frequently and honestly. Everyone who participates in group activities needs to be encouraged to tell the event coordinator if they are not feeling well. Event planners must be empowered to limit attendance to those who are healthy and have no active signs and symptoms of infection or to cancel a program if necessary. See the checklist provided on the CD-ROM.

LTCF, school, and childcare staff must be diligent in preventing the spread of infection during intergenerational activities. Infants and children up to 3 years old who are still in the "oral" phase of development are too young to participate in respiratory etiquette programs and require close supervision when in the LTCF.[7,13,14] This includes young children who may be "teething." Blankets and other floor coverings may be needed to prevent children from crawling on floors and carpets.[3,13]

Preventing the transmission of respiratory illness is particularly challenging during intergenerational activities. Respiratory illnesses in both the young and the old are a major cause of illness and death. Immune-compromised individuals and people over 65 are at greatest risk of severe illness and death from respiratory illness.[15-19] This is especially important in long-term care because infections can be transmitted even when respiratory symptoms are not apparent.[15] Influenza is perhaps the most well-known cause, but RSV is an under-recognized illness in older adults and has been associated with LTCF outbreaks.[20,21] Adenovirus can cause cold-like symptoms in children but can cause death in older adults.[18,19] Careful consideration should be given to limiting intergenerational activities during the height of the annual influenza season.

TRANSPORTATION

Many LTCFs have their own vehicles to transport residents with limited mobility or those who require wheelchairs. Drivers of these vehicles need to have specialized driver's licenses and will also need to be considered at risk for exposure to blood and other potentially infectious materials if they transport residents and patients with no HCP present. It is important to include them in bloodborne pathogen training and Hepatitis B vaccination programs. Transport vehicles need to be equipped with first aid kits, PPE, and spill containment kits. These vehicles need to be cleaned and disinfected according to LTCF policy.

VOLUNTEERS

Volunteers may perform the same or similar tasks as LTCF staff. Therefore, volunteer training programs require structure, registrations, orientation, and inservice training. Infection control orientation and annual inservices should be part of the program. Tuberculosis screening frequency is based upon risk assessment and state regulation. Seasonal influenza vaccine should be offered to volunteers.

ANIMALS IN LONG-TERM CARE COMMUNITIES

The presence of animals in nursing homes has been promoted as a way to decrease loneliness, increase socialization, and provide companionship. Even robotic dogs have been shown to decrease loneliness in institutionalized older adults.[22]

Research on the effect of companion animals on individuals in long-term care documents both risks and benefits.[23-25] Although pets and companion animals can improve the LTCF resident's quality of life, they can also transmit pathogens such as methicillin-resistant *Staphylococcus aureus* (MRSA) and *Clostridium difficile*. A LTCF's policy and procedure for an animal program must include measures and interventions that reduce risk of transmitting organisms. Animals should be clean, fully immunized, and well-mannered with no signs or symptoms of infection. If animals are used in activity programs at the LTCF, pet therapy must be included in the annual infection prevention risk assessment and described in the LTCF infection prevention program.

Visiting Animals and Personal Pets

Residents who own animals need to have appropriate facility support to ensure that pets are healthy, vaccinated, clean, and well groomed. Pets and their human companions who visit regularly may need to be registered as volunteers. The volunteer department or reception will have the most frequent contact with visiting animals and can help maintain vaccine documentation. Each state and municipality may have different health requirements for animals, including the process for recording animal bites.

Facility Animals

Successful LTCF animal programs require thoughtful planning and an interdisciplinary team approach. This includes contingency plans when animals can no longer be included in a therapeutic program. Animals must be well-trained preferably by professional trainers. Table 12.1[26] presents factors to consider when planning a resident animal program for the LTCF.

TABLE 12.1: FACTORS TO CONSIDER FOR RESIDENT ANIMALS[26]

Animal Factors
• What species? • What age? • Source • Temperament and health testing • What preventative medicine program will be used (vaccination, deworming)? • Who will pay for veterinary care? • If the animal becomes unsuitable (e.g., behavior, disease), what will happen to it? • What will happen if the animal develops a potentially zoonotic disease? Is there a plan to temporarily re-home the animal during treatment?
Management Factors
• Where will the animal be fed and by whom? • Where will the animal defecate, and will there be any potential contact with that area by residents? • Will the animal be restricted to certain areas? If so, how will that be done? • What mechanism will be used to detect, report, and deal with any problems with the animal or residents? • How will hand hygiene be emphasized/implemented? • Will all residents have access to the animal? • What will be done if a resident or staff member is fearful or allergic? • Will residents carrying pathogens that are potentially transmissible to the animal be restricted from animal contact?

When considering an animal program for the facility, it is important to understand the benefits and risks associated with different species of animals. Although species may differ, the basic principles of infection prevention are essentially the same (see Table 12.2[24,25,27,28]). The goal of the program is to maximize the benefit and reduce the potential risks for staff, residents, and visitors. This should include at a minimum the following two requirements:

- For a bite, scratch, or injury from an animal, perform first aid, complete incident reports, and contact the appropriate individuals. A follow-up investigation will help determine if the animal is appropriate to remain in the LTCF.
- For sick animals, verify that veterinary information and emergency services are available.

See Table 12.3 for sample policy.

COMPANION, THERAPY, AND SERVICE ANIMALS

The LTCF leadership must understand the distinction between animals with different levels of training and abilities. Individuals with service animals have legal rights to public access for their specially trained dogs or miniature horses under the Americans with Disabilities Act of 1990 (ADA). These rights do not extend to companion animals or therapy animals. Check federal, state, and local laws to ensure that policies are in compliance.

Companion Animals

The American Society for the Prevention of Cruelty to Animals defines companion animal as "domesticated or domestic-bred animals whose physical, emotional, behavioral, and social needs can be readily met as companions in the home, or in close daily relationship with humans."[29] Companion animals do not have the specialized training of service animals and are not guaranteed access under ADA.[25,30,31]

Therapy Animals

Therapy animals are owned pets that have been evaluated for visiting individuals in LTCFs and other healthcare facilities and trained with their volunteer handlers. There are organizations that set standards for behavior testing and evaluation of animals over 1 year of age and have registered therapy animal programs. The test includes evaluations of the animal's behavior, including reactions to wheelchairs and crutches. Although therapy animals may be registered through certain organizations, therapy animals are not service animals.[29,32]

Service Animals

The ADA guarantees access for individuals and their service animals. As of March 11, 2011, "Service animal means any dog that is individually trained to do work or perform tasks for the benefit of an individual with a disability, including a physical, sensory, psychiatric, intellectual, or other mental disability. Other species of animals, whether wild or domestic, trained or untrained, are not service animals for the purposes of this definition." Miniature horses are also included under this law if they are also "individually trained to do work or perform tasks for the benefit of an individual with a disability."[25] Pets and support animals are not covered under the ADA as service animals, as "a pet or support animal may be able to discern that the individual is in distress, but it is what the animal is trained to do in response to this awareness that distinguishes a service animal from an observant pet or support animal."[30,31]

TABLE 12.2: ANIMAL BENEFITS AND RISKS BY SPECIES[24,25,27,28]

Benefit	Risk	
BIRDS (INCLUDING CAGED PARAKEETS, CANARIES, FINCHES, ROCK DOVES, COCKATIELS, AND PARROTS)		
• Active, colorful, personable • Smaller birds can be economical • Can be kept in cages or aviaries • Can be taught to interact with humans	• Allergies • Bites or pecking • Scratches • Infected birds can remain infectious for several months, shedding bacteria through feces and nasal discharges	• Illness caused by: – *Mycobacterium avium* complex – *Chlamydophila psittaci* (psittacosis, in parrots, ornithosis in other birds) – *Salmonella* – *Giardia*
CATS		
• Affectionate • Familiar • Interacts well with humans	• Allergies • Bites • Coats can pick up multidrug-resistant organisms	• Ringworm • Scratches • *Toxoplasma gondii*
DOGS		
• Affectionate • Familiar • Interacts well with humans	• Allergies • Bites • Coats can pick up multidrug-resistant organisms • Ringworm	• Scratches • Therapy dogs have been shown to shed MRSA and *Clostridium difficile* after exposure to healthcare environments
FISH		
• Properly maintained aquariums provide colorful diversion	• Bacterial infections	
MINIATURE HORSES		
• Affectionate • Interacts well with humans • Trained as guide animals • Can be housebroken (http://www.guidehorse.org)	• Bites • Kicking or accidental misplacement of hooves • MRSA	• *Clostridium difficile* • *Salmonella*
MONKEYS AND OTHER NONHUMAN PRIMATES		
Exclude from LTCF due to infection risk	• Allergies • Bites • Scratches • Macacine herpesvirus B • Herpesvirus	• Measles • *Salmonella* • *Giardia* • Tuberculosis • Rabies
GUINEA PIGS, PET RATS, GERBILS, MICE, HEDGEHOGS, FERRETS, CHINCHILLAS, SUGAR GLIDERS		
Exclude from LTCF due to infection risk	• Allergies • Bites • Chewing • Scratches • *Giardia*	• Leptospirosis (Weil's disease) • Rat bite fever (*Streptobacillus moniliformis* or *Spirillum minus*) • Ringworm • *Salmonella*

Table 12.2 Continued

Benefit	Risk	
RABBITS		
• Affectionate • Interacts well with humans • Can be litter-box trained	• Allergies • Bites • Chewing • Can kick	• *Encephalitozoon cuniculi* (urine contact especially in immune compromised individuals) • Scratches • Rabies
REPTILES, SNAKES, AMPHIBIANS, AND TURTLES		
Exclude from LTCF due to infection risk	• Bites • Scratches • *Salmonella*	
STRAY, WILD, OR FERAL ANIMALS, CAN INCLUDE FERAL FOXES, RACCOONS, DOG/WOLF HYBRIDS, AND STRAY CATS AND DOGS		
Exclude from LTCF due to infection risk	• Rabies • Parasites	

TABLE 12.3: SAMPLE POLICY FOR ANIMALS IN LTCFS[24,25,28]

General Statement	Exclusion	Vaccinations and Health Maintenance	Cat Care	Dog Care
The presence of companion animals in long-term care facilities may have a beneficial effect on the residents, patients, and employees. While evidence is mixed, individuals with life histories of pet interactions may have decreased loneliness as the result of the presence of companion animals.	High-risk animals such as reptiles, snakes, and insects; animals with a history of biting, and wild or feral animals will not be allowed in the facility due to the documented risk of disease transmission.	• All animals allowed into care communities must have records of appropriate vaccinations and health examinations as directed by applicable state and federal laws and guidelines. • All animals need to have appropriate and responsible care provided with veterinary oversight including oral care and nail care. • All animals need to be kept clean. • Ill animals will be excluded from visiting. • Animals should not have open wounds.	• Do not allow into food preparation areas. • Do not feed cats or other pets in the kitchen or dining areas of facilities. • Clean the cat's litter box at least daily. Clean and sanitize box daily with appropriate EPA-approved disinfectant. Use appropriate PPE. • Wash hands with soap and water after cleaning litter box. • Keep facility cat indoors and ensure visiting cats are not allowed to roam in facility. Outdoor cats are more likely to be exposed to *Toxoplasma* and shed oocysts in their stool.	• Do not allow into food preparation areas. • Do not feed dogs or other pets in the kitchen or dining areas of facilities. • Dogs should be discouraged from licking patients. • Patients and residents will not feed treats to dogs.

A customizable version of this table is available on the CD-ROM.

REFERENCES

1. National Association of Activity Professionals (NAAP). *Information.* NAAP website. 2013. Available at: http://naap.info/.

2. Boyce JM, Pittet D; Healthcare Infection Control Practices Advisory Committee; HICPAC/SHEA/APIC/IDSA Hand Hygiene Task Force. Guideline for Hand Hygiene in Health-Care Settings: Recommendations of the Healthcare Infection Control Practices Advisory Committee and the HICPAC/SHEA/APIC/IDSA Hand Hygiene Task Force. *MMWR* 2002; 51: 1-45.

3. Siegel JD, Rhinehart E, Jackson M, Chiarello L, and the Healthcare Infection Control Practices Advisory Committee. *2007 Guideline for Isolation Precautions: Preventing Transmission of Infectious Agents in Healthcare Settings.* CDC website. 2007. Available at: http://www.cdc.gov/ncidod/dhqp/pdf/isolation2007.pdf.

4. Grohskopf LA, Shay DK, Shimabukuro TT, Sokolow LZ, Keitel WA, Bresee JS, et al. Prevention and Control of Seasonal Influenza with Vaccines: Recommendations of the Advisory Committee on Immunization Practices—United States, 2013–2014. *MMWR Recomm Rep* 2013 Sept 20; 62(RR07); 1-43.

5. Centers for Medicare & Medicaid Services (CMS). *State Operations Manual. Appendix PP—Guidance to Surveyors for Long Term Care Facilities.* CMS website. 2011. Available at: http://www.cms.gov/Regulations-and-Guidance/Guidance/Manuals/downloads/som107ap_pp_guidelines_ltcf.pdf.

6. Centers for Medicare & Medicaid Services (CMS). *CMS Manual System – Provider certification.* CMS website. 2009. Available at: http://www.cms.gov/Regulations-and-Guidance/Guidance/Transmittals/downloads/r55soma.pdf.

7. World Health Organization (WHO). Hand hygiene in outpatient and home-based care and long-term care facilities: A guide to the application of the WHO multimodal hand hygiene improvement strategy and the "My Five Moments For Hand Hygiene" approach. WHO website. 2012. Available at: http://www.who.int/gpsc/5may/hh_guide.pdf.

8. Apple. *How to disinfect the Apple internal or external keyboard, trackpad, and mouse.* Apple website. 2013. Available at: http://support.apple.com/kb/HT3988.

9. Rutala WA, ed. *Disinfection, Sterilization and Antisepsis: Principles, Practices, Current Issues, New Research, and New Technologies.* Washington, DC: Association for Professionals in Infection Control and Epidemiology, 2010.

10. Centers for Disease Control and Prevention (CDC). *Incidence of Foodborne Illness.* CDC website. 2010. Available at: http://www.cdc.gov/Features/dsFoodborneIllness/.

11. National Accrediting Commission of Cosmetology Arts and Sciences (NACCAS). *Information.* NACCAS website. 2013. Available at: http://naccas.org/naccas/.

12. The Professional Beauty Association (PBA). *Information.* PBA website. 2013. Available at: http://www.probeauty.org/.

13. McDuffie WG, Whiteman JR. *Intergenerational Activities Program Handbook,* 3rd ed. Binghamton, NY: Broome County Child Development Council, Inc., 1989.

14. Langley GF. Epidemiology of respiratory syncytial virus (RSV) infections in infants and young children. CDC website. 2010. Available at: http://www.cdc.gov/vaccines/recs/acip/downloads/mtg-slides-jun10/11-2-rsv.pdf.

15. Thompson WW, Shay DK, Weintraub E, Brammer L, Cox N, Anderson LJ, et al. Mortality associated with influenza and respiratory syncytial virus in the United States. *JAMA* 2003; 289: 179-186.

16. Centers for Disease Control and Prevention (CDC). *Respiratory syncytial virus infection (RSV).* CDC website. 2013. Available at: http://www.cdc.gov/rsv/.

17. Longtin J, Marchand-Austin A, Winter A-L, Patel S, Eshaghi A, Jamieson F, et al. Rhinovirus outbreaks in long-term care facilities, Ontario, Canada. *Emerg Infect Dis* 2010 Sep; 16(9): 1463-1465.

18. van Asten L, van den Wijngaard C, van Pelt W, van de Kassteele J, Meijer A, van der Hoek W, et al. Mortality attributable to 9 common infections: significant effect of influenza A, respiratory syncytial virus, influenza B, norovirus, and parainfluenza in elderly persons. *J Infect Dis* 2012 Sep 1; 206(5): 628-639.

19. Kandel R, Srinivasan A, D'Agata EM, Lu X , Erdman D, Jhung M, et al. Outbreak of adenovirus type 4 infection in a long term care facility for the elderly. *Infect Control Hosp Epidemiol* 2010; 31(7): 755-757.

20. Caram LB, Chen J, Taggart EW, Hillyard DR, She R, Polage CR. Respiratory syncytial virus outbreak in a long-term care facility detected using reverse transcriptase polymerase chain reaction: an argument for real-time detection methods. *J Am Geriatr Soc* 2009 Mar; 57(3): 482-485.

21. Osterweil D, Norman D. An outbreak of an influenza-like illness in a nursing home. *J Am Geriatr Soc* 1990 Jun; 38(6): 659-662.

22. Banks MR, Willoughby LM, Banks WA. Animal-assisted therapy and loneliness in nursing homes: use of robotic versus living dogs. *J Am Med Dir Assoc* 2008; 9(3): 173-177.

23. Centers for Disease Control and Prevention (CDC). *Healthy Pets, Healthy People.* CDC website. 2013. Available at: http://www.cdc.gov/healthypets/health_prof.htm.

24. Schlesinger DP, Joffe DJ. Raw food diets in companion animals: A critical review. *Can Vet J* 2011 January; 52(1): 50-54.

25. U.S. Department of Justice Civil Rights Division Disability Rights Section. *ADA 2010 revision: Service Animals.* ADA website. 2011. Available at: http://www.ada.gov/service_animals_2010.htm.

26. Weese JS. Fido and Fluffy: friends or foes in long-term care facilities. *Infection Connection* Winter 2010; 5.

27. Sehulster LM, Chinn RYW, Arduino MJ, Carpenter J, Donlan R, Ashford D, et al. *Guidelines for environmental infection control in health-care facilities. Recommendations from CDC and the Healthcare Infection Control Practices Advisory Committee (HICPAC).* Chicago: American Society for Healthcare Engineering/American Hospital Association, 2003.

REFERENCES

28. Darling KT. Animals visiting healthcare facilities. In: Carrico R, ed. *APIC Text of Infection Control and Epidemiology*, 3rd ed. Washington, DC: Association for Professionals in Infection Control and Epidemiology, Inc., 2009: 68-1–68-8.

29. American Society for the Prevention of Cruelty to Animals (ASPA). *Definition of a companion animal.* ASPCA website. 2013. Available at: http://www.aspca.org/about-us/aspca-policy-and-position-statements/definition-of-companion-animal.

30. Department of Justice (DOJ). Nondiscrimination on the basis of disability by public accommodations and in commercial facilities; corrections. *Fed Reg* 2001; 76(48): 13286-13288.

31. U.S. Department of Justice Civil Rights Division Disability Rights Section. *Americans with Disabilities Act revisions.* ADA website. 2011. Available at: http://www.ada.gov/regs2010/titleIII_2010/titleIII_2010_withbold.htm.

32. Pet Partners. *How to become a registered therapy animal team.* Pet Partners website. 2013. Available at: http://www.petpartners.org/TAPinfo.

CHAPTER 13

Education and Training

Irena Kenneley, PhD, APRN-BC, CIC

KEY CONCEPTS

- The long-term care-based infection preventionist needs a basic understanding of certain advanced medical conditions of residents, the therapies or devices to treat those conditions, and associated infection risks.
- Infection prevention measures are particularly critical for residents with end-stage renal disease who are in need of dialysis treatments.
- Infection preventionists should understand the different types of infusion therapies and monitor residents receiving infusion therapy as part of the facility surveillance program.
- The infection preventionist needs to monitor resident populations with chronic wounds—particularly pressure ulcers—to ensure implementation of wound care strategies to prevent infection and skin breakdown and to heal existing wounds.

IMPORTANCE OF THE LONG-TERM CARE FACILITY EDUCATIONAL PROGRAM

One of the most important roles of the long-term care facility (LTCF) infection preventionist (IP) is to educate staff, patients, and families in basic prevention practices and the application of safety science. A comprehensive education and training program supports effective infection prevention and control practices throughout the facility.[1,2] Education and training programs will increase the ability of staff to identify problems, think critically, manage challenging situations with residents and the facility, and cope with stress.[1] All facility employees, including senior leadership and administration, must be fully engaged and committed to the development, implementation, and evaluation of the education and training program.

The education and training of healthcare personnel (HCP) is mandatory for all employees and occurs not only at new employee orientation but also as ongoing training in infection prevention and control activities.[1,2] The LTCF's infection prevention educational program should be reviewed annually and as needed. Inservices, more structured or formal education, and skills-based training are recommended based on regulatory and accrediting compliance, the results of an educational needs assessment, and requests identified by staff and/or managers. Emerging pathogens, community infectious disease threats, new technology, and medications are just a few additional criteria for the justification of the educational program.

For example, to improve HCP and resident safety, the use of Standard Precautions in preventing transmission of infectious agents is an integral component of the initial and ongoing job training and/or task-specific educational program. If compliance issues arise, follow-up, targeted training will be required. A coordinated, effective educational program will support improved adherence to best practice guidelines for infection prevention activities, including compliance with the Medicare interpretive guidelines, throughout the LTCF.[1-3]

THE EDUCATIONAL NEEDS ASSESSMENT

LTCF HCP have wide ranging backgrounds, expertise, and education (see Chapter 1). Thus, the IP's challenge is to become knowledgeable in adult education principles and use educational tools and techniques that will motivate and sustain behavioral change for a wide variety of learners. The IP must also be aware of the common educational roadblocks and understand the specific age, cultural needs, and learning style preferences of the staff. In such a diverse group, a successful program will require flexibility and the use of a variety of approaches and training techniques not only by the IP but also any staff who assist in educational support activities such as mentoring, coaching, supervised practice, and direct observation. Therefore, it's important for the IP to conduct an educational needs assessment specific to infection prevention. This assessment then serves as the foundation for recommended training activities, as well as the justification for any resources required to support them.

An educational needs assessment can be conducted using a wide variety of methods. Employee surveys are often a starting point, but are rarely sufficient to obtain a thorough understanding of actual and/or potential educational gaps that may pose a threat to resident safety and the optimum performance of the LTCF. The methods listed here can be used, and may be combined, to conduct an educational needs assessment:

- **HCP self-assessment:** The employee uses a self-achievement or assessment tool to compare his/her current status to the preferred status.
- **Focus group discussion:** Learning needs are assessed in small groups, often with 10 or fewer participants, in which members assist each other to identify and clarify needs.
- **Interest-finder surveys:** Data-gathering tools, such as checklists or questionnaires, provide feedback using yes/no responses, simple rating scales, or short narrative responses.
- **Test development:** Tests, based on specific curricula and focused objectives, can be used as diagnostic tools to identify areas of learning deficiencies. Testing may be done manually or via computer and requires a minimum level of proficiency in both language and test-taking skills.

- **Personal interviews:** The instructor consults with random or selected individuals to determine learning needs. Interviews are used to compile qualitative data usually obtained by using a predetermined question set.
- **Job analysis and performance reviews:** These methods provide detailed, task-specific information about work-related knowledge, skills, and abilities. Competency-based reviews are often included in this category.
- **Observational studies:** Direct observation of personnel working can be performed by quality management analysts or IPs. This method is often used when assessing skills such as correct hand hygiene technique or the use of contact precautions. However, studies have repeatedly shown that employees who are aware that their performance is being observed will temporarily modify their behavior and potentially skew the results obtained by this approach.
- **Review of internal reports:** Incident reports, occupational injury and illness reports, and performance improvement/QAPI studies can be reviewed to determine specific learning needs of HCP.[1]

KNOWLEDGE TRANSFER

If the business and clinical culture of the LTCF is committed to learning, the HCP will be able to transfer knowledge into practice. Similarly, the accumulated knowledge of the staff, transmitted among its many members, is effectively transferred to new circumstance and situations. The ongoing transfer of knowledge, including the consistent use of best practices, reinforces the success of both the individual employee as well as the entire organizational group.

There are five key factors to ensure that HCP will actively learn, retain what is taught, transfer this new knowledge, and support socioadaptive change:

- The material presented should have immediate usefulness to the learners.
- The material presented should be relevant to adult learner's lives.
- The training environment should be welcoming so that all learners feel safe to participate.
- The training presentation should be engaging.
- The training should be presented in a respectful manner, where learners have an opportunity to share their experiences.[4]

ENGAGING THE LEARNER

The longstanding and most widely used teaching method is the lecture/slide presentation. However, when comparing the effectiveness of lectures with other teaching methods, the results are discouraging. Discussion methods are superior to lectures because the HCP will be more likely to retain information beyond the end of the session, apply this knowledge to new situations, develop problem-solving and critical thinking skills, develop a change in attitude, and be motivated to continue learning.[1,2] Printed handouts of the same information as those presented in a lecture offer advantages as well. Handouts also offer the learner the opportunity to review what he or she did not initially understand, skip material that is irrelevant, review the material immediately, and/or refer to the information later.[3]

HCP learn more effectively if they are active rather than passive during the learning process.[3] This process is referred to as educational engagement. The discussion style of teaching is an example of active, engaged learning. Discussion techniques facilitate learning by encouraging participants to actively think about their relationship to things they know or to talk about, explain, summarize, or question the topic.[3]

Learner engagement also includes engagement with others. In a long-term care setting, learning from shared experiences is often invaluable. Every staff member has a unique set of real-life professional experiences, and these can be used as powerful teaching tools. For example, if a staff member is caring for a resident with *Clostridium difficile* infection, the IP can ask him/her to describe recent experiences with contact isolation and the use of personal protective equipment (PPE) during an 8-hour shift. Sharing may also include anecdotes of how the staff member encouraged the use of contact precautions by visitors, family members, and potentially other residents. Using personal experiences can make a discussion "come alive" for the staff, engaging them at a level not readily achievable using less active methods.

FIGURE 13.1: THE LEARNING PYRAMID*

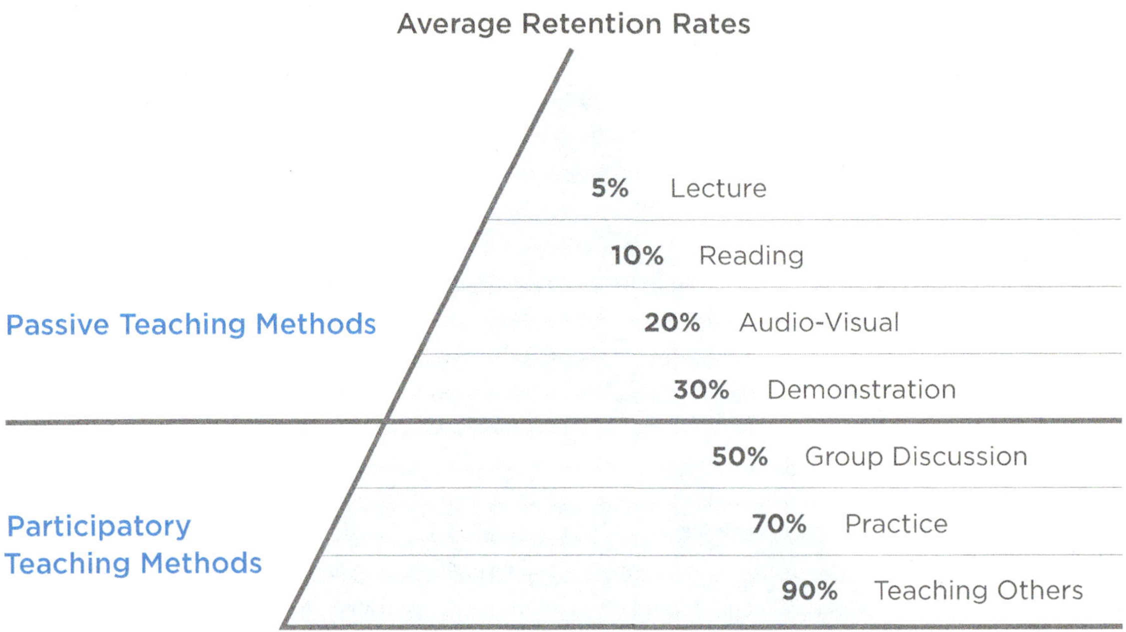

*Adapted from National Training Laboratories. Bethel, Maine

In addition, technological advances in communication now make video and telephone conferencing opportunities readily accessible and expand the number of technology-supported training systems used across the healthcare continuum.[2,3]

EDUCATIONAL MODELS AND CLASSIFICATION SYSTEMS

Not all teaching methods will have the same impact. The impact will vary not only according to the skill of the trainer and the ability or motivation of the learner, but also by the method used. The effectiveness of the different teaching methods is summarized in Figure 13.1, the "learning pyramid." In this version of the pyramid, expected retention rates are described for the most commonly used teaching methods.[3]

As shown in Figure 13.1, the lecture method has the lowest retention rate because the information is committed to short-term memory and is soon forgotten.[1-3] The teaching methods at the bottom of the pyramid have higher retention rates and most often result in behavioral changes that are more sustainable than the passive methods.

It is helpful to consider Figure 13.1 in conjunction with Bloom's taxonomy, an educational classification system first introduced in 1956 and later modified for a variety of settings. Bloom's taxonomy (Table 13.1) describes the various levels of cognitive domains. The three lowest levels of Bloom's taxonomy are knowledge, comprehension, and application. The three highest levels are analysis, synthesis, and evaluation. Each level builds on the level below it.[5] The higher levels of Bloom's taxonomy are achieved with the use of active learning methods and enhance learner retention.[3]

TABLE 13.1: BLOOM'S TAXONOMY[5]

Level	Desired Capacity/Outcome
Knowledge (Recall)	Define, list, name, recall, record
Comprehension	Describe, explain, discuss, recognize
Application	Use, demonstrate, illustrate, practice
Analysis	Distinguish, calculate, test, inspect
Synthesis	Design, organize, formulate, propose
Evaluation	Judge, appraise, evaluate, compare

The taxonomy terminology provides an excellent and widely accepted means for planning, designing, assessing, and evaluating the effectiveness of the teaching method. It offers a simple, clear, and effective model that can be easily applied to the training activities in any LTCF. The essential terminology the IP must understand includes the following:

- **Knowledge (recall)** - measures learner recognition of specific factual information; learner performs by rote memorization
- **Comprehension** - requires learner to understand the meaning, interpretation, and translation of a problem; learner should be able to explain, predict, or paraphrase the objective
- **Application** - requires learner to comprehend and manipulate data or concepts; the learner must be able to interpret, demonstrate, or illustrate the objectives
- **Analysis** - requires learner to compare, contrast, criticize, differentiate, or solve
- **Synthesis** - builds a structure from a pattern of diverse elements; learner should be able to categorize, compile, devise, explain, plan, rewrite, or summarize
- **Evaluation** - learner must be able to make judgments; learner should be able to apprise, compare and contrast, defend, describe, evaluate, or justify

INSTRUCTIONAL METHODS

To achieve educational objectives and goals, it is important for the IP to understand that adults' learning comprehension increases when a variety of methods are used. When these teaching and learning methods are employed, compliance increases as personnel are then able to operate at the higher levels of Bloom's taxonomy (i.e., analysis, synthesis, and evaluation).[1,5] For additional information on developing goals and objectives, see Chapter 3.

The best instructional methods are those that encourage active learner engagement and are aligned with the needs and preferences of those participating in the session. The IP should expect that these training variables are dynamic, sometimes unpredictable, and require the instructor to be prepared to adjust his or her methods as variables change.

Table 13.2 summarizes the instructional methods the IP should be prepared to use.

THE TEACHABLE MOMENT

In LTCFs, the IP is often in resident care and common areas, in meetings, or on rounds. These activities provide unlimited opportunities to provide on-the-spot education and coaching to staff, as well as residents, family members, and other visitors. This process is referred to as the "teachable moment." It is an unplanned time when the IP instructor can use the situation or circumstances to facilitate a spontaneous and usually brief educational interaction of some type. Although this is the most informal type of training the IP will likely do, it can have very high impact, as the timing and spontaneity of the interaction intensifies learner engagement. For this reason, it is essential that in interactions with others, the IP recognize these types of opportunities and, when present, immediately take advantage of them. A conceptual model of a teachable moment spectrum, adapted to the LTCF, is provided in Figure 13.2.

ENHANCING THE LEARNING EXPERIENCE

Even when educational programs are mandatory for staff and/or limited resources restrict the availability of more innovative methods, it is still possible for the IP to enhance any learning experience. For example, a training exercise that focuses on the learners and has personal relevance will likely improve the perceived value of the overall activity. The IP must modify language according to the leaner's needs and use concrete, familiar examples or situations to underscore the major points. Repeating a specific point in different ways also helps learners grasp and internalize the information. In addition, the IP should foster interaction with learners through dialogue, demonstrations, and role playing. All of these techniques are low cost yet highly effective when used by a skilled trainer. Audiovisuals aids also enhance the learning experience to the extent that they are available.

A summary and review of the major points at the end of the session by the IP is essential to reinforce core content.[1]

TABLE 13.2: INNOVATIVE INSTRUCTIONAL METHODS

Method	Characteristics	Advantage
Lecture Types:		
a. Symposium	Three to six lectures	Includes open discussion by the audience.
b. Forum	One or more speakers	Engage in free and open discussion. Small group sessions are often included.
c. Panel	Usually four to seven experts	Experts present facts and ideas in an orderly fashion, for example on a controversial topic; may include opportunities for the audience to ask questions.
Computer-based training	A computer program generally done at the user's pace and private; value limited with persons that have reduced reading/comprehension ability or inadequate computer skills	Learner-friendly, can be done on the individual's schedule; immediate feedback is available; graphics and video reduce boredom. Newer programs may offer interactive components.
Games	Quizzes, word searches, puzzles, or other problem solving techniques	Learner-friendly yet intentionally challenging; graphics reduce boredom; fun and informational. Newer products may record scores and encourage competition.
Mass training	Personalized education materials using an organization's intranet; same as for computer-based training	Can achieve wide-scale institutional education; able to address various personnel background and education levels. Effective when content must be delivered consistently across a wide number of participants.
Train-the-trainer	Leaders train others who are responsible for implementing the program	Those trained provide the same training to others. Although a traditional educational approach in healthcare, this method is often associated with the "see one-do one-teach one" methods, which is highly variable in performance outcomes and often unreliable. Train-the-trainer programs require measures and metrics to ensure correct and consistent educational outcomes.
Role play or reenactment	Dramatic teaching strategy that uses situational learning experiences and the techniques of simulation	This method allows for the learners to experience a situation in a controlled environment. Activities are unrehearsed.
Case studies	Presentation of a case history such as the study of famous outbreaks or epidemics	Uses a variety of formats and learning skills; often uses narratives or storytelling devices to engage the learner at a high level. Clinical problem solving and challenge questions may be included.
Mentoring programs	Links experienced workers with those needing training	Low-cost way to cross-train employees; most mentors are volunteers; mentoring program can be effective when training/orienting new employees or staff re-entering the workforce after a prolonged absence.
Simulation	Provides learning experiences from real experiences	Similarity to real situations tends to personalize the learning process. May be done using manikins, as in CPR training, or via computer.
Educational cart	Contains different types of information about various topics	A portable "library" that can be taken directly to the area of the LTCF where personnel can access the information with no interruptions in their work schedule.
Video, CD	Different types of information at various educational levels	Learner-friendly, can be done on the individual's schedule; graphics reduce boredom; topics can be very specific to the population of the LTCF being addressed. May include an interactive component.
Self-instructional modules	Can be written booklets, pamphlets, or multi-media	Self-paced approach to allow learner to gain new information.
Distance learning	Audio, and video-conferencing systems with or without a computer	Allow for exchange of information from one location to another through electronic communications. Newer approaches include computer-based instruction.

FIGURE 13.2: THE TEACHABLE MOMENT SPECTRUM

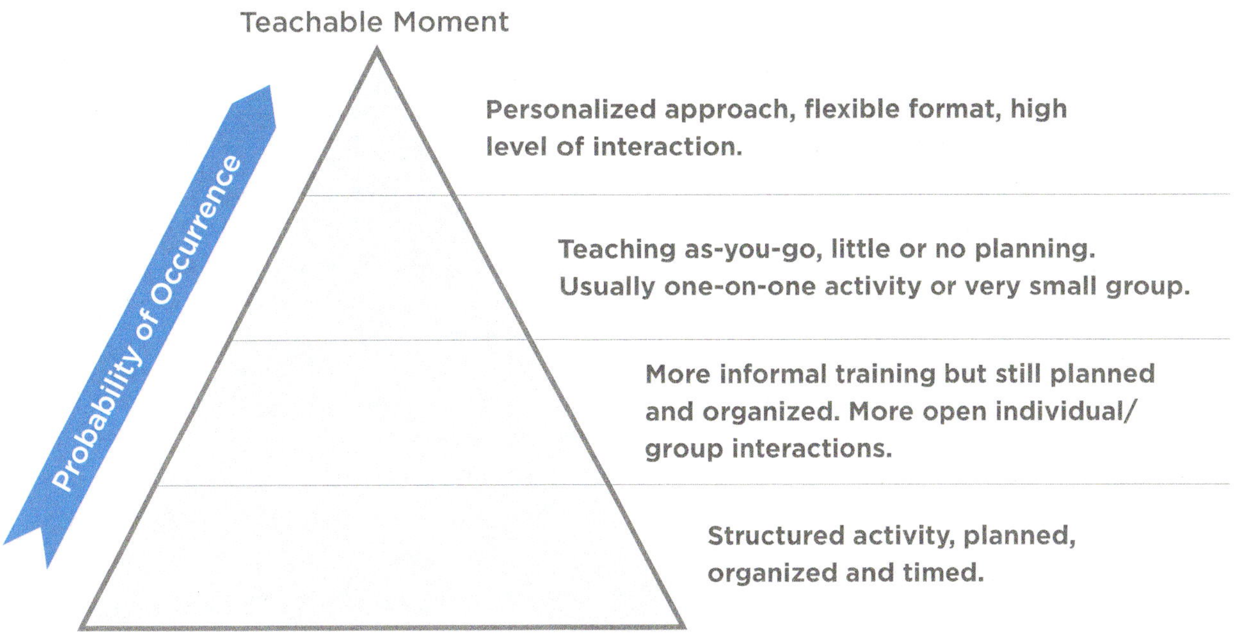

*Adapted from The Teachable Moment Spectrum. Ddeubel.edublogs.org/file/2010/11/07

Listed below are questions the IP should ask when choosing content and educational strategies:

- Does this content/strategy provide the best context for learning?
- Will this content/strategy be interesting?
- Is the content up-to-date?
- How will learners be engaged?
- Does the strategy provide deeper insight for the group? Are the take-away messages realistic?
- Is the content relevant for the learner?
- Will the content/strategy generate thought-provoking questions?
- Can clear decisions/conclusions be derived from the content presented?
- Is the content/teaching method brief? How long will it take to implement?
- Will the approach help the instructor/IP recognize and follow-up on teachable moments?

EVALUATION

An evaluation of the learning experience is essential to determine if goals and objectives have been achieved. Information can be gleaned as to the appropriateness of the program design, adequacy of teaching and resources, as well as knowledge, skills, and attitudes of the participants. A formative evaluation is conducted during the educational session to provide immediate feedback and allow appropriate changes to be made. After the program is completed, an evaluation that summarizes results will help determine the impact and overall effectiveness.[1] In LTCF, most evaluations are completed at the conclusion the program. Common methods for collecting data used in the program evaluation process include:

- Pretest and posttest
- Direct observation of performance
- Questionnaires
- One-on-one interviews
- Supervisor observation

The approach to evaluation, like all other components of the educational activity, must be appropriate for both the content as well as the audience. Although there is no absolute or preferred approach, the IP should select a method that offers the highest probability of providing meaningful results. The data obtained from the evaluation are then used to improve the activity, refine educational objectives, measure results, and better understand the impact of the facility's overall educational program.

The major goals of teaching are to improve job skills and infection prevention competence. But goal attainment can only be fully understood when the IP also tracks performance outcomes and correlates these results to training goals. Even though the process is often challenging, the positive impact of educational programs must be demonstrated in some measurable way. The IP should incorporate the use of benchmarks to analyze the impact of the educational program. Benchmarks may be internal, derived from facility data and trend analyses, or external, from reliable professional or community groups monitoring similar activities.

Checklists provide a popular means of evaluation and documentation, as they reinforce the importance of correct and consistent performance. There are many configurations for checklists; one example is provided in Figure 13.3. The IP or a designated person specifically trained should visually observe personnel for compliance. Noncompliance should be addressed immediately. Checklists may be retained as part of the LTCF's educational records and/or included in competency-based assessment activities. Because of their popularity as an evaluation tool, the IP will encounter their use throughout the LTCF. It is important to remember that summary findings from checklists can be used to improve the educational methods used to support the infection prevention program.

NEW EMPLOYEE ORIENTATION

The IP's challenge at new employee orientation sessions is conveying large amount of information in a limited period of time. A thorough orientation program will integrate both group or classroom style education and supervised practice. The IP must understand content presented to new employees, as well as any activities of other practice sessions used to reinforce the information. Common infection prevention examples include correct hand hygiene techniques, donning and removing gloves, safe disposal of lancets and other sharps, handling of soiled linen, as well as observed use of gowns, respirators, and resident care devices at risk for contamination/ disease transmission.

The orientation curriculum for infection prevention must be aligned with the LTCF's scope of service and the level of care required by residents. Essential infection prevention core topics at general orientation will include but are not limited to the following:

- Occupational Safety and Health Administration (OSHA) bloodborne pathogens and safe injection practices
- Standard Precautions
- Transmission-based Precautions
- The chain of infection
- Respiratory hygiene/cough etiquette
- Influenza and Hepatitis B vaccination
- Healthcare-associated infections (HAIs)
- Multidrug-resistant organisms (MDROs)

All orientation programs should document the date, topic, names of attendees (usually via a sign-in sheet), and evaluations. Program topics, other than those listed above, should be timely and relevant to infection prevention and control. Surveillance data should be included where appropriate.[1] The IP should plan to follow up periodically with new employees, according to the orientation plan designated by the manager, to monitor performance, provide timely coaching, encourage questions, and foster an ongoing sense of teamwork and collaboration between departments.

EDUCATION AND INFECTION PREVENTION OUTCOMES

It is important for the IP to recognize that although education and training support improvements, their causal relationship is at best ambiguous. In cases where in depth training/behavior change programs have led to measurable improvements in key performance areas such as hand hygiene compliance, the improvements declined over time, often returning to the baseline measurement. Knowing that a task should be done does not necessarily result it in being carried out. Tests of knowledge may

FIGURE 13.3: HAND HYGIENE SKILLS CHECKLIST

Date Observed: ____ / ____ /____ Observer: ______________________________ Shift Observed: 1 2 3

HCP Name	HCP Position	Nursing Unit or Ancillary Department	Hand Hygiene Random, Unannounced Observations	Person Compliant with Hand Hygiene Policy?
1.				☐ Yes ☐ No
2.				☐ Yes ☐ No
3.				☐ Yes ☐ No
4.				☐ Yes ☐ No
5.				☐ Yes ☐ No
Use the numbers to the right to fill in information above. *Comments:* For the purpose of observation, consider contact with the resident and the resident's immediate (e.g., bed room and bathroom; dining room and chair and table; activities room chair and table) environment as a single, contiguous contact.	1. RN/LVN 2. Nurse Aid/CNA 3. Physician 4. Phy. Assistant 5. Nurse Practitioner 6. Volunteer 7. Dietary 8. Visitor 9. Student 10. Respiratory Therapist 11. Radiology Tech 12. IV Therapist 13. Other	1. Unit A 2. Unit B 3. Dietary 4. EVS 5. Rehab SVC 6. Dining room 7. Activities room 8. Other	1. Enter Room 2. Leave Room 3. Touch Resident 4. Touch Equipment 5. Remove Gloves 6. Before Med Pass 7. After Med Pass 8. Before Feeding 9. After Feeding 10. Other	

Questions		Total Number Assessed and/or Observed	Total Number Failed Random Observation	Percent Failure Rate
Hand hygiene verbal skills assessed?	☐ Yes ☐ No			%
Hand hygiene with an alcohol-based product return demonstration skills assessed?	☐ Yes ☐ No			%
Hand hygiene random, unannounced observations performed?	☐ Yes ☐ No			%
Were visitors or volunteers observed for compliance with hand hygiene?	☐ Yes ☐ No			%
Data reported to Quality Improvement Committee?	☐ Yes ☐ No			%

Recommended Actions:

Also available on the CD-ROM.

Courtesy of Aureden K, Burdsall D, Harris M, Rosenbaum P. *Guide to the Elimination of Methicillin-Resistant* Staphylococcus aureus (MRSA) *in Long-Term Care Facility.* Washington, DC: Association for Professionals in Infection Control and Epidemiology, Inc.; 2009.

produce high scores among learners, but those same individuals may perform poorly when skills are observed.

The challenge for the IP is therefore a balance between providing excellent training and understanding its inherent limitations. This can be especially problematic when managing organizational expectations, where training programs may be viewed as an immediate solution to behavioral issues. In these situations, the IP must work with LTCF leadership to obtain a more complete understanding of the underlying issues. Often cultural change and stronger leadership involvement are needed to support the long-term impact and outcomes associated with the educational program.

REFERENCES

1. Schreck M, Watson S. Education and training. In: Carrico R, ed. *APIC Text of Infection Control and Epidemiology,* 3rd ed. Washington, DC: Association for Professionals in Infection Control and Epidemiology, Inc., 2009: 11-1–11-10.
2. Bryan RL, Kreuter MW, Brownson RC. Integrating adult learning principles into training for public health practice. *Health Promot Pract* 2009; 10(4): 557-563.
3. Goodlad, J. *Principles of adult learning.* WCWPDS website. 2005. Available at: http://wcwpds.wisc.edu/related-training/mandated-reporter/resources/adult_learning.pdf.
4. Northwest Center for Public Health Practice. *Effective adult learning: a toolkit for teaching adults.* NWCPHP website. 2012. Available at: http://www.nwcphp.org/documents/training/Adult_Education_Toolkit.pdf.
5. Forehand M. *Bloom's taxonomy.* EPLLT website. 2005. Available at: http://epltt.coe.uga.edu/index.php?title=Bloom%27s_Taxonomy.

CHAPTER 14

Transitions in Care

Irena Kenneley, PhD, APRN-BC, CIC
Marilyn Hanchett, RN, MA, CPHQ, CIC

KEY CONCEPTS

- Transferring facilities should have strategies in place to maintain optimum infection prevention and control for residents, personnel, and families throughout the transition process. Both the sender and receiver are stakeholders in the transition process and must play an active role.
- Communication and management of multidrug-resistant organisms and other known risk factors are essential when coordinating care transitions.
- Transition processes can be supported by formal models or programs that should include infection prevention and risk mitigation among both the strategies used and the outcomes measured.

Care transitions refer to the movement of patients or residents from one healthcare setting, level of care, or caregiver team to another. For example, a long-term care facility (LTCF) resident experiencing an acute change of condition may be transferred to the emergency department (ED), admitted to the hospital, and then discharged from the hospital back to the original LTCF.

In the past, discharge and transfer of LTCF residents from one healthcare setting to another was a relatively uncommon event. Today, a chronic disease model of care has emerged, shaped by a rapidly aging population with multiple morbidities and sustained by medications and interventions that were inconceivable even a decade ago. As a result, LTCF residents experience years of chronic disease marked by repeated admissions to various healthcare settings.

Transfers from LTCFs constitute 8.5 percent of all Medicare admissions to acute care hospitals. Approximately 40 percent of these hospitalizations occur within 90 days of LTCF admission. Of these, 84 percent are discharged from the hospital back to the original LTCF.[1,2] More than one million LTCF residents return to their homes each year.[3] Due to the inherent vulnerabilities of the long-term care population, transfer of residents between care settings can be a challenge to both the sending and receiving facilities. To avoid transmission of infection or lapses in quality of care, it is critical that LTCFs have procedures in place that ensure open communication and accountability before, during, and after transitions in care.

PLANNING FOR TRANSITIONS IN CARE

Transitions in care can be planned or unplanned. For example, if a resident is hospitalized for surgery, the LTCF is able to anticipate and plan for the resident's return. Unplanned transitions may result from unexpected incidences such as resident falls, exacerbation of illness, adverse drug events, and infections. Unplanned transitions related to infectious conditions often pose potential problems, especially if they are at time when the infection preventionist (IP) is unavailable. For this reason, the IP should include processes for both planned and unplanned transitions when developing the facility's infection prevention plan. The IP should also provide inservices and training to acquaint healthcare personnel (HCP) with infection prevention and control practices that must occur during either planned or unplanned transitions. The training should include procedures for communicating important infection-related information such as multidrug-resistant colonization or infection to the ambulance attendants as well as the receiving facility.

Planning must also include careful consideration of the resident's individual needs. Some diagnoses or other clinical criteria are associated with more frequent transitions, including cardiovascular conditions, diabetes, and age greater than 85 years. Ethnicity may also be factor.[4] In one study, older adults recovering from hip fracture experienced an average of four transitions in the year following repair. Common problems included weight loss, delirium, depression, pressure ulcers, falls, and urinary incontinence.[5] Current research focuses primarily on unplanned transitions related to serious events (e.g., adverse reaction to medication, falls) as well as exacerbation of chronic health problems (e.g., renal disease, respiratory conditions, diabetes, pain). The role of infection in triggering care transitions can only be inferred based on general incidence statistics reported in LTCFs and more studies are needed.

The effectiveness of the transition planning is also dependent on an awareness of increased risks following hospital discharge. This process involves not only a physical transfer, but also a transfer in responsibility from the inpatient provider to post-acute care or LTCF provider.[6] The period following hospital discharge is an especially vulnerable time for patients. For example, following hospital discharge, nearly half (49 percent) of patients experience at least one medical error due to lack of communication and lack of the coordination of care.[7] Ineffective planning and care coordination can undermine patient safety, facilitate adverse events, and contribute to more frequent hospital readmissions.[6] The presence of multidrug-resistant organisms (MDROs) is a well-

FIGURE 14.1: CONCEPTUAL MODEL FOR TRANSITIONS CARE[11]

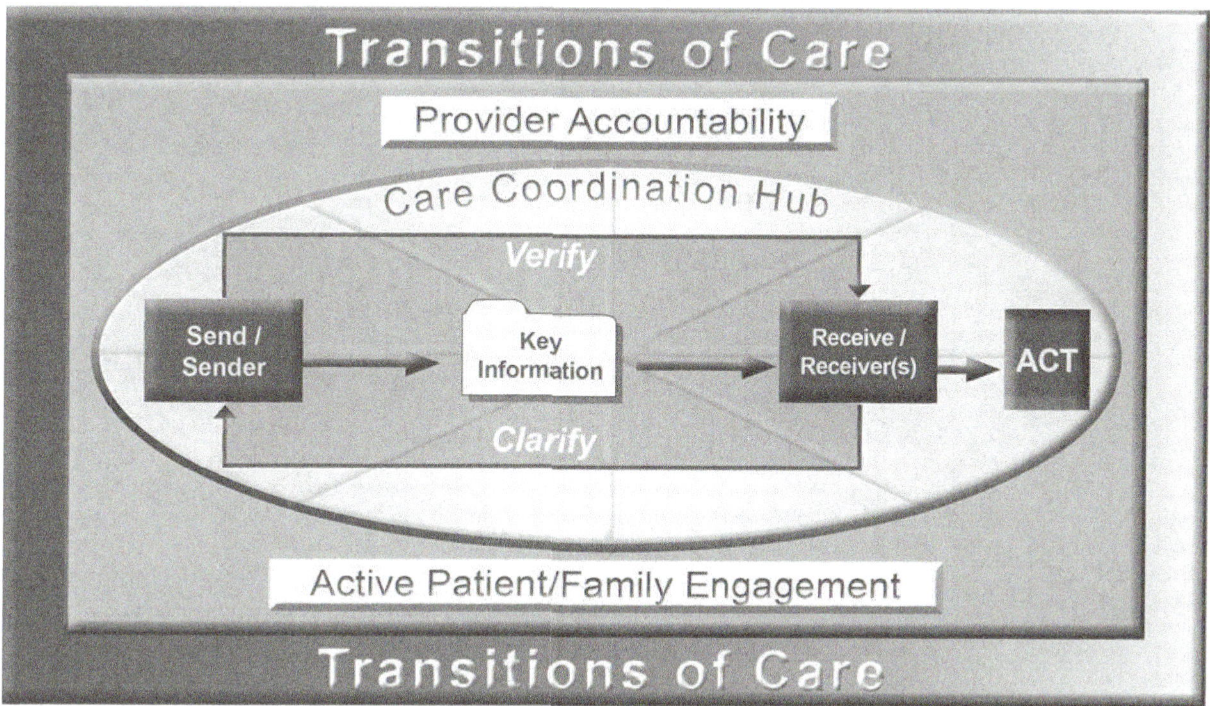

Reprinted with permission from National Transitions of Care Coalition, 750 First St, NE, Suite 700, Washington, DC 20002, www.ntocc.org.

known clinical risk. However, little is known regarding MDROs transmission, potential or actual, at the point of hospital discharge and/or during the transition process. The problem has become apparent in the increasing rate of MDRO infection and colonization spreading among different types of post-acute providers, as well as emerging MDRO strains now being identified in the community.[8]

THE TRANSITION PROCESS

The classic framework of structure, process, and outcome, commonly used in quality monitoring systems, can be applied to the essential infection prevention processes during transitions of care (Figure 14.1). The care transition process involves clear communication between both the sender and the receiver of critical medical and health-related information.[9-11]

- The sender must ensure that the key information transferred to the receiver is complete and timely. Key information may include diagnostic testing, microbiology reports, consultations, antibiotics, transition/discharge summary, history and physical assessment, clinical notes from the interdisciplinary team, and any patient/caregiver instructions prior to transfer. The sender should verify that the information was received by the intended recipient.
- The receiver must acknowledge the receipt of all information from the sender, review the information, and contact the sender with any questions in a timely manner.
- The sender should be available to clarify information or answer any questions that the receiver may have regarding the information received.
- The receiver must act on the information received. The receiver should evaluate the information received and determine if and how the plan of care for the resident needs to be altered before implementing.[11]

Gaps in communication both among HCP and during transitions between healthcare settings threaten not only patient safety but HCP as well.[9] Recent findings indicate there is a general lack of quality communication between acute- and post-acute care, emphasizing the need for standardization of the discharge planning process, for sufficient notice of discharge, and for clarification and education regarding HCP roles.[11,12]

TABLE 14.1: TRANSITION CHECKLIST: INFECTION PREVENTION ACTION ITEMS FOR LTCF ADMISSIONS BASED ON THE NTOCC CARE TRANSITION BUNDLE

Essential Intervention Categories	Infection Prevention Action Item	Completed
Medication Management	• Assess previous use of/continuing need for antibiotics (include drug, dose, route, frequency and expected end date) • Evaluate history of response of antibiotic treatment, including allergies and adverse reactions • Monitor for inappropriate use and/or opportunity to discontinue antibiotic therapies	☐ Yes ☐ No
Transition Planning	• Formally assess the resident's infection prevention needs, risks, and other related issues (may be included in an overall admission assessment if information is then relayed to the IP) • Identify any coaching, counseling, or other support for prevention practices needed by the family and other visitors • Evaluate the resident's and/or family's language, literacy, religious, and cultural needs as they pertain to infection prevention	☐ Yes ☐ No
Resident/Family Engagement and Education	• Provide education in a format aligned with resident and family needs and level of comprehension • Confirm that the resident and family understand treatment for ongoing infection, signs that the condition may be worsening, and how to communicate changes to the nursing care staff • Assess resident's understanding of prevention practices by asking him/her to explain essential steps in his/her own words	☐ Yes ☐ No
Information Transfer	• Share infection-related information in a way that supports clear and consistent communication among the resident, family, and the LTCF care team • Confirm that LTCF communication systems, including medical records, support the sharing of infection prevention and control information • Verify that care coordination and handoff processes include pertinent infection prevention and control information	☐ Yes ☐ No
Follow-up Care	• Introduce IP to resident and family following admission (time frame to be determined by the LTCF and resident care needs) • Conduct regular face-to-face or telephone communications with the resident and family when ongoing treatment of infection is needed • Assess for unintended consequences when isolation systems are needed following admission	☐ Yes ☐ No
Healthcare Provider Engagement	• Clearly identify the physician managing treatment of the infectious disease • Ensure use of infection prevention best practices, protocols, and guidelines when managing infectious diseases or infection risks • Support the IP role as the hub of facility's prevention and control coordination activities • Include infection prevention and control reports and other updates in interdisciplinary and administrative reports and communications	☐ Yes ☐ No
Shared Accountability	• Verify that infection prevention information is shared effectively and consistently between the transferring facility and the LTCF • Assess LTCF responsiveness to act on infection-related resident needs before, during, and immediately following admission • Determine that communication systems are in place and used as necessary to clarify infection related questions with the transferring facility • Document contact information for the IP at the transferring facility in LTCF records	☐ Yes ☐ No

Also available on the CD-ROM.

This basic process has been expanded by the National Transitions of Care Coalition (NTOCC) to designate seven essential interventions that must be included in a comprehensive approach. All interventions are based in the shared engagement and accountability of both the sender and receiver. These interventions are part of the care transition bundle and include:

- Medication management
- Transition planning
- Patient and family engagement
- Information transfer
- Follow-up care
- Healthcare provider engagement
- Shared accountability across provider organizations[13]

Table 14.1 lists a series of action items for each of the above bundled interventions that the IP can complete when admitting/readmitting a resident from another healthcare facility (also available on the CD-ROM that accompanies this book).

> Detailed information about the bundle interventions, as well as other resources, is available in the NTOCC Transitions of Care Compendium at **www.ntocc.org**.

CONCEPTUAL MODELS

Various models have been developed to establish conceptual frameworks to support both program development and outcome measurement. Conceptual models seek a visual representation of how transitions impact the overall delivery of healthcare across a diverse continuum of services. This is challenging because the types of transitions, as well at the various points at which they occur, are extremely heterogeneous. Although transitions have traditionally been viewed as exercises in communication and "hand offs," contemporary work conducted in the past 15 years acknowledges that the process is a complex one that must be part of an overarching safety culture and that requires integrated systems and a high level of engagement and accountability among the many participants.

Another key feature of the emerging models is the inclusion of a measurement component. These measures now extend beyond patient/resident/caregiver satisfaction and the accuracy/completion of requisite documentation by sending and receiving facilities. In some cases, newer measures are specific; in others, the scope of measurement is more broadly determined by the investigator. In spite of these variations, all models have been designed to improve the quality of the care transition experience not only for the patient/resident, but for all stakeholders in the process. Common topics for measurement include an increase in the level of patient and family involvement, more effective care coordination, improved communications, and reduced the risk of preventable problems and hospital readmissions. Major models are summarized in Table 14.2.

In addition to highly specific models, components of the transitions process may be integrated into other, larger community and primary care programs. For example, the Guided Care program, developed by Johns Hopkins University, has been adopted by large health systems across the United States. One of its components addresses the importance of an integrated care delivery system. Research shows that in an integrated system, patients in a the Guided Care program experienced, on average, 52 percent fewer skilled nursing facility days, 47 percent fewer skilled nursing facility admissions, 49 percent fewer hospital readmissions, and 17 percent fewer ED visits.[14] Guided Care is also part of ongoing university-led research projects on comprehensive and chronic care.

IPs should also investigate transitions projects and programs being developed at the state level. In 2010, 16 states had received federal funding to initiate transitions of care projects, most based on the models identified above. In a rapidly aging society, it is likely that this trend will continue. If so, it presents many new opportunities for wide IP engagement in mitigating infectious risks and preventing cross contamination during the transitions process. Figure 14.2 presents the examples of how care transition models can be integrated into the infection prevention program activities as well as potential impact in the future as the model adopted by the LTCF continues to evolve.

TABLE 14.2: MODELS OF TRANSITIONAL CARE

Essential Components	Measures and Metrics
TRANSITIONAL CARE MODEL (TCM)	
• Designed by Dr. Mary Naylor and a multidisciplinary team at the University of Pennsylvania • Addresses the negative effects associated with common breakdowns in care when older adults with complex needs transition from an acute care setting to their home or other care setting • Prepares patients and family caregivers to more effectively manage changes in health associated with multiple chronic illness	• Multiple clinical trials have consistently demonstrated the positive impact of the TCM on older adults' outcomes while reducing total costs of healthcare: 1. Avoidance of hospital readmissions for primary and complicating conditions 2. Improvements in health outcomes after hospital discharge 3. Enhancement in patient and family caregiver experience with care • Published studies: Yes
Contact: www.transitionalcare.info	
BRIDGE PROGRAM	
• Developed by the Illinois Transitional Care Consortium (ITCC) • Connects existing systems to facilitate services and support between older adults and their caregivers • Includes three essential intervention phases to ensure collaboration across care settings for safe transitions: • Before discharge • Shortly after discharge • Follow-up once the client is settled in	• Studies focus on care coordination post hospital discharge, follow-up communications with physicians, impact of telephonic follow-up • Analysis includes evaluation of psychosocial needs and patient/caregiver stress • Published studies: Yes
Contact: www.transitionalcare.org	
CARE TRANSITIONS INTERVENTIONISTS®	
• Funded by the John A. Hartford Foundation and The Robert Wood Johnson Foundation, the Care Transitions Intervention® was designed by Eric Coleman, MD, MPH, in response to the need for a patient-centered, interdisciplinary intervention that addresses continuity of care across multiple settings and practitioners • Goal is to improve care transitions by providing patients with tools and support that promote knowledge and self-management as they move from hospital to home	• Measure development supported by The Commonwealth Fund, The Robert Wood Johnson Foundation, and the Paul Beeson Faculty Scholars in Aging • The Care Transitions Measure (CTM®) assesses the quality of care transitions • Provides a measure set that is both substantively and methodologically consistent with the concept of patient-centeredness, and useful for the purpose of performance measurement and subsequent public reporting • Uses a 15-item list of unidimensional measures • Published Studies: Yes
Contact: www.caretransitions.org	
BETTER OUTCOMES BY OPTIMIZING SAFE TRANSITIONS (BOOST)	

• Developed by the Society for Hospital Medicine and supported by the John A Hartford Foundation
• Optimize the discharge process at your institution
• Based the on principles of quality improvement, evidence-based medicine, as well as personal and institutional experiences
• Offers numerous resources and mentoring
• One of several "Mentored Implementation" programs
	• Supports use of key metrics :
	  • **Key metric #1:** Care Transitions Outcome Measures such as readmission rates, average length of stay, and patient satisfaction
	  • **Key metric #2:** Care Transitions Process Measures such as how well are patients prepared for discharge or caregivers prepared in caring for the patient post-discharge, what proportion of follow-up clinicians receive communication regarding the patient's hospitalization, and follow-up issues at time of discharge
	• Published studies: Yes

Contact: http://www.hospitalmedicine.org/ResourceRoomRedesign/RR_CareTransitions/html_CC/01HowtoUse/00_Howtouse.cfm	

Table 14.2 Continued

Essential Components	Measures and Metrics
GERIATRIC RESOURCES FOR ASSESSMENT AND CARE OF ELDERS	
• Focused on a nurse practitioner and a social worker who care for low-income seniors in collaboration with the patient's primary care physician and a geriatrics interdisciplinary team • Foundational principles are based on best practices for care of chronic conditions, including specific targeting of at-risk older adults, availability of collaborative expertise in geriatrics, integration of the program into primary care, coordination of care across all sites of care, the use of an electronic medical record to support physician practices and facilitate monitoring of clinical parameters, and institutionally endorsed clinical practice guidelines	• Initial measures include chronic and preventive care costs, acute care costs, and total costs, and measurement of specific interventions in both predefined high-risk and low-risk groups • Published studies: Yes

MEDICATION MANAGEMENT AND CONTINUITY

Although much attention has been given to the misuse and overuse of antibiotics in LTCFs, much less is known about antibiotic adherence and disruptions in infection treatment during care transitions. Yet the importance of medication reconciliation as the patient/resident moves between facilities is identified as a core element in a safe, effective transitions process.[15-17]

Because healthcare providers vary in methods of data collection, interfacility communication, and documentation systems, there is no standard or preferred format for medication reconciliation. However, NTOCC has suggested common data elements that the IP may want to consider when monitoring the use and continuity of anti-infective medication use. The categories for data collection include:

Assess When Accessing Healthcare Facility (Hospital, LTCF)

- Patient/resident demographic information
- Allergy/sensitivity/intolerance to medications
- List of all current medications, including maintenance medications
- Other products (e.g., over-the-counter drugs, herbal remedies, vitamin, supplements, and other nutritional products)

Additional Assessment Criteria

- Patient/resident language and cultural issues related to medication use
- Patient/resident compliance and level of caregiver/family involvement
- Medication history and response to any previously identified issues, including adverse events (if known)
- Patient/resident's primary care provider and method and frequency of communication regarding medications, especially maintenance medications[13]

Medication reconciliation is problematic across all healthcare settings, including upon admission to the LTCF. In a study that examined medications in patients admitted to skilled nursing or sub-acute care, 21.3 percent of all medication reviewed indicated a discrepancy and 71.4 percent of skilled nursing facility admissions reflected similar problems. Antibiotics were among the categories of drugs that accounted for more than 50 percent of the discrepancies identified.[18] Another study that tracked medication usage throughout three transition care points in a large healthcare system reported all that patients experienced some form of discrepancy and 86 percent had at least one unintentional discrepancy.[19]

Delays in medication availability and omission of prescribed drugs following admission to the LTCF have also been reported. In one study, all patients transferred from the hospital to the LTCF experienced more than a 12-hour delay in receiving medications. In the same study, the mean number of missed doses was at least three per resident during the transitional period.[20]

The inclusion of a pharmacist coordinator or consultant within the transitional care team has been proposed

FIGURE 14.2: RELATIONSHIP OF CARE TRANSITIONS MODEL TO LTCF INFECTION PREVENTION PROGRAM

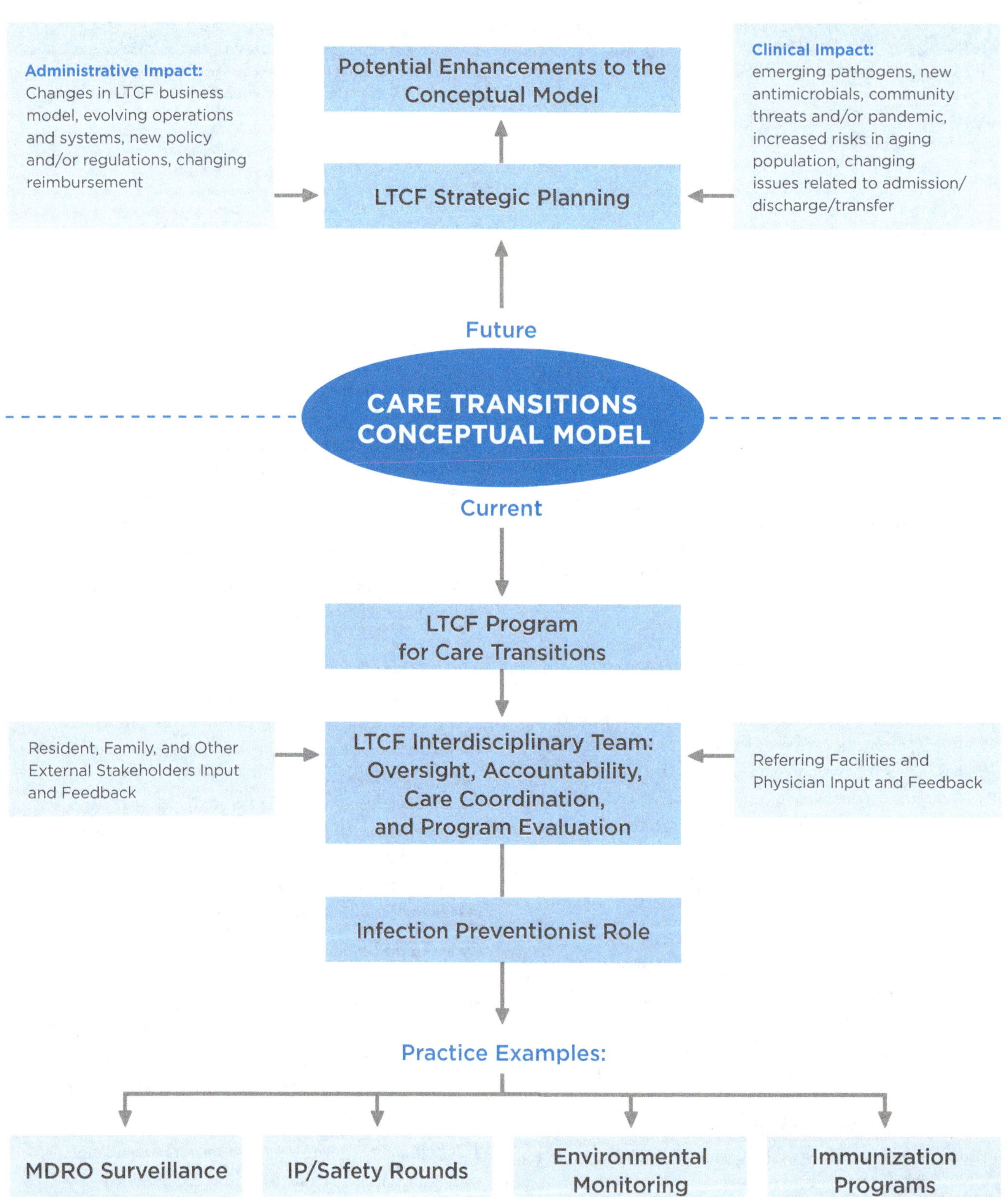

as a means of improving medication continuity. This is consistent with other studies where multicomponent interventions have been more effective in preventing rebound hospital readmissions than single component interventions.[21] One study analyzed the quality of prescribing in LTCFs in which a pharmacist transition coordinator was included. Although pain control and hospital usage (defined in this study as ED visits and/or hospital readmission) improved, there was no measurable benefit in terms of adverse drug events, worsening mobility and/or behaviors, and increased confusion.[22] Overall, there is insufficient clinical research to either propose the best method of medication reconciliation and continuity in LTCF or the optimum role of the pharmacist.[23]

Even when medication reconciliation has been conducted, it is still possible for lapses to occur. LTCFs may document these types of incidents using generic forms. However, there is a tool specifically for tracking and resolving medication discrepancies available through a program developed by Eric A. Coleman, MD, MPH. The Care Transitions Program® offers a Medication Discrepancy Tool (MDT) to help capture details and facilitate improvements. This tool differentiates noncompliance as intentional, nonintentional, and/or due to a performance deficit. The MDT is available through the Care Transitions Program® website at www.caretransitions.org.[24] The IP should be part of the LTCF's medication management program and be prepared to analyze documentation, including both reconciliation and discrepancy data, to determine if problems exist and/or trends may be developing, particularly related to the administration of antimicrobial therapies.

CULTURAL COMPETENCE DURING TRANSITIONS

Cultural competence is the process by which "individuals and systems respond respectfully and effectively to people of all cultures, languages, classes, races, ethnic backgrounds, religions, and other diversity factors in a manner that recognizes, affirms, and values the worth of individuals, families, and communities and protects and preserves the dignity of each."[25]

NTOCC and other leaders in the field of care transitions are increasingly recognizing that cultural competency is essential to successful, client-centered care.[26] In addition, cultural competency is recognized as a significant part of service design because it impacts interprofessional collaborative practice with the potential to enhance positive outcomes.[27] Although this competency includes sensitivity and skills related to language, ethics, values, and cross-cultural knowledge, issues that may impact the healthcare workforce, especially those having direct contact with patients/residents, can include the effect of immigrant cultures and languages, different intergenerational cultural constructs, and culturally derived attitudes about aging and dementia.[28] The impact of cultural competence for IPs during care transitions has not been specifically addressed in the scientific literature and is an important field for future study.

INTERFACILITY TRANSFERS

An example of an interfacility transfer form developed by the Centers for Disease Control and Prevention (CDC) can be found on the CD-ROM. This tool was developed by the Utah Healthcare-associated Infection Working Group and shared with CDC and state partners courtesy of the Utah State Department of Health.[29] This tool can be modified and adapted for use by long-term care providers. As in the use of any clinical resource, individual accountability for effective implementation must be supported by a facility-wide culture that places a high priority on safe transitions and considers them to be everyone's responsibility.[29]

The following information explains the most common types of interfacility transfers and key communication and prevention activities associated with each. Because the specific tasks pertaining to a transfer are often numerous and interrelated, the IP should have a thorough understanding of the processes in place at his or her LTCF.

Admission to Long-term Care Facility

Prior to admission, the LTCF should request clinical information from the transferring facility to verify the arriving resident's history or acute and/or chronic infection, including MDROs. If colonization is unknown, the IP should evaluate any known risk factors associated with the acute care episode that may increase the risks of an undetected MDRO, especially methicillin-resistant *Staphylococcus aureus* (MRSA). The facility should review all other pertinent clinical information, including the most recent history and physical exam reports accompanying the resident upon admission to the LTCF.[12,30]

Transfer to the Hospital or a Different LTCF

When transferring a resident to a hospital or another LTCF, the facility coordinating the discharge should prepare a transfer form to accompany the resident (see end-of-chapter appendix for a sample transfer form). The transfer form should include information regarding the resident's health status while at the LTCF, chronic medical diagnoses, symptom management, status of infectious disease (particularly MDROs), recent culture reports and associated antibiotic therapy, and vaccination history. The discharging facility should notify the admitting hospital or LTCF if laboratory data is received after the resident's discharge. Clinical information may include:

- Results of diagnostic testing (complete blood count, lipid panel, blood chemistries, enzymes, coagulation studies, etc.)
- Results of cultures
- Potential or actual exposure of the resident to an infectious disease and/or an outbreak in the LTCF prior to transfer

The LTCF should follow up promptly with the admitting facility when an MDRO or communicable disease has been identified. This communication fosters cooperation among healthcare settings and expedites tracking patients/residents to reduce potential communicable disease transmission. All information exchanged must ensure the resident's confidentiality. Transfer agreements between facilities provide efficient mechanisms to formalize the appropriate content and methods for patient/resident information exchange.[30,31]

TRANSITIONS FROM CURATIVE CARE TO PALLIATIVE OR HOSPICE CARE

Transitions of care refer to the movement of patients not only between healthcare locations, but to different levels of care that may or may not be available in the same location. Included within the long-term care continuum of services is compassionate, palliative care at the end of life.

The IP should be familiar with the use of antimicrobials in palliative and hospice care settings, including if, when, and to what extent these therapies are implemented. There are many factors to consider when deciding on the best antimicrobial treatment regimen in palliative or hospice care programs. The goal of treatment must be clear: the eradication of infection (curative therapy) or palliation (noncurative therapy) of symptoms. Some of the ethical concerns about the use of antimicrobials at the end of life include:

- Delaying transition to hospice
- Prolonging the dying process
- Prescribing regimens incongruent with a short life expectancy and goals of care
- Increasing the reservoir of potential multidrug-resistant pathogens[32]

There are instances in which the use of antimicrobials can palliate symptoms. For example, a female resident with symptomatic urinary tract infection can be treated effectively (palliation of symptoms) with a short course of oral antibiotics, aimed at improving comfort and reducing pain and fever. However, for many types of pneumonia, there are management therapies other than antimicrobial therapy. The use of opioids or anxiolytics has been effective in improving dyspnea symptoms and is consistent with the hospice treatment paradigm.[33]

The primary responsibility of clinicians is to the resident. However, there is a secondary responsibility to other residents within the LTCF community, especially when infectious disease threats have been identified.

For example, when highly contagious diseases, such as tuberculosis or severe acute respiratory syndrome exist, then the facility has an immediate obligation to protect its community, including HCP, that may temporarily supersede end of life care.[32,33] Current evidence indicates that for the treatment of infections in hospice residents with advanced cancer, there is no significant difference in survival among individual who received antimicrobials compared to those who did not.[33]

SUMMARY

Care transitions today are recognized as an integral component of safe and effective healthcare. As provider settings have diversified and expanded across the healthcare continuum, there is an emerging sense of urgency to address the challenges posed by frequent patient/resident interfacility movement. The ongoing concern about and attention to healthcare-associated infections as a major threat has underscored the need to include infectious risk mitigation and effective infection prevention practices within any care transitions model.

Avoidable hospitalizations and re-hospitalizations among long-stay LTCF residents are important and costly indicators of poor care transitions. A large proportion of these hospitalizations may be due to infections especially urinary tract infections and sepsis. However, the scope and role of the IP in LTCF transitions has not been studied, and the possibility for improved outcomes with a targeted transition infection risk reduction program remains an area for future analysis. Until that is accomplished, the IP should participate as an active member of the LTCF's care transitions program and vigilantly incorporate transitions monitoring, surveillance, and follow-up as part of the facility's overall infection prevention plan.

REFERENCES

1. Brown-Williams H, Neuhauser L, Ivey S, Graham C, Poor S, Tseng W, et al. *From Hospital to Home: Improving Transitional Care for Older Adults.* Health Research for Action website. 2006. Available at: http://www.healthresearchforaction.org/sites/default/files/REPORT_PUBS_H2H%20FNL.pdf.

2. Centers for Medicare & Medicaid Services (CMS). CMS-1533-P, Medicare Program; Proposed Changes to the Hospital Inpatient Prospective Payment Systems and Fiscal Year 2008 Rates (Proposed Rule). *Fed Regist* 2007; 72(85): 24680-25135.

3. Boling PA, Parsons P. A research and policy agenda for transitions from nursing homes to home. *Home Health Care Serv Q* 2007; 26(4): 121-131.

4. Parrish MM, O'Malley K, Adams RI, Adams SR, Coleman EA. Implementation of the care transitions intervention: sustainability and lessons learned. *Prof Case Manag* 2009 Nov-Dec; 14(6): 282-293.

5. Popejoy LL, Dorman Marek K, Scott-Cawiezell J. Patterns and problems associated with transitions after hip fracture in older adults. *J Gerontol Nurs* 2013 Sep 1; 39(9): 43-52.

6. Coleman EA, Mahoney E, Parry C. Assessing the quality of preparation for post hospital care from the patient's perspective: the care transitions measure. *Medical Care* 2005; 43(3): 246-255.

7. Forster AJ, Murff HJ, Peterson JF, Gandhi TK, Bates DW. The incidence and severity of adverse events affecting patients after discharge from the hospital. *Ann Intern Med* 2003 Feb 4; 138(3): 161-167.

8. Centers for Disease Control and Prevention (CDC). Antibiotic Resistance Threats in the United States, 2013. CDC website. 2013. Available at: http://www.cdc.gov/drugresistance/threat-report-2013/pdf/ar-threats-2013-508.pdf.

9. HMO Workgroup on Care Management. *One Patient, Many Places: Managing Health Care Transitions.* America's Health Insurance Plans website. 2004. Available at: http://www.ahip.org/content/default.aspx?bc=38|72|69|5743.

10. Coleman EA. Falling through the cracks: Challenges and opportunities for improving transitional care for persons with continuous complex care needs. *J Am Geriatr Soc* 2003 Apr; 51(4): 549-555.

11. National Transitions of Care Coalition (NTOCC) Work Group. Transitions of Care Measures. NTOCC website. 2008. Available at: http://www.ntocc.org/Portals/0/PDF/Resources/TransitionsOfCare_Measures.pdf.

12. Boutwell A, Griffin F, Hwu S, Shannon D. *Effective Interventions to Reduce Rehospitalizations: A Compendium of 15 Promising Interventions.* Cambridge, MA: Institute for Healthcare Improvement, 2009.

13. National Transitions of Care Coalition (NTOCC). *Improving on Transitions of Care: How to Implement and Evaluate a Plan.* NTOCC website. 2008. Available at: http://www.ntocc.org/Portals/0/PDF/Resources/ImplementationPlan.pdf.

14. Boult C, Reider L, Leff B, Frick KD, Boyd CM, Wolff JL, et al. The effect of guided care teams on the use of health services: results from a cluster-randomized controlled trial. *Arch Intern Med* 2011 Mar 14; 171(5): 460-466.

15. Dedhia P, Kravet S, Bulger J, Hinson T, Sridharan A, Kolodner K, et al. A quality improvement intervention to facilitate the transition of older adults from three hospitals back to their homes. *J Am Geriatr Soc* 2009 Sep; 57(9): 1540-1546.

16. Jeffs L, Law MP, Straus S, Cardoso R, Lyons RF, Bell C. Defining quality outcomes for complex-care patients transitioning across the continuum using a structured panel process. *BMJ Qual Saf* 2013 Jul 12 [epub ahead of print].

17. Bell CM, Brener SS, Comrie R, Anderson GM, Bronskill SE. Quality measures for medication continuity in long-term care facilities, using a structured panel process. *Drugs Aging* 2012 Apr 1; 29(4): 319-327.

18. Tjia J, Bonner A, Briesacher BA, McGee S, Terrill E, Miller K. Medication discrepancies upon hospital to skilled nursing facility transitions. *J Gen Intern Med* 2009 May; 24(5): 630-635.

19. Sinvani LD, Beizer J, Akerman M, Pekmezaris R, Nouryan C, Lutsky L, et al. Medication reconciliation in continuum of care transitions: a moving target. *J Am Med Dir Assoc* 2013 Sep; 14(9): 668-672.

20. Ward KT, Bates-Jensen B, Eslami MS, Whiteman E, Dattoma L, Friedman JL, et al. Addressing delays in medication administration for patients transferred from the hospital to the nursing home: a pilot quality improvement project. *Am J Geriatr Pharmacother* 2008 Oct; 6(4): 205-211.

21. Scott IA. Preventing the rebound: improving care transition in hospital discharge processes. *Aust Health Rev* 2010 Nov; 34(4): 445-451.

22. Crotty M, Rowett D, Spurling L, Giles LC, Phillips PA. Does the addition of a pharmacist transition coordinator improve evidence-based medication management and health outcomes in older adults moving from the hospital to a long-term care facility? Results of a randomized, controlled trial. *Am J Geriatr Pharmacother* 2004 Dec; 2(4): 257-264.

23. Chhabra PT, Rattinger GB, Dutcher SK, Hare ME, Parsons KL, Zuckerman IH. Medication reconciliation during the transition to and from long-term care settings: a systematic review. *Res Social Adm Pharm* 2012 Jan-Feb; 8(1): 60-75.

24. Coleman EA. The Care Transitions Program®. Care Transitions website. n.d. Available at: http://www.caretransitions.org/index.asp.

25. National Association of Social Workers (NASW). *Indicators for the achievement of NASW standards for cultural competence in social work practice.* NASW website. 2007. Available at: http://www.socialworkers.org/practice/standards/naswculturalstandardsindicators2006.pdf.

26. National Transitions of Care Coalition (NTOCC). *Cultural Competence: Essential Ingredient for Successful Transitions in Care.* NTOCC website. n.d. Available at: http://www.ntocc.org/Portals/0/PDF/Resources/CulturalCompetence.pdf.

REFERENCES

27. Oelke ND, Thurston WE, Arthur N. Intersections between interprofessional practice, cultural competency and primary healthcare. *J Interprof Care* 2013 Sep; 27(5): 367-372.

28. Davis BH, Smith MK. Developing culturally diverse direct caregivers for care work with older adults: challenges and potential strategies. *J Contin Educ Nurs* 2013 Jan; 44(1): 22-30.

29. Centers for Disease Control and Prevention (CDC). *Interfacility Infection Control Transfer Form for states establishing HAI prevention collaborative using ARRA funds.* CDC website. 2010. Available at: http://www.cdc.gov/HAI/toolkits/InterfacilityTransferCommunicationForm11-2010.pdf.

30. Jack BW, Chetty VK, Anthony D, et al. A reengineered hospital discharge program to decrease rehospitalization: A randomized trial. *Ann Intern Med* 2009; 150(3): 178-187.

31. Coleman EA, Parry C, Chalmers S, Min SJ. The care transitions intervention: Results of a randomized controlled trial. *Arch Intern Med* 2006; 166(17): 1822-1828.

32. Hooton TM, Bradley SF, Cardenas DD, Colgan R, Geerlings SE, Rice JC, et al. Diagnosis, prevention, and treatment of catheter-associated urinary tract infection in adults: 2009 International Clinical Practice Guidelines from the Infectious Diseases Society of America. *Clin Infect Dis* 2010 Mar 1; 50(5): 625-663.

33. Ferrell B, Connor SR, Cordes A, Dahlin CM, Fine PG, Hutton N, et al. The National Agenda for Quality Palliative Care: The National Consensus Project and the National Quality Forum. *J Pain Symptom Manage* 2007 Jun; 33(6): 737-744.

CHAPTER 15

Emergency and Disaster Preparedness

Dolly Greene, RN, CIC
Steven W. Hilley, RN

KEY CONCEPTS

- The infection preventionist plays an essential role in disaster planning, response, and recovery.
- Successful disaster preparedness requires having internal and external procedures in place and designated leaders who are trained to manage residents, visitors, and staff during disaster and post-event recovery.
- Infection prevention during disasters is part of an interdisciplinary facility program that is aligned with local, state, and federal regulations.

Death and injury are natural outcomes of any major disaster, whether manmade or natural. A long-term care facility's (LTCF) preparedness for such events as hurricanes, earthquakes, wildfires, infectious disease outbreaks, bioterrorism, chemical emergencies, or other type of disaster mandates a comprehensive disaster preparedness plan. Although the infection preventionist (IP) may not have primary responsibility for developing the LTCF's emergency action plan, the IP must understand the outcomes and impact from each possible emergency situation. An effective infection prevention plan must include comprehensive policies and procedures that address all potential emergencies.[1]

The facility administrator, or other designee, should develop an emergency action plan that provides for the safety and protection of residents, staff, and visitors in any emergency, whether internal or external. This plan should be coordinated with the state department of public health and environment and the local office of emergency management as well as local fire and other emergency response agencies. Procedures should be developed to ensure that all residents are properly informed about the nature of the emergency, the facility's response, and action required. Special measures must be put in place to ensure that those who have physical or other impairments understand procedures and are adequately prepared.

The IP has the following roles in disaster preparedness:

- To participate in disaster planning, response, and recovery planning and training.
- To develop alternate policies related to infection prevention and control during an emergency event.
- To create a surveillance program to ensure that appropriate indicators are used. Surveillance is a critical component of emergency management to control infectious disease occurrences.
- To assess readiness and develop emergency management plans to mitigate potential disease transmission and mass casualties.
- To control the impact of infectious disease casualties in the event of such an event.
- To be prepared to guide, manage, and supervise responders during a disaster.
- To have protocols in place for triage to minimize risk of disease transmission during surges of injured or infected individuals.
- To manage the physical environment and be able to assess potential risks of higher levels of bioburden resulting from a shortage of available environmental services staff.
- To educate and train other critical personnel and potential respondents on infection prevention and control strategies.[1]

FEDERAL REGULATION REQUIREMENTS

Disasters, natural or manmade, have been shown to affect the elderly disproportionately, especially those residing in LTCFs.[2] Limited mobility, frailty, decreased sensation, and possible cognitive impairment are among the factors that increase this population's vulnerability. In addition, preexisting medical conditions can be exacerbated during a disaster.[3] For this reason, LTCFs must develop an emergency preparedness plan that can respond to the needs of their residents and staff. In the wake of recent disasters, such as Hurricane Sandy and Hurricane Katrina, federal regulations are still limited. However, some states have placed greater focus on disaster preparedness and response to ensure protection for vulnerable populations.[4]

The Code of Federal Regulations (CFR) states:

CFR 483.75(m) disaster and emergency preparedness

1. The facility must have detailed written plans and procedures to meet all potential emergencies and disasters, such as fire, severe weather, and missing residents.
2. The facility must train all employees in emergency procedures when they begin to work in the facility, periodically review the procedures with existing staff, and carry out unannounced staff drills using those procedures.[5]

PHASES OF EMERGENCY PREPAREDNESS

Pre-Emergency Planning Phase

A LTCF's emergency plan must ensure that all systems relating to facility operations, organizational structure, emergency response teams, and staff and residents' families are accurate. Regular review is required to keep this information up to date. All administrative personnel should know where and how to turn off electricity, water, gas, or specific equipment. All facilities should have an alternative powered weather notification system to stay abreast of emergency weather situations.

A LTCF's emergency action plan should be coordinated with the local emergency management agencies and their management plans, including having in place Memoranda of Understanding (MOU) or Mutual Aid Agreements with local and regional healthcare partners. Such agreements allow all participating healthcare facilities to work together during an emergency to provide physical facilities and temporary shelter, and share staff, beds, equipment, supplies, and services during a disaster.[6] Suggested steps for pre-emergency preparedness include:

1. Review and update inventory/resource lists.
2. Ensure the availability of manpower needed to execute emergency procedures.
3. Work with the local office of emergency management (OEM) to identify and obtain available personnel, equipment, supplies, and other resources.
4. Identify staff who may need child care, transportation, or other special assistance and arrange for these services.
5. Determine code name for each emergency (i.e., Code Red, Code Black, etc.) with a scripted announcement to be made in emergency situation.
    a. *Example:* "Code Black—A biological attack has occurred. All staff, visitors, and families remain calm and in the facility until further notice from local authorities."
    b. Some states and facilities are going to a "clear text" (also "plain language") notification during emergencies (i.e., "plain language" or using language that can be easily understood by staff, residents, and visitors).[7]
6. Develop organizational chart for disaster response activities, using the Incident Command System (ICS). According to the U.S. Federal Emergency Management Agency (FEMA), the Incident Command System is a "standardized, on-scene, all-hazards incident management approach that allows for the integration of facilities, equipment, personnel, procedures and communications operating within a common organizational structure; enables a coordinated response among various jurisdictions and functional agencies, both public and private; and establishes common processes for planning and managing resources."[8] The FEMA website (www.fema.gov) provides detailed information on the ICS Core Competencies and many training resources, including free online independent study modules.
7. Designate a disaster coordinator with possible alternate staff to fill the role.
8. Designate a command center location within the facility to serve as the focal point for coordinating operations during an emergency. Consider designating an alternate location outside the facility for use if evacuation becomes necessary. This location should have computer and phone access.
9. Plan for evacuation and relocation of residents:
    a. Define the triggers for the evacuation of the facility.
    b. Define roles and responsibilities.
    c. Describe the procedures for evacuation of residents.
    d. Identify who is responsible for implementing facility evacuation procedures.
    e. Identify residents who may require specialized transportation (designate by functional limitations and/or diagnosis).
    f. Identify the facilities the LTCF has entered into an MOU (include contract in the plan) where the residents will be transferred.
    g. Identify evacuation routes with alternate route should the primary route be impassable.
    h. Specify procedures that will ensure facility staff will accompany evacuating residents.
    i. Develop a procedure and tracking system (log) that will be used to track residents who are relocated.
    j. Determine which items each resident will be permitted to take with them.
    k. Establish procedures for ensuring that all residents are accounted for. Ensure that all residents have proper identification.
10. The facilities should provide basic emergency procedure information to the residents and their families such as emergency contact information

for the facility and key staff members. This information should include specifics of how residents will be evacuated and where they will be taken to aid in reconnecting residents with concerned loved ones.

11. Develop an emergency communications plan. This should include supplies, communication methods, and emergency procedures. Cellular phones and fax machines will be quickly overwhelmed in a true disaster. Two-way radios will provide the best communications alternative. A cache of radios should be kept in a central location for staff to use.
12. Ensure the availability and functioning of the facility emergency warning system.
13. Test reliability of emergency telephone roster (phone tree) for contacting emergency personnel and activating emergency procedures. (This should be tested routinely with a plan for what to do if someone cannot be reached.)
14. Develop procedure for testing generators and equipment supported by emergency generators.
    a. Routine maintenance for generator should be provided. Check with manufacturer's recommendations and assistance on maintenance contract.[9]
    b. Recommend a 7- to 10-day supply of emergency fuel and establish an agreement for delivery with a supplier.
    c. If delivery of a generator is required, allow time to hire an electrician that will assist in installing it.
    d. Determine what the generator will power.
    e. If the LTCF already has a generator, identify and document what the generator powers (e.g., red outlets). Activate the generator under load according to the National Fire Protection Association (NFPA) requirements and state regulations.
    f. Document all testing procedures.
15. Ensure a 7- to 10-day supply of food and water for residents and staff.
    a. Arrange for an alternate contact to supply back up resources.
    b. Contact the local office of emergency management for assistance in establishing an alternate contact, as needed.
16. Schedule employee orientation and annual in-service training on the emergency operations plan.
17. Provide emergency/disaster education.
    a. Distribute personal preparedness checklists (see emergency checklists, Tables 15.1 to 15.3).
    b. Post display of evacuation routes and alarm and fire extinguisher locations.
    c. Post telephone numbers of emergency contacts in approved locations.
    d. Provide demonstrations on warning systems and proper use of emergency equipment for the staff, residents, and resident families.
18. Conduct unannounced fire drills annually according to local, state, and federal requirements.
    a. Document each drill, instruction, or event to include date, content, and participants involved. Identify and document any problems associated with the drill.
19. Corrective actions should be taken on any deficiency identified during classroom training or drills. Document drills with critiques and an after action report (AAR). The documentation should be Homeland Security Exercise Evaluation Program (HSEEP) compliant. The IP should work with facility leadership to ensure that infection prevention and control measures are appropriately documented and described in facility reports.[10-12]

Preparedness Phase

Upon receipt of an internal or external warning of an emergency, the facility administrator or appropriate designee should:

1. Activate the phone tree.
2. Notify the local communications center (county dispatch) of emergency.
3. Notify the staff in charge of emergency operations to initiate the emergency operations plan and advise personnel of efforts designed to provide resident safety.
4. If the potential disaster is weather related, closely monitor weather conditions and update department directors, as needed.
5. Inform other key agencies of any developing situation and protective actions you plan to take. This includes, but not limited to fire, law enforcement, public health, etc.

6. Review the emergency operations plan including the evacuation annex. Reevaluate the evacuation routes with staff and residents. It is important to inform resident families that the facility has a disaster plan and the plan will include contacting them. This will help in controlling calls to the facility or family members from showing up at the facility during a disaster.
7. Prepare the designated command center for operations and alert staff of impending plans to open the operations center.
8. Fill the appropriate incident command functions to include a communications branch to handle calls from family members.
9. Control facility access.
10. Confirm emergency staff available and facilitate care of their families.
11. Prearrange emergency transportation of nonambulatory residents (dialysis residents, etc.) and their medical records.
12. Check food and water supplies (7- to 10-day supply).
13. Store a supply of radios and flashlights.
14. Secure outdoor furniture.
15. Coordinate with local authorities/agencies and private contacts to confirm availability of resources, including medical services, response personnel, etc.
16. Confirm transportation agreements with emergency medical service agencies, taxies, tour bus companies, or private individuals for buses.
17. Determine if any of the residents could be discharged from the facility and go home with family members that live locally.
18. Determine how residents will be identified during an evacuation and ensure the following identifying information will be transferred with each resident:
    - Name
    - Social security number
    - Photograph, if available
    - Medicare, Medicaid, or other health insurer numbers
    - Date of birth
    - Recent history and physical (H and P)
    - Current drug prescriptions and diet regimens
    - Name and contact information for next-of-kin/ responsible party/power of attorney

    i. Determine how this information will be secured (i.e., laminated documents, water proof pouch around resident's neck, water proof wrist tag, etc.) and how medical records and medications will be transported so they can be matched with the appropriate resident.

    ii. Residents who are on isolation precautions will be cared for by staff with the personal protective equipment (PPE) appropriate to the infection and clinical condition of the resident.
19. Have a plan in place for pharmaceuticals with an alternate pharmacy or alternate source in the event of halted deliveries or need for backup.
20. Alert staff and residents and their families of the situation and immediate actions that are needed to assure the safety of everyone in the facility. Schedule extended shifts for essential staff; place alternate personnel on standby.[10-12]

Response Phase

In response to an actual emergency situation, the facility administrator or disaster coordinator will coordinate the following actions:

1. Activate the emergency operations plan and open the command center.
2. Fill the appropriate incident command roles to include the general and command staff positions.
3. Coordinate actions and requests for assistance with local emergency services and the community.
4. Determine requirements for additional resources and continue to update appropriate authorities and/or services.
5. Ensure communication with residents' families and physicians.
6. Ensure the prompt transfer of the appropriate resident records.[10-12]

Recovery Phase

Immediately following the emergency situation, the facility administrator should take the steps necessary to complete the following actions:

1. Coordinate recovery operations with the local office of emergency management, local and regional health departments, and local agencies to restore normal operations.

2. Provide crises counseling for residents, family's members, and staff as needed.
3. Compile and provide local authorities with a master list of displaced, missing, injured, or deceased residents and notify the next of kin.
4. Provide information as needed on sanitary precautions for contaminated water and food to staff, volunteers, residents, and families.
5. If necessary, arrange for alternate housing or facilities.[10-12]

The role of the IP in recovery from a disaster will vary depending on the type and scope of the event. Small incidences with no infectious disease process may likely require little IP involvement. Some facilities may have the IP as the designated technical specialist or other assigned roles in the command structure. Responsibilities that may be delegated to the IP may include:

- Surveillance to monitor and track residents' conditions to prevent spread of infectious diseases;
- Monitoring for adequate supplies to prevent spread of infections (i.e., PPE and hand hygiene supplies);
- Ensuring proper management of trash and medical waste;
- Assessing environmental contamination after the disaster;
- Assessing for potable water;
- Ensuring isolation precautions are instituted when indicated; and
- Reporting events of disaster updates internally and externally (i.e., Public Health, OEM, Fire Department, County Emergency Operations Center, etc.).[1]

Emergency Checklist

See Tables 15.1–15.3 for hazard-specific emergency checklists. These checklists and a full emergency preparedness checklist from CMS are available on the CD-ROM. All checklists should be reviewed annually.

PANDEMIC INFLUENZA PREPAREDNESS

Planning for pandemic influenza is critical for ensuring a sustainable healthcare response. The IP's role in preparing for a pandemic due to infectious diseases (e.g., influenza, severe acute respiratory syndrome) will vary depending on the nature of the infection and the potential for disease transmission. Perform an annual hazard vulnerability assessment for pandemic preparedness. Training and resources on how to conduct a hazard vulnerability assessment are available on the FEMA website.[1,11]

The U.S. Department of Health and Human Services (HHS) and the Centers for Disease Control and Prevention (CDC) developed a checklist to help long-term care and other residential facilities develop, assess, and improve their comprehensive pandemic influenza plan (see Table 15.4 for adapted check list). The checklist identifies key areas for pandemic influenza planning and preparedness. Each LTCF should adapt this checklist to meet the facility's needs based on circumstances such as resident characteristics, facility size, scope of services, or hospital affiliation. The LTCF should also incorporate information and requirements from state, regional, and local health departments and emergency management agencies/authorities to ensure that the facility's plan is in line with other community and regional planning efforts. Additional information can be found at www.pandemicflu.gov.[13]

See the CD-ROM for original HHS and CDC checklists.

BIOTERRORISM

According to the CDC, a bioterrorism attack is the deliberate release of viruses, bacteria, or other germs (agents) used to cause illness or death in people, animals, or plants. These agents are typically found in nature, but it is possible that they could be changed to increase their ability to cause disease, make them resistant to current medicines, or to increase their ability to spread into the environment. The CDC separates bioterrorism agents into three categories depending on how easily the agents can be spread and the severity of symptoms or death they may cause.[14] Category A agents are considered high priority and high risk to public and national security. They can be easily spread or transmitted from person to person, have high death rates, may cause public panic and social disruption, and require special action from public health agencies.[14] Category A organisms and toxins in this category include but are not limited to:

- Anthrax (*Bacillus anthracis*)
- Botulism (*Clostridium botulinum* toxin)
- Plague (*Yersinia pestis*)
- Smallpox (Variola major)
- Tularemia (*Francisella tularensis*)
- Viral hemorrhagic fevers[15]

Category B agents are moderately easy to spread, have moderate morbidity and mortality rates, and require enhanced monitoring and lab capacity from CDC.[14] Category B organisms and toxins include but are not limited to:

- Brucellosis (*Brucella spp.*)
- Epsilon toxin (*Clostridium perfringens*)
- Glanders (*Burkholderia mallei*)
- Q fever (*Coxiella burnetii*)
- Ricin toxin from *Ricinus communis* (castor beans).[15]

Category C agents include emerging pathogens that have the potential to be engineered for mass dissemination due to their availability, ease of production and transmission, and potential for high morbidity or mortality rates resulting in significant public health impact. Examples include:

- Hantavirus
- Nipah virus
- Multidrug-resistant tuberculosis
- Tickborne encephalitis viruses
- Tickborne hemorrhagic fever viruses
- Yellow fever
- Influenza (pandemic)[15]

The IP plays an essential part in planning and preparing for biological disasters. When planning a disaster involving agents of bioterrorism, the plan should be expanded to include all of the following components. It is essential that the IP be familiar with all of the following:

- Facility assessment for bioterrorism response
- Assessment of the emergency operations plan
- Participation in development of relevant policies
- Participation in disaster drills involving biologic agent
- Education on biological agents
- Strategies for receiving and posting health alert messages within the facility
- Screening and triage protocols
- Syndromic surveillance[16]
- Outbreak investigation coordination
- Patient management (crisis management)
- Food safety
- Water management and safety
- Development of crisis standards of care that affect infection transmission
- Prioritization of limited supplies of anti-infective therapy
- Environmental decontamination
- Sanitation control[1]

> Additional information on bioterrorism is available in **APIC's *Ready Reference for Microbes,*** 3rd edition.

Reporting Requirements and Contact Information

Healthcare facilities may be the initial site of recognition and response to a bioterrorism event. If a bioterrorism event is suspected, local emergency response systems should be activated. Notification should include the facility IP, director of nursing services, and the administrator. In addition, there should be prompt communication with the local and state health departments, FBI field office, local police, CDC, and medical emergency services. Each facility readiness plan should include a list of the following telephone notification numbers:

Internal contacts:

- IP
- Director of Nursing
- Administrator
- Medical Director

External contacts:

- Local health department
- State health department
- FBI field office
- CDC Division of Bioterrorism Preparedness and Response: 404-639-0385
- CDC Emergency Response Office: 770-488-7100[16]

Identifying and Managing a Bioterrorism-related Outbreak

The IP should follow epidemiologic principles to assess whether a resident's presenting illness (signs and symptoms) is typical of an endemic disease or is an unusual event that should raise concern. Residents in LTCFs who are symptomatic with suspected or confirmed bioterrorism-related illnesses should be managed using Standard Precautions (SPs). SPs are designed to reduce transmission from both recognized and unrecognized sources of infection in healthcare facilities and are recommended for all residents receiving care, regardless of their diagnosis or presumed infection status.[16] A facility may be notified by federal or state authorities of an attack or a threat in a specific geographic region based on their finding of outbreak characteristics. Once notified, signs that should alert the facility's IP to the possibility of a bioterrorism-related outbreak include:

1. A rapidly increasing disease incidence in a normally healthy population (i.e., within hours or days).
2. An epidemic curve that rises and falls during a short period of time. The epidemic curve is a graphical depiction which shows the progression of an outbreak over time.
3. An unusual increase in the number of residents and staff seeking care, especially with fever, respiratory, or gastrointestinal complaints.
4. An endemic disease rapidly emerging at an uncharacteristic time or in an unusual pattern.
5. Higher attack rates among people who had been indoors, especially in areas with filtered air or closed ventilation systems, compared with people who had been outdoors.
6. Large number of rapidly fatal cases.
7. Any person presenting with a disease that is relatively uncommon and has bioterrorism potential (pulmonary anthrax, tularemia, or plague).[17]

Prompt identification of a bioterrorism related outbreak requires a rapid response. Due to the rapid progression to illness and potential for dissemination of some of these agents, it may not be advisable to wait for diagnostic laboratory confirmation. Instead, it may be necessary to initiate a response based on the recognition of high-risk syndromes.[16,18]

CHEMICAL EMERGENCIES

A chemical emergency can occur accidentally or as part of a bioterrorism event. The signs and symptoms of a chemical emergency will most likely include a large number of staff or residents experiencing watery eyes, twitching, choking, difficulty breathing, or loss of coordination. Dead birds and/or animals can also indicate a possible chemical emergency. Chemical emergencies often impact not only the LTCF, but also the surrounding community.

Experts often categorize hazardous chemicals by the type of chemical or by the side effects a chemical would have on people exposed to it. The following are the categories/types used by the CDC:

a. **Biotoxins** - poisons that come from plants or animals.
b. **Blister agents/vesicants** - chemicals that severely blister the eyes, respiratory tract, and skin on contact.
c. **Blood agents** - poisons that affect the body by being absorbed into the blood.
d. **Caustics (acids)** - chemicals that burn or corrode the skin, eyes, and mucous membranes (lining of the nose, mouth, throat, and lungs) on contact.
e. **Choking/lung/pulmonary agents** - chemicals that cause severe irritation or swelling of the respiratory tract (lining of the nose, throat, and lungs).
f. **Incapacitating agents** - drugs that make people unable to think clearly or that cause an altered state of consciousness (possibly unconsciousness).
g. **Long-acting anticoagulants** - poisons that prevent blood from clotting properly, which can lead to uncontrolled bleeding.
h. **Metals** - agents that consist of metallic poisons.
i. **Nerve agents** - highly poisonous chemicals that work by preventing the nervous system from working properly.
j. **Organic solvents** - agents that damage the tissues of living things by dissolving fats and oils.
k. **Riot control agents/tear gas** - highly irritating agents normally used by law enforcement for crowd control or by individuals for protection (e.g., mace).
l. **Toxic alcohols** - poisonous alcohols that can damage the heart, kidneys, and nervous system
m. **Vomiting agents** - chemicals that cause nausea and vomiting.[19]

PROCEDURES FOR BIOTERRORISM AND CHEMICAL EMERGENCY RESPONSE

Administration

1. Preparedness planning for a bioterrorism or chemical emergency event should include collaborating with local hospitals. A plan should be developed on a process to receive patients from the acute care hospital as they may reach their capacity, as well as a plan to discharge the long-term care resident to the community to accommodate for the increase in admissions from the acute care facility. Prepare a list of vacant beds and any possible areas to set up emergency beds.
2. If a bioterrorism or chemical emergency event is suspected, the local emergency response system will be activated. Notification will include the infection preventionist, or designee, and the facility's administration.
3. The facility's administration along with the medical director will communicate with local and state health departments, law enforcement, CDC, and emergency medical services (EMS). Refer to the facility's disaster plan for contact phone numbers and information for these agencies.

Management

1. Take immediate action:
    a. Make the following announcement on the facility's overhead pager: "all staff members, residents, and visitors please remain in the facility until further notice."
    b. Close all windows, air vents, and dampers.
    c. Turn off all fans, air conditioners, and forced air heating systems.
    d. Seal all windows, doors, and air vents with plastic sheeting (large plastic trash bags may be used).
    e. When it is deemed safe, the administrator or person in charge will announce "all clear."
2. Communicate with local and/or state authorities. The local and/or state authorities will provide guidance to the facility regarding staff members leaving and returning to the facility as well as visitors and residents leaving and returning to the facility. It may take time to determine the agent used in the attack, how it should be treated, and who is in danger. Watch television, listen to the radio, or check the Internet for official news and information including signs and symptoms of the disease, areas in danger, if medications or vaccinations are being distributed, and where you should seek medical attention if needed. It will be important to follow official instructions via radio, television, and emergency alert systems.
3. Standard Precaution principles will be applied for the management and cleaning of the environment, linen, and resident care equipment. If smallpox is the suspected agent, airborne isolation of the resident will be needed. (Refer to Isolation Chapter 5 and follow airborne isolation precautions.)
4. Biohazardous waste will be collected, stored, and discarded in accordance with local medical waste management regulations.
5. Bioterrorism-related infection control guidelines:
    a. Plan to manage the residents in the facility if possible. If residents must be transferred to an acute care setting or a lesser care setting, the facility will communicate with the receiving facility to define and explain the type and extent of Transmission-based Precautions required.
    b. If a resident expires while being treated for a bioterrorism-related infection, the facility will communicate to the mortuary the type and extent of Transmission-based Precautions utilized prior to death.
    c. Follow current guidelines for the care and treatment as developed by CDC.
    d. Follow the guidance of the local, state, or federal health and/or law enforcement officials for:
        A. Decontamination
        B. Post-exposure immunization and prophylaxis
        C. Triage and management of exposures and suspected exposures
        D. Laboratory testing and confirmation
        E. Psychological aspects of bioterrorism
        F. Resident, visitor, staff member, and public information
    g. Follow the disaster manual for food, water, evacuation, sheltering in place, and staff management plans.

6. Chemical exposure guidelines (for resident, visitor, or staff):
    a. The need for decontamination depends on the suspected exposure and in most cases will not be necessary. Decontamination would only be considered in instances of gross contamination. This decision should be made in conjunction with the local health department.[16]
    b. Notify local authorities if it is determined there is a need of HAZMAT decontamination team. Follow their directions.
    c. Remove all clothing and jewelry and shower immediately. When showering, caution should be taken to avoid scrubbing the chemicals into the skin.
    d. Dispose of contaminated clothing and other items in bag and seal. Place bag in biohazardous waste container. Those healthcare personnel handling contaminated items should be wearing PPE.
    e. If the eyes are affected, flush with saline eye wash for 10 to 15 minutes, or as instructed by the local or state medical authority. If you wear contact lenses, remove them and dispose of them with the clothing.
    f. Notify the resident's attending physician for further guidance.
    g. PPE for staff will be needed for decontamination process. N95 respirator masks should be available in the event they are required. If facemasks are required (as directed by authorities), outfit caregivers first and then provide masks to the residents and visitors as the supply allows.[16,20]

TABLE 15.1: FIRE

Completed	Initial	Action
☐ Yes ☐ No	____	**Post location of fire alarms**
☐ Yes ☐ No	____	**Post location of fire extinguishers**
☐ Yes ☐ No	____	**Train employees on use of alarm system**
		Train employees on the use of fire extinguishers using the PASS Procedure:
☐ Yes ☐ No	____	1. Pull the fire extinguisher pin to activate the trigger.
☐ Yes ☐ No	____	2. Aim the fire extinguisher at the base of the flame.
☐ Yes ☐ No	____	3. Squeeze the trigger.
☐ Yes ☐ No	____	4. Sweep the fire extinguisher spray back and forth at the base of the flame.
☐ Yes ☐ No	____	**Post directions on how to utilize emergency equipment.**
		Train employees on RACE procedures:
☐ Yes ☐ No	____	1. Rescue residents in immediate danger.
☐ Yes ☐ No	____	2. Alarm—sound nearest alarm if not already activated.
☐ Yes ☐ No	____	3. Confine the fire to the extent possible.
☐ Yes ☐ No	____	4. Evacuate to a safe area.

Signature ____ Date ____ / ____ / ____

Also available on the CD-ROM.

Adapted from Missouri Department of Health & Senior Services (Health MO). *Disaster Preparedness Plan Template for Use in Long Term Care Facilities*. Health MO website. 2007. Available at: http://health.mo.gov/emergencies/readyin3/pdf/emergencyactionplan.pdf.

TABLE 15.2: NATURAL DISASTERS

Completed	Initial	Action
		Severe Electrical Storm:
☐ Yes ☐ No	______	1. Relocate to the inner areas of facility as possible per LTCF policy and procedures.
☐ Yes ☐ No	______	2. Keep all staff and residents away from glass windows, doors, skylights, and appliances.
☐ Yes ☐ No	______	3. Refrain from using landline phones or televisions or from taking showers.
☐ Yes ☐ No	______	4. Stay away from computers.
		Tornado (Watch Issued):
☐ Yes ☐ No	______	1. Listen to local radio and TV stations for updates. Check that radio batteries are available and charged.
☐ Yes ☐ No	______	2. Be alert to changing weather conditions.
☐ Yes ☐ No	______	3. Secure equipment, outdoor furniture, and articles that act as projectiles.
☐ Yes ☐ No	______	4. Alert staff for possible sheltering of residents.
		Tornado (Warning Issued):
☐ Yes ☐ No	______	1. Seek shelter in designated area per LTCF policy and procedures (e.g., safe room, basement first floor interior hallways, restrooms, or other enclosed areas).
☐ Yes ☐ No	______	2. Check restrooms or vacant rooms for visitors or stranded residents and escort them to the shelter area.
☐ Yes ☐ No	______	3. Take position of greatest safety: a. If possible, crouch down on knees with head down and hands locked at back of neck; or b. Protect head/body with pillows or mattress. c. If bedridden residents cannot be moved to central corridors, close window blinds or curtains and protect the residents as much as possible. Additional blankets may be used as shields.
		Winter Storms:
☐ Yes ☐ No	______	1. Secure facility against frozen pipes.
☐ Yes ☐ No	______	2. Check emergency and alternate utility sources.
☐ Yes ☐ No	______	3. Check emergency generator to ensure it functions and that there is fuel. Identify what the generator powers.
☐ Yes ☐ No	______	4. Conserve utilities by maintaining low temperature, consistent with health needs.
☐ Yes ☐ No	______	5. Equip vehicles with chains and snow tires.
☐ Yes ☐ No	______	6. Keep sidewalks clear.
		Flooding (External Sources):
☐ Yes ☐ No	______	1. Shut off water main to prevent contamination. Fill clean bathtubs, large pans, and buckets with fresh water and store in case water services are interrupted or become contaminated.
☐ Yes ☐ No	______	2. Pack refrigerators/food lockers with dry ice if available.
☐ Yes ☐ No	______	3. Fill and use sandbags to ward off floodwaters.
☐ Yes ☐ No	______	4. Prepare to evacuate residents.

Table 15.2 Continued

Completed	Initial	Action
		Flooding (Internal Sources):
☐ Yes ☐ No	____	1. Turn off building electricity.
☐ Yes ☐ No	____	2. Move residents as required.
☐ Yes ☐ No	____	3. Generators can be rendered inoperable by flooding. Mount outdoor generators on an elevated platform above the highest expected water level and get a generator enclosure for additional protection. If feasible, place generator on upper building floor or rooftop.[9]
		Earthquake:
☐ Yes ☐ No	____	1. Evaluate facility for potential dangers and resolve any problems before earthquake occurs (e.g., secure furniture, store heavy items low to the ground, bolt and strap water heater to the wall and ground, affix pictures and mirrors securely, and brace overhead light fixtures).
☐ Yes ☐ No	____	2. Train employees on "Drop, Cover, and Hold." • Drop to the ground. • Take cover under a sturdy table or piece of furniture. • Hold on until the shaking stops.
☐ Yes ☐ No	____	3. During earthquake: • Drop, Cover and Hold, then • Inspect facility for safety. Evacuate if building is not safe using RACE system. Put out small fires if possible and evacuate the area or building as appropriate.
☐ Yes ☐ No	____	4. Check on residents, staff, and visitors. Check restrooms or vacant rooms for visitors or stranded residents.
☐ Yes ☐ No	____	5. Take care of injured or trapped persons. Provide first aid and potential injury assessment as needed. Call 9-1-1 only for life threatening emergencies.
☐ Yes ☐ No	____	6. Turn off gas only if gas fumes are detected. (Natural gas line cannot be turned on again except by the gas company.)
☐ Yes ☐ No	____	7. Be prepared for aftershocks and reevaluate building safety after additional seismic activities.

Signature ______________________________ Date ____ / ____ / ____

Also available on the CD-ROM.

Adapted from Missouri Department of Health & Senior Services (Health MO). *Disaster Preparedness Plan Template for Use in Long Term Care Facilities.* Health MO website. 2007. Available at: http://health.mo.gov/emergencies/readyin3/pdf/emergencyactionplan.pdf.

TABLE 15.3: WATER, ELECTRICAL OUTAGE, OR GAS LINE BREAK

Completed	Initial	Action
		Preparedness:
☐ Yes ☐ No	______	1. Stock a 7- to 10-day supply of food and water for residents and staff and a 7- to 10-day supply of fuel.
☐ Yes ☐ No	______	2. Keep an accurate blueprint of all utility lines and pipes associated with the facility and grounds.
☐ Yes ☐ No	______	3. Develop procedures for emergency utility shutdown.
☐ Yes ☐ No	______	4. List all Emergency Utility contact phone numbers for 24/7 coverage.
☐ Yes ☐ No	______	5. List names and numbers of all maintenance personnel for emergency notification.
		Response—Electric Power Failure:
☐ Yes ☐ No	______	1. Call #______________________________(power company).
☐ Yes ☐ No	______	2. Notify the facilities maintenance staff.
☐ Yes ☐ No	______	3. Consider evacuation if necessary.
☐ Yes ☐ No	______	4. Keep refrigerated food and medicine storage units closed to retard spoilage.
☐ Yes ☐ No	______	5. Turn off power at main control point if short is suspected.
☐ Yes ☐ No	______	6. Follow repair procedures.
		Response—Water Main Break:
☐ Yes ☐ No	______	1. Call #______________________________(city water or local water authority).
☐ Yes ☐ No	______	2. Notify facility maintenance personnel.
☐ Yes ☐ No	______	3. Shut off valve at primary control point.
☐ Yes ☐ No	______	4. Relocate articles which may be damaged by water
☐ Yes ☐ No	______	5. Call #______________________________(predesignated assistance groups) if flooding occurs.
☐ Yes ☐ No	______	6. Determine water needs and implement Emergency Utilities Plan.
☐ Yes ☐ No	______	7. When there is a significant water disruption or an emergency occurs, follow the local advisory to boil water, which may be issued by municipal water utility.
☐ Yes ☐ No	______	8. Alert residents, families, staff, and visitors not to consume water from drinking fountains, ice, or drinks made from municipal tap water while the advisory is in effect unless that water has been disinfected by boiling or treating with bleach.21 For further information, www.cdc.gov/ncidod/dhqp/gl/environinfection.html.
		Response—Gas Line Break:
☐ Yes ☐ No	______	1. Evacuate the building immediately. Follow evacuation procedures.
☐ Yes ☐ No	______	2. Keep a list of phone numbers for maintenance staff, administrator, local public utility department, gas company, and police and fire departments. Notify immediately.
☐ Yes ☐ No	______	3. Shut off the main valve.
☐ Yes ☐ No	______	4. Open widows.
☐ Yes ☐ No	______	5. Re-enter buildings only at the direction of the local fire authorities and utility officials.

Signature ____ Date ____ / ____ / ____

Also available on the CD-ROM.

Adapted from Missouri Department of Health & Senior Services (Health MO). *Disaster Preparedness Plan Template for Use in Long Term Care Facilities.* Health MO website. 2007. Available at: http://health.mo.gov/emergencies/readyin3/pdf/emergencyactionplan.pdf.

TABLE 15.4: PANDEMIC INFLUENZA PLANNING CHECKLIST[13]

PLANNING AND COORDINATION			
Tasks	Not Started	In Progress	Completed
Identify a pandemic coordinator and response team. The team should include the facility administrator, medical director, nursing administration, infection preventionist, occupational health, staff developer, environmental services, engineering and maintenance services, dietary, pharmacy, rehab team, transportation services, purchasing agent, facility staff representative, and other members as appropriate (e.g., clergy, community representatives, department heads, risk management, family representatives). List names of team members in plan.	☐	☐	☐
Local and state health departments and provider/trade association points of contact have been identified for information on pandemic influenza resources. Insert name, title and contact information for each below: Local Health Dept. contact __________ State Health Dept. contact __________ State LTC Trade Association contact __________	☐	☐	☐
Local, regional, or state emergency preparedness groups, including bioterrorism/communicable disease coordinators' points of contact have been identified. Insert name, title, and contact information for each: City __________ County __________ Other Regional __________	☐	☐	☐
The LTC facility's emergency preparedness coordinator has contacted other pandemic influenza planning groups to obtain information on coordinating the facility's plan with other influenza plans.	☐	☐	☐

DEVELOPMENT OF A WRITTEN PANDEMIC INFLUENZA PLAN			
Tasks	Not Started	In Progress	Completed
Copies have been obtained of relevant sections of the HHS Pandemic Influenza Plan (available at www.hhs.gov/pandemicflu/plan/) and available state, regional, or local plans are reviewed for incorporation into the facility's plan.	☐	☐	☐
The plan identifies the person(s) authorized to implement the plan, the triggers that would initiate the plan, and the organizational structure that will be used.	☐	☐	☐
The pandemic plan recommends the LTCF implement a "Mandatory Vaccination" policy for all staff working in the LTCF.	☐	☐	☐

Table 15.4 Continued

ELEMENTS OF AN INFLUENZA PANDEMIC PLAN			
Tasks	Not Started	In Progress	Completed
A plan is in place for surveillance and detection of the presence of pandemic influenza in residents and staff.	☐	☐	☐
A person has been assigned responsibility for monitoring public health advisories (federal and state) and updating the pandemic response coordinator and members of the pandemic influenza planning committee when pandemic influenza has been reported in the United States and is nearing the geographic area. For more information see www.cdc.gov/flu/weekly/fluactivity.htm. Insert name, title, and contact information of designate responsible person ____________________________________	☐	☐	☐
A written protocol has been developed for weekly or daily monitoring of seasonal influenza-like illness in residents and staff. For more information, see www.cdc.gov/flu/professionals/diagnosis/. Having a system for tracking illness trends during seasonal influenza will ensure that the facility can detect stressors that may affect operating capacity, including staffing and supply needs during a pandemic.	☐	☐	☐
A protocol has been developed for the evaluation and diagnosis of residents and/or staff with symptoms of pandemic influenza.	☐	☐	☐
Assessment for influenza is included in the evaluation of incoming residents. There is an admission policy or protocol to determine the appropriate placement and isolation of residents with an influenza-like illness. (Author's note: The 2012 CDC/SHEA surveillance definitions for LTC may be applied during pandemic influenza. Revised definition of influenza has removed criteria of seasonality to define influenza. Influenza or influenza-like illness can be considered a diagnosis throughout the year.)[22]	☐	☐	☐
A system is in place to monitor for, and internally review transmission of, influenza among residents and staff in the facility. Information from this monitoring system is used to implement prevention interventions (e.g., isolation, cohorting).This system will be necessary for assessing pandemic influenza transmission.	☐	☐	☐
A facility communication plan has been developed. For more information, see www.hhs.gov/pandemicflu/plan/sup10.htm.	☐	☐	☐
Key public health points of contact during an influenza pandemic have been identified. Insert name, title, and contact information for each: Local health department contact ____________________ State health department contact ____________________ Designated person responsible for communications with public health authorities during a pandemic ____________________ Designated person responsible for communication with staff, residents, and their families regarding the status and impact of influenza in the facility. ____________________________________	☐	☐	☐
Contact information for family members or guardians of facility residents is up to date.	☐	☐	☐
A list has been created of other healthcare facilities and their points of contact (e.g., other LTCFs, local hospital, emergency medical services, relevant community organizations) with whom it will be necessary to maintain communication during a pandemic (insert location of contact list and attach a copy to the pandemic plan).	☐	☐	☐
A facility representative has been involved in the discussion of local plans or interfacility communication during a pandemic.	☐	☐	☐

Table 15.4 Continued

ELEMENTS OF AN INFLUENZA PANDEMIC PLAN CONTINUED			
Tasks	Not Started	In Progress	Completed
A plan is in place to provide education and training to ensure that all personnel, residents, and family members of residents understand the implications of, and basic prevention and control measures for, pandemic influenza.	☐	☐	☐
A person has been designated with responsibility for coordinating education and training on pandemic influenza (e.g., identifies and facilitates access to available programs, maintains a record of personnel attendance). Insert name, title, and contact information ______________________	☐	☐	☐
Current and potential opportunities for long-distance (i.e., web-based) and local (i.e., health department or hospital-sponsored) programs have been identified. See www.cdc.gov/flu/professionals/training/.	☐	☐	☐
Language and reading-level appropriate materials have been identified to supplement and support education and training programs (i.e., available through state and federal public health agencies such as www.cdc.gov/flu/groups.htm and through professional organizations), and a plan is in place for obtaining these materials.	☐	☐	☐
Education and training includes information on infection control measures to prevent the spread of pandemic influenza.	☐	☐	☐
The facility has a plan for expediting the credentialing and training of nonfacility staff brought in from other locations to provide resident care when the facility reaches a staffing crisis.	☐	☐	☐
Informational materials (e.g., brochures, posters) on pandemic influenza and relevant policies (e.g., suspension of visitation, where to obtain facility or family member information) have been developed or identified for residents and their families. These materials are language and reading-level appropriate, and a plan is in place to disseminate these materials in advance of the actual pandemic. For information, see www.cdc.gov/flu/professionals/infectioncontrol/index.htm and www.cdc.gov/flu/groups.htm.	☐	☐	☐
An infection control plan is in place for managing residents and visitors with pandemic influenza. (For information on infection control recommendations for pandemic influenza, see www.hhs.gov/pandemicflu/plan/sup4.html.)	☐	☐	☐
An infection control policy that requires direct care personnel to use Standard (www.cdc.gov/ncidod/dhqp/gl isolation standard.html) and Droplet Precautions (www.cdc.gov/ncidod/dhqp/gl isolation droplet.html).	☐	☐	☐
A plan for implementing Respiratory Hygiene/Cough Etiquette throughout the facility. (See www.cdc.gov/flu/professionals/infectioncontrol/resphygiene.html.)	☐	☐	☐
A plan for cohorting symptomatic residents, using one or more of the following strategies: 1. Confining symptomatic residents and their exposed roommates to their room, 2. Placing symptomatic residents together in one area of the facility, or 3. Closing units where symptomatic and asymptomatic residents reside (e.g., restricting all residents to an affected unit regardless of symptoms). The plan includes a stipulation that, where possible, personnel who are assigned to work on affected units will not work on other units.	☐	☐	☐
Criteria and protocols for closing units or the entire facility to new admissions when pandemic influenza is in the facility have been developed.	☐	☐	☐
Criteria and protocols for enforcing visitor limitations have been developed.	☐	☐	☐

Table 15.4 Continued

ELEMENTS OF AN INFLUENZA PANDEMIC PLAN CONTINUED			
Tasks	Not Started	In Progress	Completed
An occupational health plan for addressing staff absences and other related occupational issue has been developed that includes the following: 1. A liberal nonpunitive sick leave policy that addresses the needs of symptomatic personnel and facility staffing needs. The policy considers: a. The handling of personnel who develop symptoms while at work. b. When personnel may return to work after having pandemic influenza. c. When personnel who are symptomatic, but well enough to work, will be permitted to continue working. d. Personnel who need to care for family members who become ill. A plan to educate staff to self-assess and report symptoms of pandemic influenza before reporting for duty. A list of mental health and faith-based resources that will be available to provide counseling to personnel during a pandemic. A system to monitor influenza vaccination of personnel. A plan for managing personnel who are at increased risk for influenza complications (i.e., pregnant women, immunocompromised workers) by placing them on administrative leave or altering their work location.	☐	☐	☐
A vaccine and antiviral use plan has been developed.	☐	☐	☐
CDC and state health department websites have been identified for obtaining the most current recommendations and guidance for the use, availability, access, and distribution of vaccines and antiviral medications during a pandemic. For information, see www.hhs.gov/pandemicflu/plan/sup6.html and www.hhs.gov/pandemicflu//sup7.html.	☐	☐	☐
HHS guidance has been used to estimate the number of personnel and residents who would be targeted as first and second priority for receipt of pandemic vaccine or antiviral prophylaxis. For more information, see www.hhs.gov/pandemicflu/plan/sup6.html and www.hhs.gov/pandemicflu/plan/sup7.html.	☐	☐	☐
A plan is in place for expediting delivery of influenza vaccine or antiviral prophylaxis to residents and staff as recommended by the state health department.	☐	☐	☐

Adapted from U.S. Department of Health and Human Services and Centers for Disease Control and Prevention. Long-term care and other residential facilities: Pandemic influenza planning checklist. Flu.gov website. 2006. Available at: www.flu.gov/planning-preparedness/hospital/longtermcare.pdf.

REFERENCES

1. Rebmann T; 2008 APIC Emergency Preparedness Committee. APIC state-of-the-art report: The role of the infection preventionist in emergency management. *Am J Infect Control* 2009; 37(4): 271-281.
2. Centers for Disease Control and Prevention (CDC). *CDC's Disaster Planning Goal: Protect Vulnerable Adults.* CDC website. n.d. Available at: http://www.cdc.gov/aging/pdf/disaster_planning_goal.pdf.
3. Harvey SA. *Natural Disasters are Especially Hard for Seniors.* Cornell Chronicle website. 2013. Available at: http://www.news.cornell.edu/stories/2013/03/natural-disasters-are-especially-hard-seniors.
4. University of Minnesota. *NH Regulations Plus—Administration—Disaster and Emergency Preparedness.* University of Minnesota website. 2011. Available at: http://www.hpm.umn.edu/nhregsplus/NH%20Regs%20by%20Topic/Topic%20Administration%20-%20Disaster%20and%20Emergency%20Preparedness.html.
5. Code of Federal Regulations. *Public Health: Requirements for states and long-term care facilities: Administration.* 42 CFR 483.75(m), 2011. Government Printing Office website. 2011. Available at: http://www.gpo.gov/fdsys/pkg/CFR-2011-title42-vol5/pdf/CFR-2011-title42-vol5-sec483-75.pdf.
6. Federal Emergency Management Agency (FEMA). *Preparedness.* FEMA website. 2013. Available at: http://www.fema.gov/preparedness-0.
7. Federal Emergency Management Agency (FEMA). *NIMS and Use of Plain Language.* NIMS Alert. FEMA website. 2006. Available at: http://www.fema.gov/pdf/emergency/nims/plain_lang.pdf.
8. Federal Emergency Management Agency (FEMA). *Incident Command System.* FEMA website. 2013. Available at: http://www.fema.gov/incident-command-system.
9. Hamilton R. *Lessons in emergency power preparedness: Planning in the wake of Katrina.* Cummins Power website. 2007. Available at: http://cumminspower.com/www/literature/technicalpapers/PT-7006-Standby-Katrina-en.pdf.
10. Allied Healthcare Facilities Work Group, Santa Clara County Emergency Medical Services Agency. *Emergency preparedness and planning toolkit for long-term care providers.* California Association of Health Facilities website. 2007. Available at: www.cahfdownload.com/cahf/dpp/AHFWGBinder6.12.09complete.pdf.
11. Missouri Department of Health & Senior Services (Health MO). *Disaster Preparedness Plan Template for Use in Long Term Care Facilities.* Health MO website. 2007. Available at: http://health.mo.gov/emergencies/readyin3/pdf/emergencyactionplan.pdf.
12. Centers for Medicare & Medicaid Services (CMS). Emergency preparedness checklist: Recommended tool for effective healthcare facility planning. CMS website. 2007. Available at: http://www.cms.gov/Medicare/Provider-Enrollment-and-Certification/SurveyCertEmergPrep/Downloads/SandC_EPChecklist_Provider.pdf.
13. U.S. Department of Health and Human Services and Centers for Disease Control and Prevention. *Long-term care and other residential facilities: Pandemic influenza planning checklist.* Flu.gov website. 2006. Available at: www.flu.gov/planning-preparedness/hospital/longtermcare.pdf.
14. Centers for Disease Control and Prevention (CDC). *Emergency preparedness and response: Bioterrorism overview.* CDC website. 2007. Available at: www.bt.cdc.gov/bioterrorism/overview.asp.
15. Brooks K. *Ready Reference for Microbes,* 3rd ed. Washington, DC: Association for Professionals in Infection Control and Epidemiology, 2012: 61-68.
16. Bioterrorism readiness plan: A template for healthcare facilities. *ED Manag* 1999; 11(11): suppl 1-16.
17. South Central Public Health District. *Epidemiologic Features of a Possible Bioterrorism Event.* South Central Public Health District website. 2008. Available at: http://www.phd5.idaho.gov/Emergency/bioterrorism.htm.
18. Kaufman AF, Pesik NT, Meltzer MI. Syndromic surveillance in bioterrorist attacks. *Emerg Infect Dis* 2005; 11(9): 1487-1488.
19. Centers for Disease Control and Prevention (CDC). Emergency preparedness and response. CDC website. 2012. Available at: http://emergency.cdc.gov/chemical/overview.asp.
20. Rebmann T. Infectious disease disasters: bioterrorism, emerging infections, and pandemics. In: Carrico R, ed. *APIC Text of Infection Control and Epidemiology,* 3rd ed. Washington, DC: Association for Professionals in Infection Control and Epidemiology, Inc., 2009: 118-1–118-37.
21. Centers for Disease Control and Prevention (CDC), HICPAC. Guidelines for environmental infection control in health-care facilities, 2003. CDC website. 2013. Available at: http://www.cdc.gov/ncidod/dhqp/gl/environinfection.html.
22. Stone ND, Ashraf MS, Calder J, Crnich CJ, Crossley K, Drinka PJ, et al. SHEA/CDC Position Paper: Surveillance definitions of infections in long-term care facilities: revisiting the McGeer Criteria. *Infect Control Hosp Epidemiol* 2012; 33(10): 965-977.

Glossary

Absolute risk: The incidence of a disease in a certain population.

Active learning: Active learning is a process whereby students engage in activities such as reading, writing, discussion, or problem solving that promote analysis, synthesis, and evaluation of class content. Cooperative learning, problem-based learning, and the use of case methods and simulations are some approaches that promote active learning.

Active surveillance culture (ASC): A program whereby all residents admitted to the facility who are at high risk for developing infections are screened through performing cultures on admission. ASCs are used to identify the reservoir for multidrug-resistant organisms such as methicillin-resistant *Staphylococcus aureus*, vancomycin-resistant enterococci, etc.

Activities/life enrichment: A type of sociotherapy in long-term care communities where social interaction, spiritual gatherings, games, group outings, and individual or group activities, art, music, and interactive media are used to enhance personal experience and quality of life.

Activities of daily living (ADL): Usually refers to dressing, bathing, grooming, and eating.

Adult day services: Programs that support community living for older adults with daily social interaction and activities, meals, hygiene, and medication management.

Airborne Isolation/Precautions: Airborne Isolation Precautions prevent transmission of infectious agents that remain infectious over long distances when suspended in the air. This type of isolation requires a single-patient room that is equipped with special air handling and ventilation. Healthcare personnel caring for residents on Airborne Isolation Precautions should wear a respirator mask prior to entering the room of the isolated resident.

Alcohol-based hand rub (ABHR): A 60 to 95 percent ethanol- or isopropyl-containing preparation base designed for application to the hands to reduce the number of viable microorganisms. Sometimes referred to as alcohol hand rub (AHR).

Analytic bias: Having a preconception of what is causing the problem and letting the preconceived notions affect the data analysis.

Antibiogram: An aggregate report prepared in the laboratory that analyzes susceptibility and resistance patterns for clinically significant pathogens among a set of isolates.

Antifungal: A medication used to treat fungal infections such as athlete's foot, ringworm, or candidiasis.

Antigen: Any substance (e.g., a toxin or the surface of a microorganism or transplanted organ) recognized as foreign by the human body and that stimulates the production of antibodies.

Anti-infective: A group of medications used to treat infections.

Antimicrobial stewardship program (ASP): A program that promotes effective management and utilization of antibiotics prescribed for residents. The program should be designed to measure and optimize the appropriate use of antimicrobials, which is achieved by selecting the appropriate dose, duration of therapy, and route of administration.

Antiseptic: Chemical agent that kills microorganisms on living skin or mucous membranes.

Arteriovenous fistula (AV fistula): A direct vascular connection between an artery and vein used in hemodialysis.

Arteriovenous graft (AV graft): A vascular connection that is created by indirectly connecting an artery to a vein by a synthetic vessel tubing, which supports blood flow.

Automatic positive airway pressure (APAP): A device used to automatically deliver the minimum pressure needed to keep the upper airway open during sleep.

Bactericidal: Chemicals or products that kill bacteria.

Bacteriostatic: Chemicals that retard the growth of bacteria but do not necessarily kill them.

Bacteriuria: A condition in which a resident is free of any clinical symptoms of an infection but may contain microorganisms in the urine revealed in culture. May be symptomatic or asymptomatic.

B cell: Also known as B lymphocytes. Produced in the bone marrow of humans, B cells develop into antibody producing plasma cells or into memory cells.

Bias: A perspective, way of thinking, or way viewing a situation that may interfere with considering factors or circumstances that may be equally valid in a particular situation.

Bilateral positive airway pressure (BPAP): A respiratory treatment that delivers inspiratory and expiratory positive pressure without the use of mechanical ventilation.

Bioburden: The number and types of viable microorganisms with which an item is contaminated; also may be referred to as bioload or microbial load.

Biofilm: Communities of microorganisms that are attached to a surface. They can detach and frequently resist penetration by antimicrobials.

Bioterrorism: A deliberate release of biological agents to cause illness or death.

Bloodborne pathogen (BBP): A microorganism capable of causing an infectious disease through exposure to blood and other specific body fluids.

Carrier status: Exists when an individual has been colonized with a potentially infectious pathogen but shows no sign of active infection.

Chain of infection: A concept that describes how infections occur. To develop an infection, there must be a reservoir, a portal of exit, a mode of transmission, a portal of entry, and a susceptible host.

Chemical terrorism: Intentional release of hazardous chemicals with the potential for harming the health or well-being of people, animals, or plants.

Cleaning: Physical removal, usually with detergent and water or enzyme cleaner and water, of adherent visible soil, blood, protein substances, microorganisms, and other debris from the surfaces, crevices, serrations, joints, and lumens of instruments, devices, and equipment by a manual or mechanical process that prepares the items for safe handling and/or further decontamination.

Cohorting: The practice of grouping residents infected or colonized with the same agent to confine their care to one area and prevent contact with susceptible residents and staff (cohorting residents).

Colonization: Colonization refers to when microorganisms live on or in a host organism but do not invade tissues or cause damage. Residents who are referred to as "colonized" are those without signs or symptoms of an infection.

Community-associated infection: Infections that are present or incubating at the time of admission or generally develop within 72 hours of admission to the long-term care facility.

Contact Isolation/Precautions: Contact Precautions are intended to prevent transmission of infectious agents that are spread by direct/indirect contact with the resident or the resident's environment. Healthcare personnel caring for residents on Contact Isolation/Precautions must wear a gown and gloves for all interactions.

Contact time: The amount of time required for the disinfectant to kill the intended organisms. Also refers to the duration of time the surface should remain wet after applying the disinfectant.

Contaminated: The actual or potential presence of pathogenic organisms.

Continuous ambulatory peritoneal dialysis (CAPD): An alternative to hemodialysis in which the peritoneum is used as an artificial kidney.

Continuous positive airway pressure (CPAP): A form of respiratory therapy that maintains a continuous level of positive airway pressure to keep the airway open.

Critical items: Objects that enter sterile tissues and the vascular system. Critical items present a high risk of infection if the item is contaminated with any microorganisms. Reprocessing critical items involves cleaning followed by sterilization.

Cultural sensitivity: Awareness of cultural differences associated with social behaviors, values, and expectations that can impact the delivery of care.

Decolonization: The use of an antimicrobial product to eliminate the carrier state of a potential pathogen.

Decontamination: The use of physical or chemical methods to remove, inactivate, or destroy bloodborne pathogens on a surface or item to the point where they are no longer capable of transmitting infectious particles and the surface or item is rendered safe for handling, use, or disposal.

Detergent: Products capable of removing, separating, and dispersing solid or liquid contamination from a surface. A cleaning agent that makes no antimicrobial claims on the label.

Dialysis: The mechanical removal of excess fluid, electrolytes, metabolic waste, and toxins that would be normally cleared by the kidneys.

Disinfection: The thermal or chemical destruction of pathogenic and other types of microorganisms. Disinfection is less lethal than sterilization because it destroys most recognized pathogenic microorganisms but not necessarily all microbial forms (e.g., bacterial spores). There are three disinfection levels: low, intermediate, and high.

Droplet Isolation/Precautions: Actions designed to reduce/prevent the transmission of pathogens spread through close respiratory or mucous membrane contact with respiratory secretions. Healthcare personnel who care for residents on Droplet Isolation Precautions should wear a mask (a respirator is not necessary) prior to entering the room of the isolated resident.

Early detection: Purposeful awareness of an epidemiologically significant event at the onset of the event.

Endemic: Present in or restricted to a particular community, region, or people.

End-stage renal disease (ESRD): Chronic, irreversible kidney failure requiring dialysis.

Engineered sharp safety device: A medical device that protects the user from an accidental puncture. Passive devices protect the user without an additional action after the device is used. Active devices require the user to engage the safety mechanism.

Engineering controls: Engineering controls are activities and processes designed to eliminate or reduce exposure to a chemical or physical hazard through the use or substitution of engineered machinery or equipment.

Epidemic: An epidemic is the occurrence of atypically large number or more cases of a disease than would be expected in a community or region during a given period of time.

Epidemic curve: A graphical depiction that shows the progression of an outbreak over time.

Event-related sterility: Concept that items are considered sterile unless the integrity of the packaging is compromised (i.e., torn, soiled, or wet or there is evidence of tampering). Shelf life is indefinite.

Formative evaluation: A method for judging the worth of a program while the program activities are in progress. This part of the evaluation focuses on the process.

Hand hygiene: A general term that refers to any one of the following: (1) hand washing with plain (non-antimicrobial) soap and water; (2) antiseptic hand wash; (3) antiseptic hand rub (waterless antiseptic product); or (4) surgical hand antisepsis (antiseptic hand wash or antiseptic hand rub performed preoperatively by surgical personnel to eliminate transient hand flora and reduce resident hand flora). A major component of Standard Precautions and one of the most effective methods to prevent transmission of pathogens associated with healthcare.

Healthcare-associated infections (HAIs): (a.k.a. "nosocomial" and "facility-acquired" infection) An infection that generally occurs after 72 hours from the time of admission to a healthcare facility and is associated in some way with receiving care.

Healthcare personnel: Someone who works in a healthcare facility either directly or indirectly with patients or residents. Also called healthcare worker.

Hepatitis B virus (HBV): A communicable virus capable of causing liver failure.

Hepatitis C virus (HCV): A communicable virus capable of causing liver failure.

Herd immunity: Protecting a community from an infectious agent through the immunity of a large number of immune individuals within the group or community, decreasing the likelihood that any susceptible person will come in contact with an infected person.

High-level disinfectant: A product capable of killing bacterial spores when used in sufficient concentration under suitable conditions. It is expected to kill all other microorganisms. Examples include glutaraldehyde and ortho-phthalaldehyde.

Histamine: An amine (organic nitrogen compound) released by mast cells in response to injury or infection or ingested in certain types of fish. A "mediator of inflammation." Physiological responses to histamine release include swelling, dilation of blood vessels causing flushing, gastrointestinal symptoms, hives, and generalized itching.

Hospital disinfectant: Disinfectant registered for use in hospitals, clinics, dental offices, and any other medical-related facility. Efficacy is demonstrated against *Salmonella choleraesuis*, *Staphylococcus aureus*, and *Pseudomonas aeruginosa*.

Human immunodeficiency virus (HIV): A communicable virus that attacks the immune system.

Hydrogen peroxide disinfectant: Chemical disinfectant used for resident care items and equipment.

Hypodermoclyis: The infusion of solution into subcutaneous tissue.

Iceberg concept of disease: The concept that different individuals express colonization and infection in different ways. One individual may be colonized with pathogens that do not cause them infection but may cause infection in other individuals.

Immunosenescence: The decreasing ability of the immune system to maintain health and respond to threats as a person ages.

Implanted port: A device surgically inserted under the skin, usually on the upper chest, for venous access to administer medication and fluids.

Inanimate surface: Nonliving surfaces such as floors, walls, and furniture.

Incidence rate (intensity): Measure of new cases of illness or a condition in a particular period of time.

Infection: Clinical manifestation of symptoms with host invasion, and presence of a pathogen on culture in large numbers. Infections may be caused by a microorganism that naturally resides in the body (endogenous) or by a pathogen introduced from the outside world (exogenous).

Infection definition for clinical diagnosis: ICD-9 and ICD-10 diagnoses assigned by licensed provider such as physician or advanced practice nurse or physician's assistant. The clinical diagnosis is based on symptoms and diagnostic testing and provides a basis for clinical treatments and approaches.

Infection definitions for surveillance: Constant characteristics that meet specific criteria. All characteristics must be met to be defined as an infection for surveillance purposes.

Infection preventionist: (a.k.a. infection control professional) A healthcare professional with specialized training in infection prevention and control and who is primarily responsible for a facility's infection prevention program.

Infection prevention and control program: Refers to a program (including surveillance, investigation, prevention, control, and reporting) that provides a safe and sanitary environment to help prevent the development and transmission of infection.

Infectious microorganisms: Microorganisms capable of producing disease in appropriate hosts.

Infusion therapy: The administration of fluids and medications through a catheter into a vein.

Intensified Interventions: The Centers for Disease Control and Prevention defines Intensified Interventions as the additional measures taken when there is (1) a new or unusual pathogen circulating in the community, or (2) if a resident continues to get re-infected even when all measures are used to curtail the infection, or (3) when a common pathogen develops an unusual resistance pattern.

Interdisciplinary team (IDT): Representatives from various departments of the long-term care facility who coordinate and implement their joint efforts in support of resident care and safety.

Intergenerational programming: Planned and unstructured programs that involve people of all ages coming together for meaningful activities.

Intermediate-level disinfectant: Agent that destroys all vegetative bacteria, including tubercle bacilli, lipid, and some nonlipid viruses, and fungi, but not bacterial spores. Most phenolic disinfectants are considered intermediate disinfectants.

Kennedy terminal ulcer: A pressure ulcer that some residents develop during the dying process.

Kill-time: Same as "contact-time." The amount of time required for the disinfectant to kill the intended pathogenic organism. The duration of time that the surface should remain wet after applying the disinfectant.

Leukocytosis: Increase in the number of white blood cells.

Low-level disinfectant: Agent that destroys all vegetative bacteria (except tubercle bacilli), lipid viruses, some nonlipid viruses, and some fungi but not bacterial spores. Products containing quaternary ammonium compounds (Quats) are low-level disinfectants.

Medical waste: Any solid waste that is generated in the diagnosis, treatment, or immunization of human beings or animals and in research pertaining to, or in the production of, testing of biologicals (e.g., blood-soaked bandages, sharps).

Methicillin-resistant *Staphylococcus aureus*: *Staphylococcus aureus* bacteria that is resistant to treatment with semi-synthetic penicillins (e.g., oxacillin/nafcillin/methicillin).

Microorganisms: Animals or plants of microscopic size. As used in healthcare, generally refers to bacteria, fungi, viruses, and bacterial spores.

Midline catheter: A vascular device inserted via the antecubital veins and advanced into the upper arms, but not extending past the axilla, to administer fluids and medication.

Morbidity: Objective or subjective change from a state of physiological or psychological health and wellness to illness.

Multidose vial: The container of fluid used in healthcare that contains a preservative to inhibit microbial growth. The fluid can be used on multiple patients but each entry into the vial must be done with a new, sterile, unused syringe and needle. Most multidose vials must be used with a specified time frame that varies based on the manufacturer's directions.

Multidrug-resistant organism (MDRO): Microorganisms that have inherent or acquired resistance to antimicrobial agents. (e.g., MRSA, VRE, ESBL)

N95 respirator: A particulate filtering face piece resembling a mask that is used when caring for an individual with a disease transmitted via the airborne route.

National vaccine injury compensation program (VICP): U.S. government program that provides compensation to people who may have been unavoidably injured by vaccines.

Noncritical items: Items that come in contact with intact skin but not mucous membranes (e.g., bedpans, blood pressure cuffs).

Obstructive sleep apnea (OSA): An acronym for obstructive sleep apnea is a respiratory disorder where a person will stop breathing while sleeping.

Occupational exposure: Being in contact with a potential infectious disease in the course of work.

Occupational Safety and Health Administration (OSHA): An U.S. government agency that oversees personnel safety and imposes regulatory requirements on healthcare facilities.

One-step disinfection process: Simultaneous cleaning and disinfection of a noncritical surface or item.

Outbreak: The occurrence of more cases of disease than normally expected within a specific place or group of people over a given period of time.

Pandemic: An outbreak of a disease that occurs over a wide geographic area and affects an exceptionally high proportion of the population. Refers to a disease epidemic that is widespread and often global.

Performance improvement (PI): The systematic approach to identifying, analyzing, responding to, and evaluating the outcomes for potential and actual long-term care facility (LTCF) challenges. This may apply to resident care or to LTCF operational issues. Also known as performance improvement projects (PIP).

Peripheral catheter: A venous catheter usually placed into a peripheral vein to administer fluids and medication.

Peripherally inserted central catheters (PICC): A central venous catheter inserted into an extremity, with the tip being positioned in the superior vena cava, to administer fluids and medication.

Peritoneal dialysis: A dialysis technique where the abdominal cavity is used as a filter for waste removal.

Personal protective equipment (PPE): Protective items or garments specified by OSHA or NIOSH that must be used or worn when exposure to blood and body fluids is likely.

Phagocytosis: A defensive mechanism where white blood cells (leukocytes; first neutrophils, then macrophages) engulf and destroy microorganisms to prevent infections.

Polypharmacy: The use of multiple medications for which the use is unnecessary to maintain or restore health. Older adults are particularly vulnerable to the use of cumulative medications not coordinated by a single healthcare provider.

Positive airway pressure (PAP): A generic term applied to all sleep apnea treatments that use a stream of compressed air to support the airway during sleep.

Potable water: Water that is safe enough to be used with low risk of immediate harm to humans.

Presenteeism: Attending work while sick.

Pressure ulcer: A wound caused by constant pressure (e.g., prolonged lying or sitting positions) that deprives the tissue of oxygen and nutrients, resulting in ischemia, cellular death, and damage.

Prevalence: The percentage or proportion of a population who have a specific condition at a specific point in time (point prevalence) or specific period of time (period prevalence).

Prions: Transmissible pathogenic agents that cause a variety of neurodegenerative disease of humans and animals, including sheep and goats, bovine spongiform encephalopathy in cattle, and Creutzfeldt-Jakob disease in humans.

Prodrome: An early symptom indicating the onset of an attack or a disease (prodromal symptoms).

Quality assurance (QA): QA is a process of measuring a long-term care facility's performance against standards established by regulatory, accrediting, or other authoritative sources.

Quality assurance and performance improvement (QAPI): QAPI is a data-driven, proactive approach to improving the quality of life, care, and services in nursing homes.

Quaternary ammonium compound (Quat): A surface-active, water-soluble disinfecting agent used for low-level disinfection.

Respirator: A specially designed mask used to protect the wearer from breathing in infectious microorganisms; requires the user to have a medical evaluation and fit testing before use.

Reusable medical equipment: Equipment intended to be used with multiple residents after appropriate cleaning/disinfection.

Root cause analysis (RCA): A systematic process to identify the underlying cause of a problem.

Sanitation: A process whereby microorganisms on inanimate object are decreased to a level below that of infectious hazard (e.g., dishes and eating utensils are sanitized).

Semicritical items: Objects that touch mucous membranes or skin that is not intact. These items require a high-level disinfection process that kills all microorganisms and most spores.

Sensitivity: The ability of a test, case definition, or surveillance system to identify true cases (persons who have the health condition of interest).

Shelf life: Length of time a product can remain active and safe to use as specified by the manufacturer's expiration date on the label.

Single dose vial: The container of sterile fluid used in healthcare with no preservative that can only be accessed one time for one patient.

Socioadaptive change: Modifications in behavior and/or attitudes in response to a particular social challenge.

Spaulding classification: The system for classifying a medical device on the basis of risk to patient/resident safety from contamination. The system identifies three categories of classification (critical, semicritical, or noncritical) and three levels of germicidal activity (sterilization, high-level disinfection, and low-level disinfection) for each.

Specificity: The ability of a test, case definition, or surveillance system to exclude persons who do not have the health condition of interest.

Standard Precautions (formerly Universal Precautions): Infection prevention practices that apply to all residents, regardless of suspected or confirmed diagnosis or presumed infection status. Standard Precautions is a combination and expansion of Universal Precautions and Body Substance Isolation (a practice of isolating all body substances such as blood, urine, and feces).

Sterilization: A process by which all viable forms of microorganisms (including spores) are destroyed.

Summative evaluation: A method of facility or program evaluation based on both its processes and related outcomes.

Surveillance: The ongoing, systematic collection, analysis, interpretation, and dissemination of data to identify infections and infection risks to try to reduce morbidity and mortality and to improve resident health status.

Syndrome-based criteria: Criteria that are based on recognition of a group or cluster of symptoms indicating a specific clinical condition.

T cell: Also known as T lymphocytes. Produced in the thymus, T cells have a variety of immune functions, including helping other leukocytes perform immune activities, regulating immune function, destroying tumor cells and cells containing viruses, and cytokine.

Terminal cleaning: The process of environmental cleaning and disinfection used after a resident is discharged or transferred to a different room or facility.

Transmission-based Precautions: (a.k.a. "Isolation Precautions") The actions (precautions) implemented, in addition to Standard Precautions, that are based on the means of transmission (airborne, contact, and droplet) in order to prevent or control infections.

Tuberculocide: An EPA-classified hospital disinfectant that also kills *Mycobacterium tuberculosis* (tubercle bacilli).

Tunneled catheter: A central venous catheter that is passed under the skin from the insertion site to a separate exit site from which the access port emerges.

Vaccine adverse event reporting system (VAERS): A passive reporting system that accepts reports from the public on adverse events associated with vaccines licensed in the United States.

Vaccine information sheet (VIS): An information sheet explaining the risks and benefits of a vaccine to recipients.

Vaccines: Any preparation intended to produce immunity to a disease by stimulating the production of antibodies.

Virucide: An agent that destroys viruses.

Index

D

E

F

G

H

I

P

Q

R

S